vabnf W9-BAZ-868 VAL
615.1 PAGE

Page, Clive, author
Dale's pharmacology condensed
33410016708010   11-25-2020

DALE'S
Pharmacology
CONDENSED

Valparaiso Public Library
103 Jefferson Street
Valparaiso, IN 46383

THIRD EDITION

DALE'S
Pharmacology
CONDENSED

Clive Page OBE, PhD

Director, Sackler Institute of Pulmonary
 Pharmacology,
Institute of Pharmaceutical Science
King's College London,
London, United Kingdom

Simon Pitchford BSc, PhD

Sackler Institute of Pulmonary Pharmacology
Institute of Pharmaceutical Science
King's College London
London, United Kingdom

ELSEVIER

Copyright © 2021 by Elsevier LTD. All rights reserved.
Previous editions copyrighted 2004 and 2009

The right of Clive Page and Simon Pitchford to be identified as authors of this work has been asserted by them in accordance with the Copyright, Designs and Patents Act 1988

No part of this publication may be reproduced or transmitted in any form or by any means, electronic or mechanical, including photocopying, recording, or any information storage and retrieval system, without permission in writing from the publisher. Details on how to seek permission, further information about the Publisher's permissions policies and our arrangements with organizations such as the Copyright Clearance Center and the Copyright Licensing Agency, can be found at our website: www.elsevier.com/permissions.

This book and the individual contributions contained in it are protected under copyright by the Publisher (other than as may be noted herein).

Notice

Practitioners and researchers must always rely on their own experience and knowledge in evaluating and using any information, methods, compounds or experiments described herein. Because of rapid advances in the medical sciences, in particular, independent verification of diagnoses and drug dosages should be made. To the fullest extent of the law, no responsibility is assumed by Elsevier, authors, editors or contributors for any injury and/or damage to persons or property as a matter of products liability, negligence or otherwise, or from any use or operation of any methods, products, instructions, or ideas contained in the material herein.

ISBN: 978-0-7020-7818-7

Content Strategist: Alexandra Mortimer
Content Development Specialist: Rae Robertson/Kevin Travers
Publishing Services Manager: Shereen Jameel
Senior Project Manager: Kamatchi Madhavan
Design: Patrick Ferguson
Marketing Manager: Heidi Splane

Printed in Poland

Last digit is the print number: 9 8 7 6 5 4 3 2 1

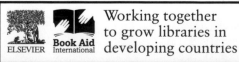

Contents

DALE'S
Pharmacology
CONDENSED

Pharmacology Condensed has been written as a companion volume to Rang and Dale's *Pharmacology*. Each theme has been condensed to a few pages to enable students to retrieve the most pertinent concepts and facts quickly. We consider an understanding of pharmacology is best gained by appreciating the integrative nature of body systems, and thus we have arranged the chapters here to represent this learning context that is nicely represented in further detail in Rang & Dale's *Pharmacology* and *Integrated Pharmacology* by Page et al. As such, chapter headings, and some figures and tables, where pertinent, have been utilized from these textbooks to make their cross-reference obvious and intentional.

We have made some minor changes to this edition to highlight at the front of the book the processes a research team has undertaken to discover and develop a drug. We have also highlighted the safety and toxicology assessment of any new drug, regulatory law, and pharmacovigilance once approved. By doing this we hope the reader understands that pharmacology is a dynamic, live discipline and the application of the principles of pharmacology are requisite to the continued successful introduction of efficacious and safe drugs for use as medicines. This occurs through the continual challenge of predicting drug tolerability via the prism of the *therapeutic index*. Any research into the number of US Food and Drug Administration (FDA) approvals for novel chemical entities and biologicals over the last 25 years will prove to the reader that this period of drug discovery is as buoyant and exciting as any time preceding it. Biologicals, and specifically antibodies, are a very important and expanding therapeutic consideration and therefore a topic that pharmacologists must embrace so that the characteristics of these molecules can be predicted and assessed just as small chemical entities are. We have given the subject of antibody discovery and development the same prominence at the front of the textbook (rather than the back) as that of traditional small molecules, especially given the expansion of biologics from inflammatory and autoimmune disorders to cancer therapy and beyond: for example, the current interest in inflammation and neurodegeneration, or the worrying issue of increased antibiotic resistance. A pharmacologist in the twenty-first century therefore needs to understand immunology and antibody design to the same extent that pharmacologists are knowledgeable about physiology and drug actions on the nervous system.

Pharmacology is an applied discipline that has mathematical principles based on the physics of molecular interactions (the Hill-Langmuir equation) at the core. We encourage readers of this book to remember that whilst pharmacology, as a biological subject, is based on experimentation via scientific method to observe actions, the concepts and predictive qualities are based firmly on logic, and to embrace this will serve to improve understanding of receptor theory (molecular physics), signalling processes (functional selectivity and biased agonism), and modelling of tissue and whole body integrated responses (quorum sensing of cell populations).

As with the previous edition of *Pharmacology Condensed*, our aim is to pinpoint the essential aspects of pharmacology in a precise manner so that the reader has the confidence to recall or research more detailed material. This approach might be useful for anyone preparing for examinations, or for scientists in need of reprisal of distant and forgotten topics.

Clive Page and Simon Pitchford, London, December 2019

Pharmacology is derived from the ancient Greek word for a drug, *pharmakon,* and is the study of how drugs and xenobiotics affect body function and also how the body will act on the drug. The use of chemicals to induce a response on the body is as old as time itself, whether through the use of herbal remedies as the earliest forms of medicine, or perhaps the dubious creation of poisons to rid individuals of enemies. Thus the (unintentional) practice of pharmacology might have been considered earlier in history as magic. The intentional formation of pharmacology as a scientific discipline has evolved from our need to apply scientific principles to create better medicines to improve clinical practice, emanating from an understanding of physiology and pathology, and the earlier exploits of apothecaries to the present creation of a pharmaceutical industry (Fig. 2.1). Pharmacology requires an understanding of other disciplines such as pathology, physiology, biochemistry, synthetic chemistry and molecular biology, and it is underpinned by fundamental physical concepts of mass action and mathematics.

DRUG NAMES

As with the emergence of any scientific discipline, there are a set of codifying rules and an identifiable taxonomy to allow drugs with similar clinical uses, or actions on classes of receptors, to be grouped and classified together via the use of a common naming system.

Drugs will have brand names that are identifiable to consumers and follow no consistent naming pattern. Furthermore, brand names for the same drug may vary from country to country and from manufacturer to manufacturer and therefore should generally not be used. On the other hand chemical names are exact and follow the strict criteria based on their molecular structure by the International Union of Pure and Applied Chemistry (IUPAC). Chemical names are necessary because they allow scientists to interpret the exact structure of a chemical, needed during their synthesis by chemists and by regulatory agencies. Drugs approved for marketing and pharmacological tools used in research will also often have another non-chemical generic name that identifies their pharmacological classification usually by one of the criteria set out below:

- Therapeutic action
- Pharmacological or molecular mechanism of action
- Chemical nature or source

Of course, not all compounds have a therapeutic indication, as many are used as research tools, and some compounds might not have a known molecular mechanism of action. However, using the different classifications above, salmeterol would be classed as a bronchodilator/sympathomimetic, β_2 adrenoceptor agonist, or a phenylethanolamine. Most β_2 adrenoceptor agonist names end in *rol*. The registered brand commercial name for salmeterol is Serevent, a name that provides distinctiveness in the marketplace. Its IUPAC name on the other hand is 2-(hydroxymethyl)-4-[1-hydroxy-2-[6-(4-phenylbutoxy)hexylamino]ethyl]phenol. Perhaps

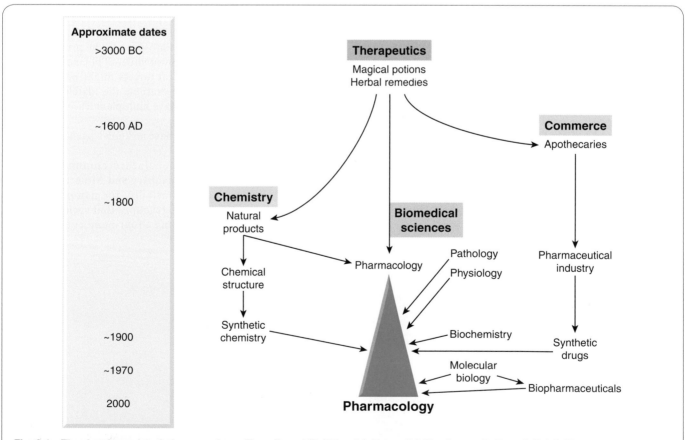

Fig. 2.1 The development of pharmacology. (From Rang HP, Ritter JM, Flower RJ, Henderson G. *Rang & Dale's Pharmacology*. 8th ed. Philadelphia: Elsevier; 2016.)

Table 2.1 Common endings to official names which indicate the pharmacological classification of a drug

Ending	Classification	Prototype for class
-olol	B adrenoceptor blocking drug	Propranolol
-caine	Local anaesthetic	Cocaine, procaine
-dipine	Calcium channel blocker of the dihydropyridine type	Nifedipine
-tidine	H_2 histamine receptor antagonist	Cimetidine
-prazole	Proton pump inhibitor	Omeprazole
-quine	Antimalarial drugs	Chloroquine
-ane	Halogenated hydrocarbon general anaesthetics	Halothane
-zosin	α adrenoceptor blockers (not all)	Prazosin
-profen	One class of nonsteroidal anti-inflammatory drugs (NSAIDs)	Ibuprofen
-clovir	Antiviral (herpes) drugs	Acyclovir
-mycin	Macrolide-aminoglycoside antibiotics	Erythromycin/streptomycin
-cycline	Tetracycline-derived broad spectrum antibiotics	Tetracycline
-ium	Competitive neuromuscular blockers	Decamethonium (but the true pharmacologic prototype is *d*-tubocurarine)
-zolam -zepam	Benzodiazepine sedatives	Diazepam

From Page C, Curtis M, Sutter M, Walker M, Hoffman B. *Integrated Pharmacology*. 2nd ed. Philadelphia: Elsevier; 2002.

the most useful classification of all these names is the use of β_2 adrenoceptor agonist: from this we understand the type of receptor salmeterol acts on, and therefore its primary pharmacological effect. The use of *rol* in salmeterol also informs us of this precise pharmacological action.

Some examples of pharmacological drug classifications are listed in Table 2.1. The naming of antibodies is also codified, based on structure, and the taxonomy of 'biologics' is shown in Figure 8.5 (Chapter 8).

RECEPTORS, ION CHANNELS AND ENZYMES

Pharmacological targets are divided into sections based on structure. The molecular aspects of drug action and classes of receptors, carriers, ion channels and enzymes are discussed in Chapter 4. Similar to the compounds that act on them, the targets also have their own nomenclature and taxonomy. Groupings of similar structures or function are agreed by the International Union of Basic and Clinical Pharmacology Committee on Receptor Nomenclature and Drug Classification (http://www.guidetopharmacology.org/nciupharPublications.jsp) to include the following seven sections:

- 7-transmembrane spanning receptors (or GPCRs): around 800 exist.
- Ion channels, including voltage operated and ligand gated, represent the second largest target for existing drugs.
- Catalytic receptors, including integrins.

- Nuclear receptors: around 50 identified in the human genome.
- Kinases: around 500 identified in the human genome.
- Transporters: the second largest family of membrane proteins after GPCRs.
- Enzymes: more numerable than receptors, but relatively few are drug targets.
- Other protein targets.

Subtypes of pharmacological targets are denoted usually with an alphanumeric symbol, and this is often, but not always, a subscript. For example, purinergic receptors (P2Y) are designated $P2Y_1$, $P2Y_2$, $P2Y_4$, $P2Y_6$, $P2Y_{11}$, $P2Y_{12}$, $P2Y_{13}$ and $P2Y_{14}$. The name on its own does not inform as to the principal signal transduction mechanism or the rank order of potency of receptor agonists. Some pharmacological targets might only have one identified family member, for example the platelet-activating factor receptor (PAF-R), but have multiple intracellular signalling pathways.

Pharmacological targets that have no known ligand are referred to as *orphan* targets.

There is a separate nomenclature committee of the International Union of Biochemistry and Molecular Biology (NC-IUBMB) that has responsibility for naming enzymes. Thus, six families based on the reactions that various enzymes catalyse have been created, using a four-number code with an 'EC' prefix.

3 General principles of drug action

Pharmacology concerns the study of how drugs affect the function of host tissues or combat infectious organisms. In most cases, drugs bind selectively to target molecules within the body, usually proteins but other macromolecules as well. The main drug targets are receptors, enzymes, ion channels, transporters (carriers) and DNA. There are few instances (e.g. osmotic purgatives and antacids) of drugs acting without binding to a specific target.

It is generally desirable that a drug should have a higher affinity for its target than for other binding sites. First, it ensures that the drug's free concentration (and hence action) is not reduced by nonproductive binding to the much greater number of nontarget molecules in the body. Second, lower doses can be used, which automatically reduces the risks of unwanted actions at other sites that may cause toxicological side effects. Chapter 4 deals specifically with the consequences of drug binding to these targets. The rest of this chapter will deal predominantly with the principles of receptor pharmacology.

RECEPTORS AS DRUG TARGETS

Receptors are protein macromolecules – on or in cells – that act as recognition sites for endogenous ligands such as neurotransmitters, hormones, inflammatory/immunological mediators, etc. Many drugs used in medicine make use of these receptors. The effect of a drug may be to produce the same response as the endogenous ligand or to prevent the action of an endogenous (or exogenous) ligand. A drug (or endogenous chemical) that binds to a receptor and activates the cell's response is termed an *agonist*. A drug that reduces or inhibits the action of an agonist is termed an *antagonist*, and therefore has no biological activity per se.

Receptors are perhaps the most common 'target' for a drug, and understanding the interactions between drugs and receptors is a fundamental tenet of pharmacology. Proteins (receptors) are not rigid structures, but due to their inherent kinetic energy, will vibrate, or shimmer, to induce slight variations in shape, such that a receptor will alternate between periods of 'inactive' and 'active' conformations. Within the vicinity of the receptor, several drug molecules will surround the space. Through random motion, during time, occasionally some of those molecules will collide with the 'active pocket' of the receptor when it is in the active conformation. This active pocket is commonly known as the orthosteric binding site (Fig. 3.1). Thus when an agonist fits in the active pocket, the receptor is held in the active conformation for a period of time until the agonist is displaced, and this leads to biochemical processes occurring.

The action of an inflammatory mediator, histamine, on bronchial smooth muscle can be taken as an example. There are two aspects to this action:
- The agonist–receptor (drug–receptor) interaction
- The agonist-induced (drug-induced) response

The action of histamine could be measured at various levels: molecular, cellular, tissue and system. With the drug–receptor interaction, we will be dealing with the concepts of *affinity*, *occupancy* and *selectivity*. With the drug-induced response, we will meet the concepts of *efficacy* and *potency*:
- *Affinity*: The ability of a drug to bind to a receptor.
- *Occupancy*: The proportion of receptors to which a drug is bound.

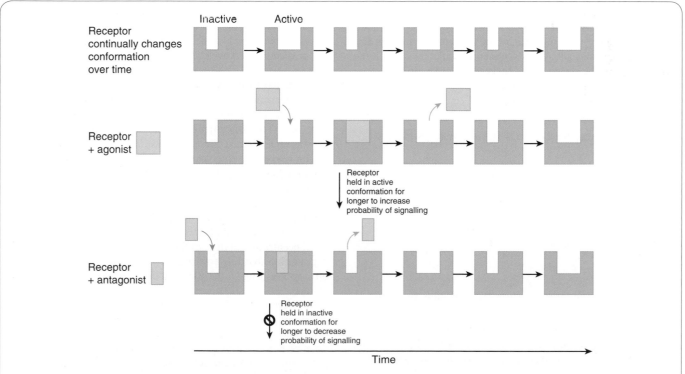

Fig. 3.1 Schematic diagram illustrating a receptor occupied by agonist or antagonist and the influence of conformation and time on the probability of a biological response.

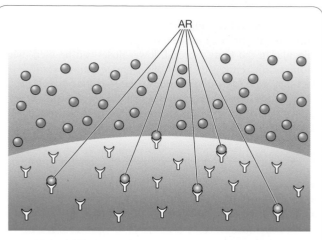

Fig. 3.2 Schematic diagram illustrating receptor (R) occupied by agonist A (e.g. histamine) on the surface of smooth muscle.

- *Selectivity*: Relative affinity or activity of a drug between different receptor types. Largely replaced the concept of specificity, since it is improbable that any drug is specific for a particular receptor.
- *Efficacy*: The ability of an agonist to elicit a response following binding.
- *Potency*: A measure of the concentration of a drug (agonist or antagonist) at which it is effective.

The agonist–receptor (drug–receptor) interaction

In Fig. 3.2 as an example of a tissue, the smooth muscle surface (which can be stimulated by histamine) is represented by the blue curved segment. The receptors (shown as cups) are representative of the total number of receptors on the muscle (R_{tot}). The histamine molecules are represented by the grey circles. When the muscle is exposed to a concentration of histamine [A] and allowed to come to a dynamic equilibrium, where the drug occupation of a number of receptors (AR) at any point is steady. We now need to consider the relationship between [A] and the occupancy of the receptors [AR]/[R_{tot}].

Drug–receptor interaction is usually freely reversible and can be represented by the following equation:

(The rate constant for the forward (association) reaction)

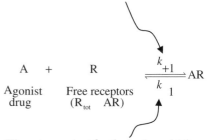

$$A + R \underset{k_{-1}}{\overset{k_{+1}}{\rightleftharpoons}} AR$$

Agonist drug   Free receptors (R_{tot} – AR)

(The rate constant for the backward (dissociation) reaction)

The Law of Mass Action (the rate of the reaction is proportional to the product of the concentrations of the reactants) can be applied to the reaction. At equilibrium the forward and reverse rates are equal, i.e.:

$$k_{+1} [A] [R] = k_{-1} [AR]$$

so that

$$\frac{[A] [R]}{[AR]} = \frac{k_{-1}}{k_{+1}} = K_A$$

k_{+1} and k_{-1} have the units $M^{-1} sec^{-1}$ and sec^{-1} respectively. K_A (equal to k_{-1}/k_{+1}) is the dissociation equilibrium constant for the binding of drug to receptor; it has the dimensions of concentration and is used by pharmacologists rather than an 'association' constant, which confusingly has the units L/mol. (It is the reciprocal of the affinity constant, i.e. the higher the affinity of the drug for the receptors, the lower the value of K_A.) A high K_A specifies a low affinity, which means that there are fewer drug–receptor complexes overall.

The relationship at equilibrium between K_A, the concentration of agonist drug, and the proportion of receptors occupied (i.e. the occupancy p_A) is given by:

This is self-evident (i.e. the concentration of receptors occupied over the total receptor concentration)

$$p_A = \frac{[AR]}{[R_{tot}]} = \frac{[A]}{K_A + [A]}$$

But this may not be obvious to every student; it is the Hill Langmuir equation

The value of K_A is equal to the concentration of the agonist drug that at equilibrium results in occupancy of 50% of the receptors. For example, if the concentration of the drug is 10 μmol/l and the K_A is 10 μmol/l, then:

$$P_A = \frac{10}{10 + 10} = 0.5$$

The relationship between occupancy and drug concentration specified by the Hill–Langmuir equation (identified above) can be represented graphically as shown in Fig. 3.3. The theoretical curves given are for occupancy. Now let us consider the agonist-induced response.

The agonist-induced (drug-induced) response

An agonist-induced response – if it is a *graded response* – can be plotted as a concentration–effect or dose–response curve (Fig. 3.4). The concentration producing a response 50% of the maximum is termed the EC_{50} (EC, effective concentration).

Can one make the assumption that responses such as these are directly proportional to occupancy at the relevant receptors?

Certainly the log concentration–response curve in Fig. 3.4 looks very like the theoretical log concentration–occupancy curve in Fig. 3.3. However, even with the simple *in vitro* response of smooth muscle to noradrenaline, it is not possible to know, with certainty, the concentration of drug at the receptors. Factors such as enzymic degradation, binding to tissue components, problems related to diffusion of drug to the site of action, and so on, complicate the picture.

The relationship between occupancy and response is in most cases unknown and, almost certainly, not linearly related to occupancy. Consequently, although concentration–response (or dose–response) curves look very similar to concentration–occupancy curves, they cannot be used to determine the agonist affinity for the respective receptors.

The dose that produced a 50% of a maximal response using *in vitro* preparations (EC_{50}), and ED_{50} for *in vivo* preparations

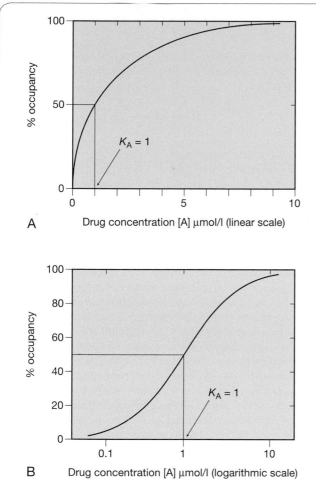

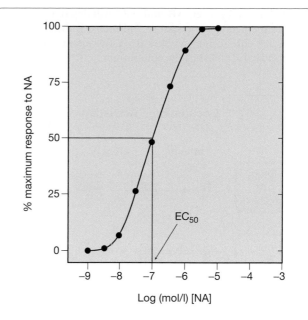

Fig. 3.4 The concentration–response curve for noradrenaline (NA)-mediated contraction of smooth muscle *in vitro*.

Fig. 3.3 Occupancy, according to the Hill–Langmuir equation, plotted against drug concentration. The graph has been drawn according to a K_A value of 1 μmol/l. When the concentration of the agonist also equals 1 μmol/l, the occupancy of receptors is 50%.

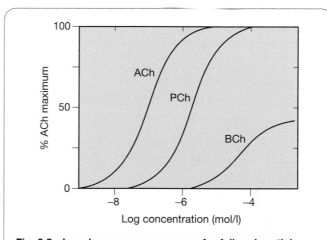

Fig. 3.5 Log dose–response curves for full and partial agonists on gastrointestinal smooth muscle. *ACh,* Acetylcholine; *PCh,* propionylcholine; *BCh,* butyrylcholine.

(ED, effective dose), or when discussing a population response ED_{50} will represent 50% of the individuals responding.

With some drugs, the maximum response produced corresponds to the maximum response that the tissue can give. These are termed *full agonists*. The action depicted in Fig. 3.4 is that of a full agonist. Other drugs, even though acting on the same receptors, may not give the maximum tissue response in any concentration (E_{max}). These are termed *partial agonists*. Therefore it is always important to have knowledge of the EC_{50} (or ED_{50}) to compare drug *potency*, and E_{max} to compare *efficacy*.

Partial agonists

The concentration–response curves of some full and partial agonists on the muscarinic receptors of smooth muscle of the gastrointestinal tract are shown in Fig. 3.5. It can be seen that both acetylcholine and propionylcholine are full agonists but propionylcholine requires a larger concentration to produce a maximum response. Butyrylcholine even in very high concentration never produces as great a response as acetylcholine – it is a partial agonist.

What is the explanation for the different responses of partial and full agonists? Experiments have shown that this is not because the partial agonists bind to fewer receptors, but that they are less

able to elicit a response from the receptors to which they do bind. They are, in fact, less potent. They are said to have less *intrinsic activity* (or *lower efficacy*).

Efficacy

Efficacy is a complex concept that, in simple terms, describes the ability of the drug (agonist), after binding to the receptor, to activate transduction mechanisms that lead to a response.

Partial agonist action can be best interpreted in terms of a two-state model of the molecular events at a single receptor on interaction with agonist A. The model envisages that an occupied receptor can exist in two states: a 'resting' state (R) and an 'activated' state (R*). This is represented in Fig. 3.6 which shows the distinction between drug binding and receptor activation.

$$A + R \underset{k_{-1}}{\overset{k_{+1}}{\rightleftharpoons}} AR \underset{\alpha}{\overset{\beta}{\rightleftharpoons}} AR^*$$

The equilibrium between AR and AR* will determine the magnitude of the maximum response. Normally, if there is no drug present, the equilibrium favours R. A full agonist would bind preferentially to, and shift the equilibrium to, R*:

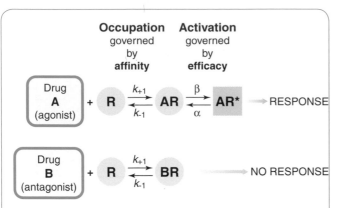

$$A + R \underset{k_{-1}}{\overset{k_{+1}}{\rightleftharpoons}} AR \underset{\alpha}{\overset{\beta}{\rightleftharpoons}} AR^*$$

An equilibrium that favours AR, with few receptors in the activated state, would make the drug A a partial agonist (i.e. a drug with low efficacy):

$$A + R \underset{k_{-1}}{\overset{k_{+1}}{\rightleftharpoons}} AR \underset{\alpha}{\overset{\beta}{\rightleftharpoons}} AR^*$$

Note that because partial agonists occupy receptors, they competitively antagonize the action of a full agonist while producing a small effect of their own. A clinical example is oxprenolol, a β-blocker (a partial agonist on β_1-adrenoceptors in the heart, causing tachycardia and increased force in its own right) that antagonizes the action of endogenous noradrenaline (full agonist).

Inverse agonists

The model of drug–receptor interaction, specified in this chapter so far, assumes that receptors are inactive in the absence of bound ligand. It is now known that some receptors can adopt the active, R*, conformation even in the absence of an agonist. They are said to show *constitutive* activity. These include receptors for benzodiazepines, cannabinoids and serotonin. Under these conditions, it may be possible for a ligand to reduce the level of constitutive activation, which results in a reverse of the biological effect. Such ligands are referred to as *inverse agonists,* to distinguish them from *neutral antagonists*, which inhibit a biological process rather than reversing the effect, as shown in Fig. 3.7. They have a higher affinity for the inactive compared with the active state of the receptor. The best examples are the β-carbolines, which are inverse agonists at the benzodiazepine binding sites on γ-aminobutyric acid (GABA)$_A$

Fig. 3.6 The distinction between drug binding and receptor activation. Ligand A is an agonist, because when it is bound, the receptor (R) tends to become activated, whereas ligand B is an antagonist, because binding does not lead to activation. It is important to realize that for most drugs, binding and activation are reversible, dynamic processes. The rate constants k_{+1}, k_{-1}, α and β for the binding, unbinding and activation steps vary between drugs. For an antagonist, which does not activate the receptor, β=0, for a partial agonist, either k_{+1} or α can be less than that of a full agonist, and k_{-1} or β can be greater than that of a full agonist. (From Rang HP, Ritter JM, Flower RJ, Henderson G. *Rang & Dale's Pharmacology.* 8th ed. Philadelphia: Elsevier; 2016.)

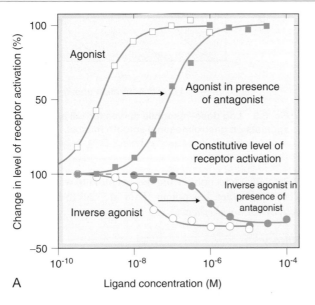

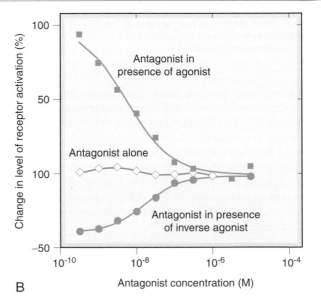

Fig. 3.7 Inverse agonism. The interaction of a competitive antagonist with normal and inverse agonists in a system that shows constitutive receptor activation in the absence of added ligands. (A) The degree of receptor activation (vertical scale) increases in the presence of agonist (open squares) and decreases in the presence of an inverse agonist (open circles). Addition of a competitive antagonist shifts both curves to the right (closed symbols). (B) The antagonist on its own does not alter the level of constitutive activity (open symbols), because it has equal affinity for the active and inactive states of the receptor. In the presence of an agonist (closed squares) or inverse agonist (closed circles), the antagonist restores the system towards the constitutive level of activity. (Modified from Newman-Tancredi A, Conte C, Chaput C, Spedding M, Millan MJ. Inhibition of the constitutive activity of human 5-HT1A receptors by the inverse agonist, spiperone but not the neutral antagonist, WAY 100,635. *Br J Pharmacol.* 1997;120(5):737-739.)

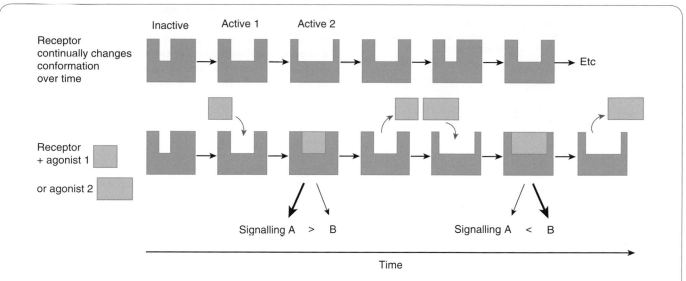

Fig. 3.8   Biased agonism. Schematic diagram illustrating a receptor occupied by agonist 1 or agonist 2 in two different active conformations, leading to differential downstream activities.

receptors. Rather than being anxiolytic, as most benzodiazepines, these agents are anxiogenic (see Ch. 12).

Biased agonism

The concept of basic agonist/antagonist relationships is understood via the two-state model of receptor theory. As is evident from inverse agonism above, the simplistic relationship between a ligand and a receptor starts to require a different conceptual understanding. It is now known that receptors are not actually restricted to two distinct states but have a much more conformational flexibility. Thus some types of receptors will have more than one resting and active conformation. The different conformations that they can adopt may be preferentially stabilized by different ligands (*biased agonists*, or *biased antagonists*) and may produce different functional effects by activating different signalling pathways, that is, they confer *functional selectivity* (Fig. 3.8). An example is the 5-HT$_{2A}$ receptor: activation via serotonin leads to phospholipase C (PLC) signalling (and inositol triphosphate accumulation), whilst activation via dimethyltryptamine leads to phospholipase A2 (PLA$_2$) signalling (and arachidonic acid production). The implications to drug discovery of biased agonism are not yet known, but a benefit might be the development of drugs with fewer side effects, or the discovery of otherwise 'silent' receptor activities that have hitherto been hidden by canonical signalling pathways.

ANTAGONISTS

In simple terms, an antagonist can be defined as a drug that reduces the action of an agonist, which may be an endogenous ligand or a drug. Many of the clinically most useful drugs are antagonists. Drug antagonism can be produced by a variety of mechanisms, the most important being competitive antagonism.

Competitive antagonism

Numerous drugs (e.g. propranolol, naloxone) exert their clinical action by competitive antagonism at receptors. A competitive antagonist binds to the receptor and prevents the binding of an agonist at the orthosteric site. If the antagonist binds reversibly, then the effect of the antagonist can be overcome by raising the concentration of the agonist so that it competes more effectively for the binding sites. For a given concentration of reversible

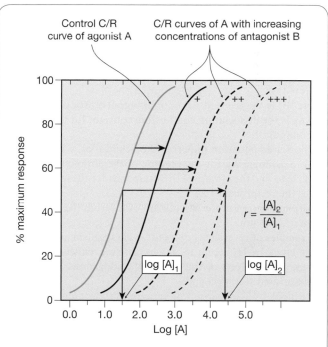

Fig. 3.9   Reversible competitive antagonism. Increasing concentrations of a competitive antagonist prazosin (indicated by +, ++, +++) produce increasing shifts of the control log concentration–response curve of agonist A (noradrenaline) to the right. The response is expressed as a percentage of maximum contraction of the rat vas deferens. The shift can be expressed as a ratio *r*. C/R, Concentration versus response.

competitive antagonist, the log concentration–response curve of the agonist drug (A) will be displaced to the right in a parallel fashion (Fig. 3.9). The shift is expressed as a ratio *r* (termed 'dose ratio' or 'concentration ratio'), which is defined as the factor by which the agonist concentration must be increased in the presence of the antagonist to restore the response to that given by agonist alone. The magnitude of the shift is given by the Schild equation:

$$r1 = \frac{[B]}{K_B}$$

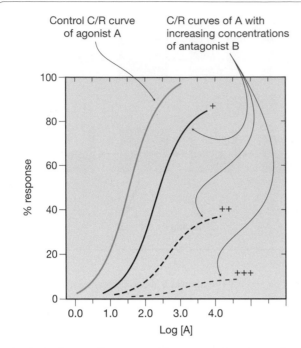

Control C/R curve
of agonist A

C/R curves of A with
increasing concentrations
of antagonist B

Fig. 3.10 Irreversible competitive antagonism. Increasing concentrations of an irreversible antagonist, B, causes progressively greater depressions of the maximum response to agonist A. *C/R,* Concentration versus response.

where [B] is the concentration of antagonist producing the shift and K_B is the dissociation equilibrium constant for the binding of the antagonist.

The Schild equation underlies the Schild plot, which is widely used to estimate K_B for the binding of the antagonist. It is thus possible to find the *affinity* of the antagonist for the receptors since this is the reciprocal of K_B.

An explanation of the calculation of K_B from the Schild plot is given in Appendix 1.

Examples of reversible competitive antagonism are:
- the block by H_2 receptor antagonists (e.g. cimetidine, used to treat peptic ulcer) of the action of endogenous histamine on gastric acid secretion and
- the block by β-adrenoceptor antagonists (e.g. atenolol, used for hypertension and other cardiovascular conditions) of the action of endogenous noradrenaline on $β_1$-adrenoceptors in the heart.

Other forms of drug antagonism
There are some other ways in which the effect of one drug can be reduced by the action of another.

Irreversible competitive antagonism
In irreversible competitive antagonism, the antagonist binds irreversibly, usually because of the formation of covalent bonds, effectively reducing the number of receptors available for binding. There may then be insufficient receptors available for the agonist to regain its maximum response as its concentration is increased (Fig. 3.10). Note: In some tissues there are spare receptors, i.e. more receptors are present than must be occupied to give a full response; under these conditions a limited exposure to an irreversible antagonist might produce a parallel shift – hinted at in Fig. 3.10.

An example is the block of $α_1$-adrenoceptors by phenoxybenzamine (used to treat pheochromocytoma), which forms a covalent bond with the receptor.

Physiological (functional) antagonism
In physiological antagonism, the 'antagonist' has the opposite biological action of the agonist, reducing the agonist effect by action on a different receptor (on which it is itself an agonist). An example of physiological antagonism is salbutamol (albuterol in the United States; used to treat the acute asthmatic attack), which, by acting as an agonist (a smooth muscle relaxant) on $β_2$-adrenoceptors in bronchiolar smooth muscle, antagonizes the bronchoconstrictor action of endogenous leukotrienes acting on leukotriene C_4 receptors.

Noncompetitive antagonism
In noncompetitive antagonism, the antagonist does not block the receptor itself but blocks the signal transduction process initiated by receptor activation, e.g. Ca^{2+} channel blockers will prevent smooth muscle contraction elicited by various agonists.

Pharmacokinetic antagonism
The antagonist reduces the free concentration of drug at its target either by reducing drug absorption or by accelerating renal or hepatic elimination. For example, induction of the cytochrome P450 drug-oxidizing system by phenobarbital can reduce the effectiveness of many drugs.

Chemical antagonism
A chemical antagonist combines with the drug (in plasma or gut lumen) to produce an insoluble and inactive complex, e.g. protamine sulphate neutralizes the action of heparin.

ALLOSTERIC MODULATION

Drug-receptor interactions have been described above as occurring via the orthosteric site on the receptor protein. Receptors may possess other binding sites that are distant from the orthosteric binding pocket, known as allosteric binding sites. Chemicals binding to an allosteric binding site might increase agonist or antagonist affinity at the orthosteric binding site and may therefore have either positive or negative allostery (i.e. the EC_{50} may be shifted, or the E_{max} affected), or even produce an effect themselves. Examples of allosteric modulation include glycine at N-methyl-D-aspartate (NMDA) receptors, benzodiazepines at $GABA_A$ receptors, cinacalcet at the Ca^{2+} receptor, and sulfonylurea drugs at K_{ATP} channels. In the future, drug development might benefit from exploiting allostery at a particular receptor by improving selectivity and potentiating effects on receptors that are being activated.

DESENSITIZATION AND TOLERANCE

There are many examples of the failure of drug action to be maintained despite continued administration. Receptors can be converted to an inactive, desensitized form either by a simple isomerization (e.g. the very rapid desensitization of nicotinic receptors) or by a slower phosphorylation, e.g. of G-protein-coupled receptors (GPCRs). There are indeed specific enzymes that mediate the phosphorylation and hence inactivation of GPCRs. Receptors can also be removed from the cell surface by internalization subsequent to agonist binding. This process of receptor downregulation may take several days to reverse.

Homeostatic mechanisms may also come into play to reduce drug action. For example, the antihypertensive effect of thiazide diuretics is blunted by a slow activation of the renin–angiotensin system.

Drugs produce effects in the body mainly in the following ways:
- By acting on *receptors*
- By inhibiting *carriers* (molecules that transport one or more ions or molecules across the plasma membrane)
- By modulating or blocking *ion channels*
- By inhibiting *enzymes*

RECEPTORS AS TARGETS FOR DRUG ACTION

Receptors are protein molecules in or on cells whose function is to interact with the body's endogenous chemical messengers (hormones, neurotransmitters, the chemical mediators of the immune system, etc.) and thus initiate cellular responses. They enable the responses of the body's cells to be coordinated. Drugs used in medicine make use of these chemical sensors – either stimulating them (drugs that do this are termed *agonists*) or preventing endogenous mediators or agonists from stimulating them (drugs that do this are termed *antagonists*).

There are four major types of receptor:
- Type 1: Receptors linked to ion channels, also termed ionotropic receptors or ligand-gated ion channels.
- Type 2: Receptors coupled to G-proteins (GPCRs): that are guanine nucleotide-binding proteins, also termed *metabotropic receptors.*
- Type 3: Receptors linked to enzymes (e.g. kinases, guanylate cyclase, etc.); these mostly initiate a kinase cascade within the cell (e.g. tyrosine kinase linked receptors).
- Type 4: Receptors that affect gene transcription (receptors for steroids).

Within these classes are also so-called orphan receptors, which currently have no well-defined ligands.

Why has evolution provided the body with these many different ways to provide cellular signalling? One answer is the timing of responses, as removing your hand from a hot surface requires an immediate response, whereas the control of cell division requires more subtle biological control over a longer period of time. This is represented in Fig. 4.1.

The structure and mechanisms of receptor activation are summarized below, adapted from detailed discussion from Rang and Dale's *Pharmacology.*

Type 1: Receptors linked to ion channels (i.e. ionotropic receptors)

Receptors linked to ion channels are located in the cell membrane and respond in milliseconds. The channel forms part of the receptor, which are assembled from four to five membrane spanning units named α, β, γ, δ. Ion channels that have a pentameric structure (rather than a quatromeric) will have one repeated subunit. The nicotinic receptor for acetylcholine (see Chapter 11) is an example, which is composed of $\alpha 2$, β, γ and δ (Fig. 4.2). This receptor type controls the fastest synaptic events in the nervous system. As an example, the action of acetylcholine acting on nicotinic receptors at the neuromuscular junction causes an increase in sodium ion (Na^+) and potassium ion (K^+) permeability and sometimes calcium ion (Ca^{2+}) permeability to result in net inward Na^+ currents at negative membrane potentials to depolarize a cell and raise the probability of an action potential. In contrast to other receptor types, no other biochemical steps are required for the immediate transduction event, and therefore this provides for a very fast cellular response.

Type 2: Receptors coupled to G-proteins

G-protein-coupled receptors (GPCRs) occur in the cell membrane and respond in seconds. They have a single polypeptide chain that has seven transmembrane helices. Signal transduction occurs by activation of particular G-proteins that are membrane resident and recognize GPCRs in their active state to then generate signalling pathways to modulate enzyme activity or ion channel function and thus produce a cellular response (Figs. 4.3 to 4.5).

The mechanics of G-protein assembly and disassembly are highly orchestrated, and the cyclical activation and inactivation of G-proteins is best represented in a diagram (Fig. 4.5). G-proteins consist of three subunits: α, β and γ. Guanine nucleotides bind to $G\alpha$, which has enzymic (GTPase) activity. Receptor activation leads to interaction with the $G\alpha$ subunit and bound guanine diphosphate (GDP) is displaced by cytoplasmic guanine triphosphate (GTP). The $G\alpha$-GTP unit then interacts with a target protein to induce its GTPase activity to catalyse GTP to GDP and activate the target protein. The β and γ subunits remain together as a $\beta\gamma$ complex ($G\beta\gamma$). Specificity of GPCR response is achieved with different classes of G-protein that show selectivity with regards to receptors and effector targets (enzymes) they couple to. Thus, there are four main classes of $G\alpha$-protein that are pharmacologically relevant: $G\alpha_s$, $G\alpha_i$, $G\alpha_o$ and $G\alpha_q$ along with $G\beta\gamma$. Targets for G-proteins include the following:
- Adenyl cyclase (cyclic adenosine monophosphate (cAMP) production).
- Phospholipase C (inositol phosphate and diacylglycerol (DAG)) formation.
- Rho A/Rho kinases (these regulate signalling pathways controlling cell growth and proliferation, contraction and motility).
- Mitogen-activated protein (MAP) kinases (these regulate many cellular functions, including cell division).
- Ion channels (direct G-protein-channel interaction through $G\beta\gamma$ of G_i and G_o proteins).

In some instances, GPCR activity can be affected by membrane proteins called receptor activity-modifying-proteins (RAMPs). Furthermore, G-protein-independent signalling can sometimes occur with GPCRs. In this regard, signalling mediated by arrestins, rather than by G-proteins, is important since arrestins can act as a link to MAP kinase cascades.

It is important to note that understanding GPCR activity can no longer be represented by the dogma that one GPCR acts on one G-protein to create one distinct response via a canonical pathway. Rather, there are various processes that can lead to qualitatively different actions:
- One GPCR protein can associate with others (GPCRs) to produce more than one type of functional receptor complex (oligomerization).
- Different agonists may affect GPCRs in different ways and elicit different responses (biased signalling or selective functionality), whether this be through G-protein, RAMP or arrestin signalling.
- The signal transduction pathway can be independent of G-proteins and can cross talk with tyrosine kinase-linked receptors (see below).

Type 3: Receptors linked to enzymes

These receptors are single transmembrane proteins with a large extracellular portion that contains the binding sites for ligands (e.g. growth factors, cytokines and some hormones) and an intracellular portion that has integral enzyme activity – usually tyrosine kinase activity (Fig. 4.6). Activation initiates an intracellular pathway involving cytosolic and nuclear transducers and eventually gene transcription. They are important for cell division, growth,

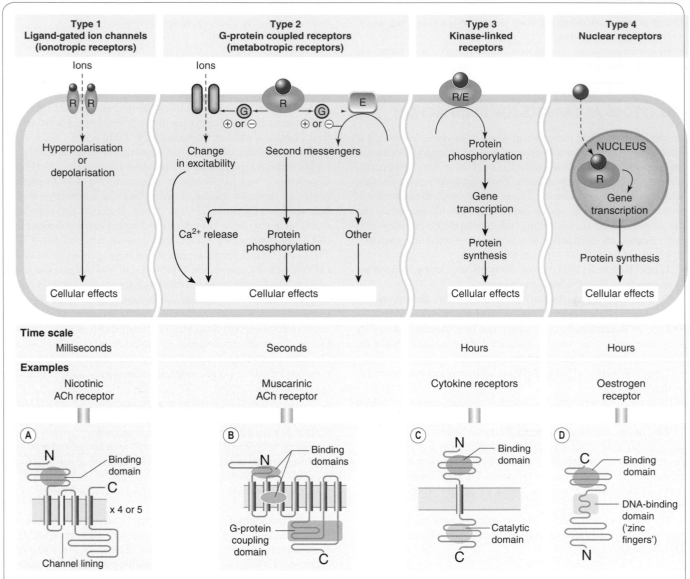

Fig. 4.1 **General structure and signalling mechanism of four receptor families.** *ACh*, Acetylcholine; *E*, enzyme; *G*, G-protein; *R*, receptor. (Modified from Rang HP, Ritter JM, Flower RJ, Henderson G. *Rang & Dale's Pharmacology*. 8th ed. Philadelphia: Elsevier; 2016.)

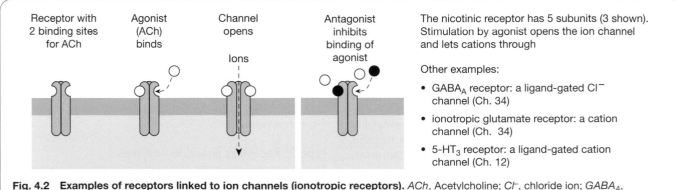

Fig. 4.2 **Examples of receptors linked to ion channels (ionotropic receptors).** *ACh*, Acetylcholine; *Cl⁻*, chloride ion; *GABAₐ*, γ-aminobutyric acid; *5-HT₃*, 5-hydroxytryptamine.

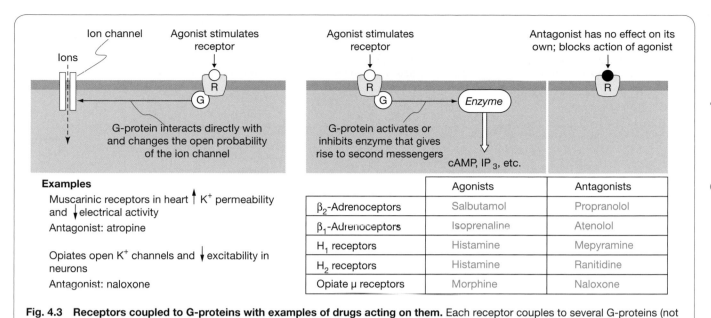

Examples

Muscarinic receptors in heart ↑ K⁺ permeability and ↓ electrical activity
Antagonist: atropine

Opiates open K⁺ channels and ↓ excitability in neurons
Antagonist: naloxone

	Agonists	Antagonists
β_2-Adrenoceptors	Salbutamol	Propranolol
β_1-Adrenoceptors	Isoprenaline	Atenolol
H_1 receptors	Histamine	Mepyramine
H_2 receptors	Histamine	Ranitidine
Opiate μ receptors	Morphine	Naloxone

Fig. 4.3 Receptors coupled to G-proteins with examples of drugs acting on them. Each receptor couples to several G-proteins (not shown), resulting in amplification of the response.

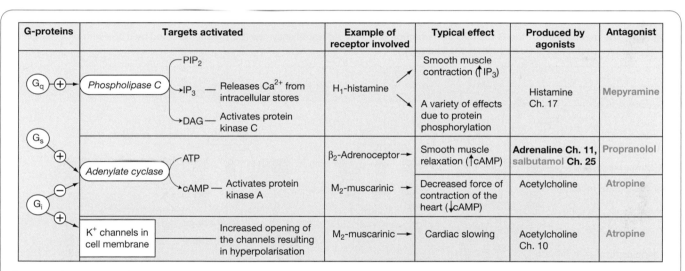

G-proteins	Targets activated		Example of receptor involved	Typical effect	Produced by agonists	Antagonist
G_q (+) Phospholipase C	PIP₂		H_1-histamine	Smooth muscle contraction (↑ IP₃)	Histamine Ch. 17	Mepyramine
	IP₃	Releases Ca²⁺ from intracellular stores				
	DAG	Activates protein kinase C		A variety of effects due to protein phosphorylation		
G_s (+) Adenylate cyclase	ATP		β_2-Adrenoceptor	Smooth muscle relaxation (↑cAMP)	**Adrenaline Ch. 11,** salbutamol **Ch. 25**	Propranolol
G_i (−)	cAMP	Activates protein kinase A	M_2-muscarinic	Decreased force of contraction of the heart (↓cAMP)	Acetylcholine	Atropine
G_i (+)	K⁺ channels in cell membrane	Increased opening of the channels resulting in hyperpolarisation	M_2-muscarinic	Cardiac slowing	Acetylcholine Ch. 10	Atropine

Fig. 4.4 Examples of G-protein-coupled actions. The pathways are shown for three different G-proteins. *cAMP*, Cyclic adenosine monophosphate; *IP₃*, inositol trisphosphate; *PIP₂*, phosphatidylinositol 4,5-bisphosphate.

differentiation, inflammation, tissue repair, apoptosis and immune responses. There are three main types:
- Receptor tyrosine kinases: these incorporate a tyrosine kinase moiety in the intracellular region.
- Receptor serine/threonine kinases: these phosphorylate serine or threonine residues.
- Cytokine receptors: these have no intrinsic enzyme activity but will activate various tyrosine kinases such as Janus kinase (Jak), named after the Greek god Janus because they act in a double-faced manner, whereby they contain two near-identical phosphate-transferring domains. One domain regulates kinase activity but is ultimately opposed by the other (Fig. 4.6).

Signal transduction usually occurs through dimerization of receptors, followed by autophosphorylation of tyrosine residues. These then act to accept SH₂ domains of intracellular proteins. Two important pathways are (1) the Ras/Raf/MAP kinase pathway and (2) the Jak/Stat pathway (mentioned above).

Note that many receptors activate *kinase cascades*. The target proteins of these cascades include (in addition to the transcription factors mentioned above) other enzymes, ion channels and transporters (see below) as well as contractile proteins and secretory mechanisms.

Type 4: Receptors linked to gene transcription

The receptors that regulate gene transcription are called nuclear receptors, although some are located in the cytosol (e.g. glucocorticoid receptors) rather than embedded in membranes, and they migrate to the nucleus after binding a ligand (Fig. 4.7). Steroid hormones, other hormones (e.g. thyroid hormone T_3) and fat-soluble vitamins (e.g. vitamin D and A) act via nuclear receptors. Unlike other receptors that are membrane bound, cytosolic nuclear receptors can interact with DNA, and they have been described as ligand-activated gene transcription factors.

The structure of nuclear receptors is made up of an *N-terminal domain* that has the greatest heterogeneity. It contains a distinct region: activation function 1 (AF1) site that can bind to other transcription factors and modify the response of the nuclear receptor. The *core domain* is highly conserved and is responsible

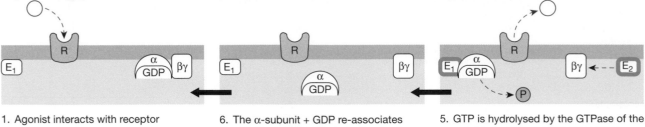

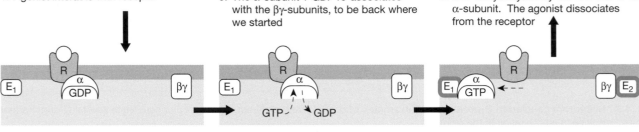

G-proteins are attached to the membrane and consist of three subunits α, β and γ, the last two being closely associated:

In the free G protein, GDP occupies the binding site on the α-subunit. The α subunit and the β/γ complex can each activate intracellular targets. **Subtypes of all three subunits exist; the particular subunit determines which targets are activated**

1. Agonist interacts with receptor

6. The α-subunit + GDP re-associates with the β/γ-subunits, to be back where we started

5. GTP is hydrolysed by the GTPase of the α-subunit. The agonist dissociates from the receptor

2. The α-subunit (+ GDP) interacts with the receptor

3. GTP replaces GDP

4. The α-subunit + GTP interacts with the enzyme, activating it. The β/γ complex also activates a target enzyme

Fig. 4.5   The mechanism of the G-protein transduction process. Activated enzymes (E_1, E_2) are indicated by a box with blue margins. *GDP*, Guanine diphosphate; *GTP*, guanine triphosphate.

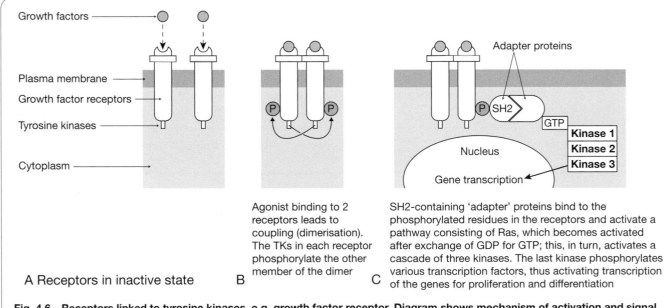

Agonist binding to 2 receptors leads to coupling (dimerisation). The TKs in each receptor phosphorylate the other member of the dimer

SH2-containing 'adapter' proteins bind to the phosphorylated residues in the receptors and activate a pathway consisting of Ras, which becomes activated after exchange of GDP for GTP; this, in turn, activates a cascade of three kinases. The last kinase phosphorylates various transcription factors, thus activating transcription of the genes for proliferation and differentiation

A Receptors in inactive state

Fig. 4.6   Receptors linked to tyrosine kinases, e.g. growth factor receptor. Diagram shows mechanism of activation and signal transduction.

for DNA recognition and binding through two *zinc fingers* that bind to *hormone response elements* (HRE) in the DNA sequence. The *C-terminal domain* contains the specific ligand binding site.

There are four classes of nuclear receptors: I, II, III and IV. Class I comprises endocrine steroid (glucocorticoid, mineralocorticoid, oestrogen, progesterone and androgen) receptors. They are found in the cytoplasm or cytoskeleton, complexed with regulatory proteins (e.g. heat shock proteins). Ligands bind after diffusion through the cell membrane as homodimers, whereupon the complex translocates to the nucleus to bind to HREs that can act to repress or activate genes. Class II receptors have ligands that are generally lipids that are already present within the cell and bind in a heterodimeric manner. Class II receptors are located within the nucleus and can be complexed to repressors, which become displaced following ligand binding. An example is the *peroxisome proliferator-activated receptor* (PPAR). Classes III and IV are less well characterized in terms of pharmacological actions.

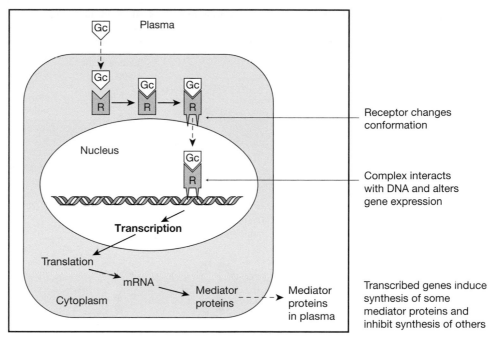

Examples are members of the steroid superfamily of receptors:
- corticosteroid receptors
- oestrogen and progestogen receptors
- thyroid hormone receptors
- Vitamin D$_3$ receptors

The Gc/receptor complexes form dimers before entering the nucleus (not shown)

Fig. 4.7   Mechanism of action of a receptor linked to gene transcription. *Gc*, Glucocorticoid; *R*, receptor.

CARRIER MOLECULES AS TARGETS FOR DRUG ACTION

In essence there are two main types of membrane transport proteins:
- Adenosine triphosphate (ATP)-powered ion pumps
- Transporters

Both are transmembrane proteins. In Rang & Dale's *Pharmacology*, these proteins are termed *carriers*.

ATP-powered ion pumps

The three principal ion pumps are the sodium pump (the Na$^+$/K$^+$ ATPase), the calcium pump and the Na$^+$/H$^+$ pump in the gastric parietal cell, which is the target for the proton pump inhibitor **omeprazole**. Here we will concentrate on the sodium pump. This is important in maintaining cellular osmotic balance and cell volume and in maintaining the membrane potential. In many cells (e.g. in the myocardium, the nephron) it is the primary mechanism for transporting Na$^+$ out of the cell (Fig. 4.8).

The K$^+$ concentration is 140 mmol/L inside cells and 5 mmol/l outside. For each molecule of ATP hydrolysed, the sodium pump pumps 3 Na$^+$ out of the cell and 2 K$^+$ in against their chemical gradients. (The pump in Fig. 4.8 has simplified stoichiometry.)

Transporters

The main transporters involved in drug action are symporters and antiporters (exchangers) (Fig. 4.9).

Symporters

These use the electrochemical gradient of one ion (usually Na$^+$) to carry another ion (or molecule or several ions) across a cell membrane. Drugs can modify this action by occupying a binding site (e.g. the action of furosemide (frusemide) on the Na$^+$/K$^+$/2Cl$^-$ symport in the nephron (Fig. 4.9). Similarly, thiazide diuretics bind to and inhibit the Na$^+$/Cl$^-$ symporter in the distal tubule.

Antiporters

These use the electrochemical gradient of one ion (usually Na$^+$) to drive another ion (or molecule) across the membrane in the opposite direction. An important example is the Ca^{2+} exchanger, which exchanges 3 Na$^+$ for 1 Ca^{2+} (see Fig. 4.9). Note that this calcium exchanger should be distinguished from the ATP-driven calcium pump and the ligand-gated and voltage-gated Ca^{2+} channels (see Fig. 4.1 in Rang & Dale's *Pharmacology*). The calcium exchanger is crucial in the maintenance of the Ca^{2+} concentration in blood vessel smooth muscle and cardiac muscle (see Chapter 14). Another example is the uptake carrier in the noradrenergic varicosity, which transports noradrenaline into the cell (see Chapter 11).

ION CHANNELS AS TARGETS FOR DRUG ACTION

Some drugs produce their actions by directly interacting with ion channels. Three examples are given in Fig. 4.10. Note that these ion channels transport ions across the plasma membrane. They are not receptors and should be distinguished from ion channels that function as ionotropic receptors (see above).

ENZYMES AS TARGETS FOR DRUG ACTION

Drugs can produce effects on enzyme reactions by substrate competition or by reversibly or irreversibly modifying the enzyme. Some examples are given in Table 4.1. Drugs mostly act as inhibitors of enzymes (e.g. aspirin), but a few act to stimulate enzyme function, for example metformin, which can stimulate adenosine monophosphate (AMP)-activated protein kinase. Enzyme inhibitors are also important for targeting enzymes in prokaryotic cells as the basis of antimicrobial activity against pathogens.

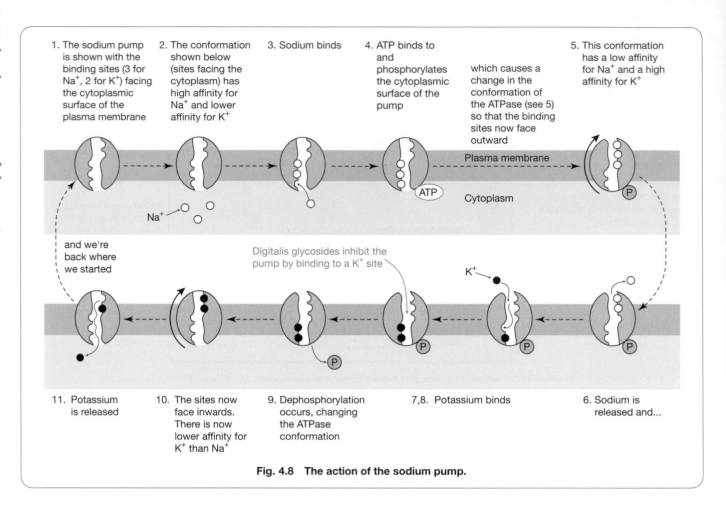

1. The sodium pump is shown with the binding sites (3 for Na⁺, 2 for K⁺) facing the cytoplasmic surface of the plasma membrane

2. The conformation shown below (sites facing the cytoplasm) has high affinity for Na⁺ and lower affinity for K⁺

3. Sodium binds

4. ATP binds to and phosphorylates the cytoplasmic surface of the pump

which causes a change in the conformation of the ATPase (see 5) so that the binding sites now face outward

5. This conformation has a low affinity for Na⁺ and a high affinity for K⁺

and we're back where we started

Digitalis glycosides inhibit the pump by binding to a K⁺ site

11. Potassium is released

10. The sites now face inwards. There is now lower affinity for K⁺ than Na⁺

9. Dephosphorylation occurs, changing the ATPase conformation

7,8. Potassium binds

6. Sodium is released and...

Fig. 4.8   The action of the sodium pump.

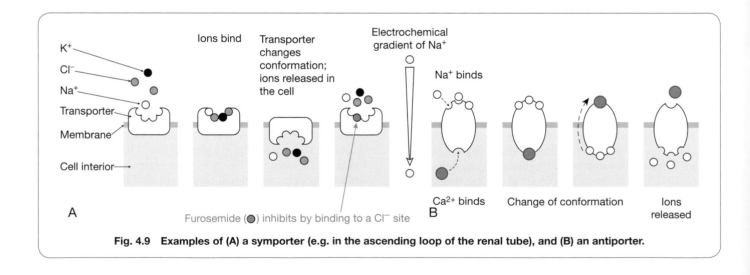

A

K⁺
Cl⁻
Na⁺
Transporter
Membrane
Cell interior

Ions bind

Transporter changes conformation; ions released in the cell

Furosemide (●) inhibits by binding to a Cl⁻ site

Electrochemical gradient of Na⁺

Na⁺ binds

Ca²⁺ binds

Change of conformation

Ions released

B

Fig. 4.9   Examples of (A) a symporter (e.g. in the ascending loop of the renal tube), and (B) an antiporter.

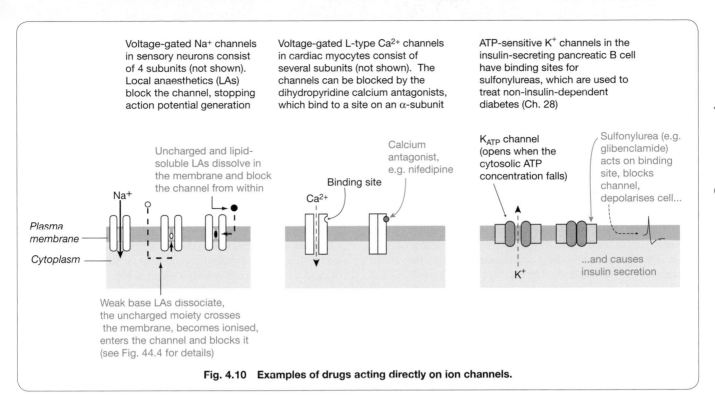

Fig. 4.10 Examples of drugs acting directly on ion channels.

Voltage-gated Na+ channels in sensory neurons consist of 4 subunits (not shown). Local anaesthetics (LAs) block the channel, stopping action potential generation

Uncharged and lipid-soluble LAs dissolve in the membrane and block the channel from within

Na+

Plasma membrane

Cytoplasm

Weak base LAs dissociate, the uncharged moiety crosses the membrane, becomes ionised, enters the channel and blocks it (see Fig. 44.4 for details)

Voltage-gated L-type Ca2+ channels in cardiac myocytes consist of several subunits (not shown). The channels can be blocked by the dihydropyridine calcium antagonists, which bind to a site on an α-subunit

Calcium antagonist, e.g. nifedipine

Binding site

Ca2+

ATP-sensitive K+ channels in the insulin-secreting pancreatic B cell have binding sites for sulfonylureas, which are used to treat non-insulin-dependent diabetes (Ch. 28)

K_{ATP} channel (opens when the cytosolic ATP concentration falls)

Sulfonylurea (e.g. glibenclamide) acts on binding site, blocks channel, depolarises cell...

...and causes insulin secretion

K+

Table 4.1 **Drugs Acting Through Alteration of Enzyme Reactions**

Substrate	Enzyme	Products	Inhibitor	Uses
Acetylcholine	Acetylcholine esterase	Choline; acetate	Neostigmine	Myasthenia gravis and to reverse neuromuscular block
Arachldonate	Cyclooxygonase	Prostanoids	Aspirin	Heart disease and inflammation
Angiotensin (AT)I	AT converting enzyme	AT II	Captopril	Hypertension, heart failure, post-infarct
Hypoxanthine	Xanthine oxidase	Uric acid	Allopurinol	Gout
β-Hydroxy β-methyl glutaryl-CoA (HMG CoA)	HMG CoA reductase	Mevalonic acid	Simvastatin	To lower blood cholesterol
Folate	Dihydrofolate reductase	Tetrahydrofolate	Trimethoprim	With cotrimoxazole as antibacterial
Thymidine	Viral reverse transcriptase		Zidovudine	Human immunodeficiency virus (HIV) infection
Deoxyribonucleotides	DNA polymerase	DNA	Cytarabine	Anticancer drug

Whilst the practice of pharmacology is to ultimately reach an end goal of understanding pharmacodynamics (what the drug does to the body), scientists and clinicians also need to understand what the body does to the drug (pharmacokinetics). This is a vitally important aspect of pharmacology both in drug development and also in the practice of medicine, where individuals, populations and ethnic groups will vary considerably in their response to drugs, and the dose and frequency will need adjusting accordingly to control the amount of drug within the 'therapeutic window'.

Pharmacokinetics therefore provides an understanding of the fate of the dose of drug administered, and the time course and levels of unbound drug in the body. This is influenced by factors determining drug disposition that is divided into four stages and is recognized by the acronym 'ADME':
• Absorption from the site of administration
• Distribution within the body
• Metabolism
• Excretion

ABSORPTION AND DISTRIBUTION OF DRUGS

It is important to know how drug concentrations in tissues change with time, i.e. to understand the pharmacokinetic aspects of drug action. The time course of drug action usually follows that of the concentration at the target site. Important exceptions are drugs that bind irreversibly (e.g. organophosphorus anticholinesterases), where the effect can outlive the concentration. Following absorption, drugs are carried to their targets in the body and their sites of elimination by the blood circulation. Well-perfused tissues, such as the lungs and kidney, can equilibrate with the plasma concentration quickly, whereas poorly perfused tissues, such as fat, will only take up and release drugs slowly. Once a drug arrives at a tissue, it must pass out of the blood capillaries and possibly cross cell membrane barriers, either to reach its target or to pass into the urine or bile. Accordingly, a drug's ability to cross cell membranes is of major concern in pharmacology.

Membrane permeation by drugs
The plasma membrane of cells constitutes a hydrophobic lipid barrier and drug permeation can occur by:
• direct diffusion through the lipid,
• carrier-mediated transport,
• diffusion through aqueous pores, or
• pinocytosis.
The first two mechanisms are most important; aqueous pores are too small to allow the passage of most drugs (which typically have molecular weights in the range 200–1000) and pinocytosis is thought to be important for only a few large molecules (e.g. insulin penetration of the blood–brain barrier).

Diffusion through membrane lipids
Diffusion of a drug depends on its concentration gradient and its diffusion coefficient. The concentration gradient established within the cell membrane depends on the drug's lipid/water partition coefficient. This is conveniently estimated by the drug's distribution between water and a simple organic solvent, such as heptane. (There is a good correlation between such partition coefficients and drug absorption.)

Ionization
Most drugs, being weak acids or weak bases, ionize to some extent in aqueous solution. The ionized form is *lipophobic*, so that ionization impedes passive membrane permeation.

The fractional ionization can be determined from the *Henderson–Hasselbalch* equation:

$$\text{for a weak acid:} \log_{10} {c_i}/{c_u} = \text{pH} - \text{pK}_a$$

$$\text{for a weak base:} \log_{10} {c_i}/{c_u} = \text{pK}_a - \text{pH}$$

Where c_i is the concentration of drug in ionized form, c_u is that in unionized form, pK_a is $-\log_{10}$ of the acid dissociation constant for the drug and pH is $-\log_{10}$ of the hydrogen ion concentration.

Ionization thus depends on the pH of the aqueous environment and the drug's acid dissociation constant (a strong acid has a low pK_a and a strong base has a high pK_a; see Fig. 5.1).

Ion trapping
Where a lipid membrane separates solutions of different pH, the difference in ionization on the two sides can lead to an uneven distribution. The ionized molecules do not readily cross the membrane and there is an effective trapping of these molecules on the side promoting ionization. For example, a weak base such as morphine, even when given intravenously, will achieve a high concentration in the acidic gastric lumen (Fig. 5.2).

Active transport
Carriers are important for membrane transport of essential nutrients that have low lipid solubility. Carriers can be classified into *solute carrier (SLC) transporters* (aid the passive transport of solutes down their electrochemical gradient) and *ATP-binding cassette (ABC) transporters* (pumps that are active and require ATP as an energy source). SLCs may be further classified as *organic cation transporters (OCTs)* and *organic anion transporters (OATs)*. Most drugs are exogenous substances of no nutritional value and are not substrates for the carriers involved in nutrient absorption or delivery to cells (exceptions include the anticancer agent 5-fluorouracil, an analogue of uracil, which can use the transporter for pyrimidines in the gut). However, SLCs

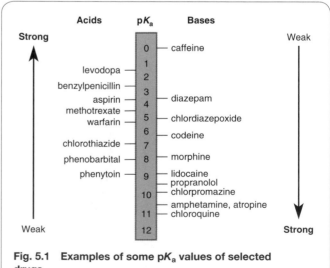

Fig. 5.1 Examples of some pKa values of selected drugs.

are important for carrier-mediated drug transport in the blood-brain barrier, gastrointestinal tract, renal tubules, biliary tract, and the placenta.

Active transport systems in the kidney and liver are, by comparison, very important in the elimination of drugs from the body. (Such carriers have probably evolved for the clearance of toxic substances that might have been ingested and whose rapid elimination would have survival value.) Active transport (via the P-glycoprotein transporter) is also an important mechanism for resistance to anticancer drugs.

Features of active drug transport are:
• uphill transport (allowing high renal clearances) and
• a finite number of transporter molecules leading to:

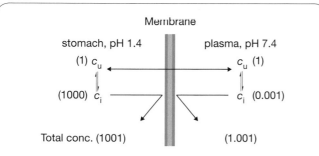

Fig. 5.2　Ion trapping. In this theoretical example, a weak base with a pK_a of 4.4 is shown concentrating in the stomach. (The numbers in brackets indicate relative concentrations in the steady state. C_u (given a value of 1) is assumed to attain the same concentration on each side of the membrane.)

– saturation and
– competition between drugs for transport, exacerbated by the low substrate specificity of many carriers.

Drug absorption
Drugs can be administered via the gut (enteral) or by other routes (parenteral), and the route will be chosen based on a number of factors concerning the chemical properties of the drug that will affect its ADME profile, the target organ and safety (Fig. 5.3).

Enteral administration
Oral absorption from the stomach or intestines, after the drug is swallowed, is the most convenient and acceptable route. An important consideration is that oral absorption will deliver the drug directly to the liver, the major site of drug metabolism, via the portal circulation; this may result in substantial *first-pass elimination*. Drugs absorbed from the mouth (*sublingual* or *buccal*) and the lower rectum do not enter the hepatic portal vein and so avoid first-pass metabolism. Sublingual glyceryl trinitrate is rapidly absorbed to provide quick relief of anginal pain (it is ineffective if swallowed). Rectal administration is suitable for some irritants and when vomiting prevents oral medication.

Factors controlling oral absorption
Lipid solubility and ionization　This is discussed above. Note that the intestine with its villi and microvilli is the main absorptive area, so that weak acids, which will be less ionized in the stomach, will, nevertheless, be mostly absorbed in the more alkaline intestine. Rapid passage of drug from the stomach to intestine is likely to speed up drug absorption.

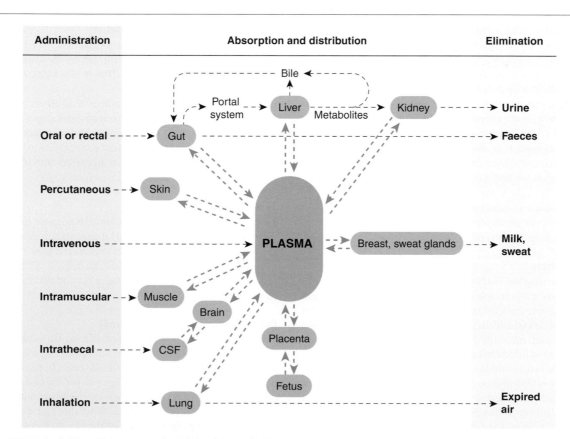

Fig. 5.3　The main routes of drug administration and elimination. (From Rang HP, Ritter JM, Flower RJ, Henderson G. Rang & Dale's *Pharmacology*. 8th ed. Philadelphia: Elsevier; 2016.)

Drug formulation Drugs must dissolve to establish a concentration gradient for absorption, the rate and extent of absorption depending on the pharmaceutical formulation. Rapid absorption of a tablet requires its disintegration into small particles that readily dissolve. Note that while a drug is more water soluble in its ionized form, it is the unionized form that is membrane permeable. *Sustained release* formulations release the drug slowly to prolong drug action and reduce the frequency of administration.

Gastrointestinal motility Stasis can slow oral absorption while diarrhoea, predictably, may allow insufficient time for complete absorption.

Interactions with other substances in the gut Food will often slow absorption by simply reducing the drug's concentration. More specific interactions can also occur; for example tetracyclines will interact with Ca^{2+} in food to form an incompletely absorbed, insoluble complex.

Bioavailability
Bioavailability is a term applied particularly to oral preparations and expresses the extent to which a dose is absorbed. The most useful definition is *the proportion of the administered dose that reaches the systemic circulation*. Incomplete release from the dosage form, destruction within the gut, poor absorption and first-pass elimination are important causes of low bioavailability. For drugs with a low therapeutic index, it is important that repeat prescriptions provide medicines of equivalent bioavailability (*bioequivalence*).

Parenteral administration
These routes are useful for:
- rapid effects (e.g. in status asthmaticus),
- drugs that are poorly absorbed from the gut (e.g. pancuronium, insulin),
- irritants (some anticancer agents), and
- localization of action (e.g. inhaled bronchodilators, mydriatics).

Intravenous (IV) injection is the most rapid route, IV infusions allowing tight control of drug concentration in the plasma. *Intramuscular* (IM) and *subcutaneous* (SC) injection have found particular utility in providing long-term therapy from *depot* preparations (e.g. contraceptive steroid implants (Ch. 17) or slowly released antipsychotic agents (Ch. 12)). *Inhalation* is used for anaesthetic gases (Ch. 27) and in treatment of bronchial asthma and chronic obstructive pulmonary disease (COPD) with bronchodilators and antiinflammatory steroids (Chs. 16 and 20).

Topical application of drugs to the skin is used mainly for local actions, but systemic absorption of very lipid-soluble substances is possible (e.g. scopolamine patches to prevent motion sickness).

Drug distribution
Most drugs entering the body do not spread rapidly throughout the whole of body water to achieve a uniform concentration within the major compartments (plasma, interstitial fluid, intracellular fluid, transcellular fluid and fat). Large molecules (heparin, insulin) cannot easily enter interstitial and intracellular spaces whereas smaller and lipid-soluble molecules can.

A drug's penetration into these compartments is indicated by its *apparent volume of distribution* (V_d): the volume of fluid that would be required to hold the amount of drug in the body at the measured plasma concentration. It can be estimated by the equation:

$$V_d = Dose/c_p$$

where c_p is the concentration of drug in the plasma after it has equilibrated in its distribution volume but before a significant fraction has been eliminated. Examples of V_d values (l/kg) include the following:
- Heparin: 0.05–0.1
- Tubocurarine: 0.2–0.4
- Ethanol: 1.0
- Propranolol: 2–5
- Nortriptyline: >20

The 'volume of distribution' is not a real 'volume', but a parameter of the amount of drug in the plasma relative to the total amount of drug in the body. V_d is determined by the binding of drug to tissue compared to plasma protein. A large V_d is suggestive of a drug tightly bound to tissues and little in the blood plasma. Thus in the examples above, heparin (which is a very large, highly charged drug) is held in blood plasma to a far greater extent than propranolol or nortriptyline. Lipid-insoluble drugs are mainly confined to plasma and interstitial fluids, whereas lipid-soluble drugs reach all compartments and may accumulate in fat.

V_d is used to determine the *loading dose* of drugs, that is the initial dose of drug administered to reach steady state more quickly, than if the *maintenance dose* was used where clearance might delay the level of drug concentration needed to reach a therapeutic level.

Binding to protein and other tissue components
Tetracyclines bind to calcium in bones and teeth (which can produce abnormalities in tooth development in children). Many drugs bind to plasma proteins of which albumin is generally the most important, although α-acid glycoprotein is of greater importance for some basic drugs (e.g. propranolol). For some drugs, more than 95% of drug in plasma may be bound to protein. Binding to plasma proteins is of finite capacity and of low specificity and has several consequences:
- The bound drug is usually inactive.
- The reduction in free drug concentration may reduce elimination (by reducing glomerular filtration) or, conversely, protein binding may serve to deliver drug to the kidney and liver, and so enhance elimination.
- One drug may prevent the binding of another, and so enhance pharmacological activity. (This is of significance only for highly bound drugs, such as warfarin (98% bound), whose displacement by just 2% would double the free concentration. Thus, changes by only a fraction will result in increased activity and thus can lead to serious side effects such as bleeding.)

Accumulation in lipid
Lipid-soluble drugs may concentrate in adipose tissue which is a large non-polar compartment. For example, halothane can concentrate in fat during long operations and its slow release can lead to prolonged CNS depression postoperatively. Certain pesticides such as DDT can also accumulate in fat and this can lead to long-term neurotoxicity.

Penetration of drugs into the brain
The endothelial cells lining brain capillaries are joined to each other by tight junctions to produce an unbroken cell membrane lining, which is the main element of the blood–brain barrier. This prevents passive entry into the brain of lipophobic/ionized molecules. An additional feature is the turnover of cerebrospinal fluid. This is produced by the choroid plexuses, flows through the ventricles and after reaching the outer surface of the brain drains into the blood at the arachnoid villi. Drugs that penetrate slowly will be removed by 'washout' in this way and achieve a steady-state concentration much below the plasma concentration.

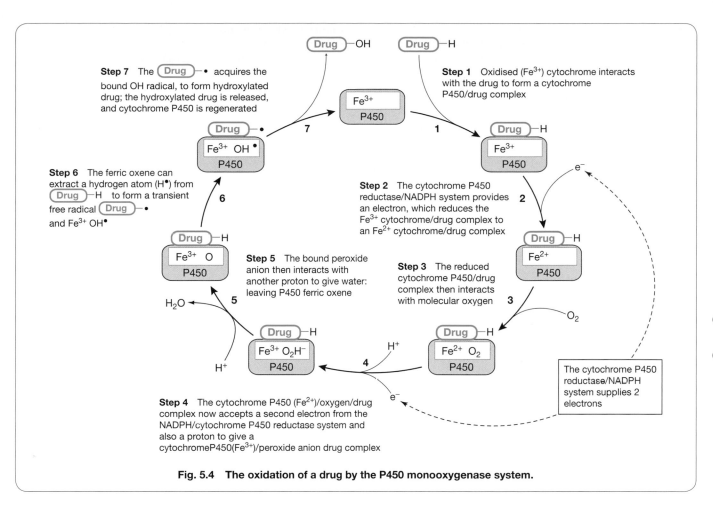

Step 7 The (Drug)— • acquires the bound OH radical, to form hydroxylated drug; the hydroxylated drug is released, and cytochrome P450 is regenerated

Step 1 Oxidised (Fe^{3+}) cytochrome interacts with the drug to form a cytochrome P450/drug complex

Step 6 The ferric oxene can extract a hydrogen atom ($H^\bullet$) from (Drug)—H to form a transient free radical (Drug)— • and $Fe^{3+} OH^\bullet$

Step 2 The cytochrome P450 reductase/NADPH system provides an electron, which reduces the Fe^{3+} cytochrome/drug complex to an Fe^{2+} cytochrome/drug complex

Step 5 The bound peroxide anion then interacts with another proton to give water: leaving P450 ferric oxene

Step 3 The reduced cytochrome P450/drug complex then interacts with molecular oxygen

The cytochrome P450 reductase/NADPH system supplies 2 electrons

Step 4 The cytochrome P450 (Fe^{2+})/oxygen/drug complex now accepts a second electron from the NADPH/cytochrome P450 reductase system and also a proton to give a cytochrome P450(Fe^{3+})/peroxide anion drug complex

Fig. 5.4 The oxidation of a drug by the P450 monooxygenase system.

Improvements in drug delivery

Pharmaceutical scientists have developed technologies to overcome some of the issues described above in order to improve drug delivery and tissue localization. Pro-drugs, biologically erodible nanoparticles, antibody-drug conjugates, packaging in liposomes, and coatable implantable devices are examples of how this may be achieved.

DRUG METABOLISM AND EXCRETION

The effects of a drug depend not only on its pharmacological actions, but also on how it is handled in the body. When a drug enters the body, it is subjected, in essence, to the processes that have been developed for dealing with any foreign molecule – it is metabolized and/or excreted. The liver is the main site of drug metabolism and the kidney the main site of excretion. Metabolism involves two main processes: first, the molecule is made more lipophobic so as to reduce the possibility of reabsorption in the renal tubules; second, it is conjugated so as to reduce its effects and aid excretion. With some drugs the metabolites share the actions of the parent drug (e.g. diazepam and its metabolite nordazepam). With other drugs the metabolite may be responsible for toxicity (e.g. paracetamol). Some drugs are prodrugs, i.e. inactive themselves but converted into an active drug within the body; for example, enalapril is hydrolysed to the active compound enalaprilat and minoxidil is activated by sulphate conjugation. Some drugs can modify their own metabolism and that of other drugs by induction of hepatic enzymes. For many drugs there are two phases of metabolism to decrease lipid solubility.

The phases of drug metabolism

Phase I comprises the following reactions to make drugs more polar:
- Oxidation (Fig. 5.4), e.g. propranolol, paracetamol
- Reduction, e.g. prednisone
- Hydrolysis, e.g. procaine, succinylcholine

Phase II comprises the following conjugation reactions which usually results in inactive products:
- Glucuronidation, e.g. morphine
- Glycosidation
- Sulphation, e.g. paracetamol
- Methylation
- Acetylation, e.g. sulphonamides, isoniazid
- Amino acid (esp. glycine) conjugation
- Glutathione conjugation, e.g. paracetamol

The phase I oxidation reactions by the hepatic P450 monooxygenase system are perhaps the most important.

The P450 monooxygenase system

The oxidation of a drug by the monooxygenase system requires:
- the cytochrome P450 haem protein: a family of isoenzymes found in the smooth endoplasmic reticulum,
- molecular oxygen,
- cytochrome P450 reductase (which is closely associated with cytochrome P450), and
- nicotinamide adenosine dinucleotide phosphate, reduced form (NADPH).

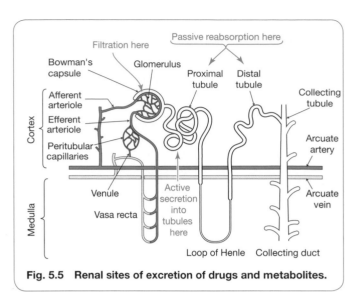

Filtration here

Passive reabsorption here

Bowman's capsule

Glomerulus

Proximal tubule

Distal tubule

Collecting tubule

Afferent arteriole

Efferent arteriole

Cortex

Peritubular capillaries

Arcuate artery

Venule

Active secretion into tubules here

Arcuate vein

Medulla

Vasa recta

Loop of Henle   Collecting duct

Fig. 5.5   Renal sites of excretion of drugs and metabolites.

Table 5.1   Examples of drugs metabolized by P450 monooxygenase oxidation reactions

Reactions	Drugs
O-dealkylation	Codeine, dextromethorphan (Ch. 13), indometacin (Ch. 16)
Aliphatic hydroxylation	Ibuprofen (Ch. 16), ciclosporin (Ch. 16)
Deamination	Amphetamines (Ch. 37)
N-dealkylation	Morphine (Ch. 13), diazepam (Ch. 12), tamoxifen (Ch. 34)
N-oxidation	Chlorphenamine (antihistamine), dapsone (Ch. 31)
S-oxidation	Cimetidine (Ch. 22), thioridazine (Ch. 12)
Aromatic hydroxylation	Propranolol (Chs. 11 and 14), phenytoin (Ch. 12)

The cytochrome P450 reductase catalyses the following reaction (cyto = cytochrome):

$$NADPH + Oxidised\ cyto + H^+ \longrightarrow Reduces\ cyto + NADP^+$$

During the reaction, two electrons – required for the oxidation reaction – are generated. Cytochrome P450 undergoes cyclic oxidation/reduction during drug oxidation, as shown in Figure 5.5. Table 5.1 gives examples of drugs metabolized by oxidation.

The activity of the cytochrome P450 system can be markedly increased by exposure to other drugs or dietary factors; such enzyme induction can reduce the effect of a drug, or conversely increase the production of toxic metabolites. Other drugs may potentiate drug action by inhibiting the P450 system.

The excretion of drugs and their metabolites

The kidney is the principal organ of excretion of drugs and their metabolites but some compounds are excreted in the bile and some by other routes such as the lungs.

Renal excretion

Renal excretion involves the following processes.

Filtration in the glomerulus

Arterial blood pressure forces an ultrafiltrate from the glomerular capillaries into the Bowman's capsule in the kidney (see Fig. 5.5). Small drug molecules ($M_r < 5000$) in both charged and uncharged states cross the glomerular membranes readily, achieving a concentration in the filtrate identical to their free concentration in the plasma. (Negatively charged sialoproteins in the capillary wall can impede the filtration of larger, negatively charged molecules.) Drug molecules bound to plasma proteins are not filtered.

Active tubular secretion

This occurs in the proximal convoluted tubule in the kidney. About 80% of drugs or metabolites pass from the glomerulus via the efferent arterioles to the peritubular capillaries that surround the proximal convoluted tubule; here the agents become available for active transport into the tubule. In the basolateral membranes of the tubule, there are low-specificity carriers for organic anions and organic cations, which transport endogenous substances and drugs from the plasma into the tubular cells from where they pass into the filtrate by facilitated diffusion (see Fig. 5.5). Some organic acids that are secreted are the **penicillins, probenecid**, some diuretics (**furosemide, thiazides**) and various conjugates (glycine, glucuronic acid, sulphate). Some organic cations that are secreted are morphine, amiloride (a K^+-sparing diuretic) and quaternary ammonium compounds such as the cholinergic agonists and antagonists. The carriers may have sufficient activity to clear the drug completely from the blood passing through the kidney. Tubular secretion of one drug may be competitively inhibited by another; in this way, for example, the half-life of penicillin is markedly increased by probenecid.

Reabsorption from the tubules

Drugs within the tubules in the unionized form and therefore lipid soluble will be reabsorbed. A weak acid, such as aspirin, will thus be more readily excreted in alkaline rather than acidic urine. The ratio of ionized to unionized acid is given by 10^{pH-pK_a}.

Taking the pK_a of aspirin as 3.4, the ratio of ionized to unionized drug in the urine at a pH value of 6.4 will be $10^{6.4-3.4} = 10^3 = 1000:1$. At pH 8.4, it will be $10^{8.4-3.4} = 10^5 = 100\,000:1$.

At both pH values, very little of the drug will be in the unionized, membrane permeant form. Nevertheless, the proportion at the lower pH will be 100 times that at the higher pH. This allows much more reabsorption at the lower pH and has a dramatic effect on the clearance of aspirin as shown in Figure 5.6. This is effectively an example of ion trapping as described earlier in this chapter. The enhanced elimination of weakly acidic drugs at high urinary pH is made use of in the process of forced alkaline diuresis.

Hepatic excretion

Bile is produced at a daily rate of 0.5–1.0 L and is a major route of excretion for a few drugs (e.g. cromoglicate) and rather more drug metabolites (e.g. morphine glucuronide). Drug excreted in bile may be reabsorbed from the intestine to undergo further cycles of biliary excretion: so-called *enterohepatic circulation*. A significant proportion of drug in the body may be held in this *enteric pool*, which may act to increase the drug's half-life. Drugs pass from blood to bile by active transport and competition may occur. The transporters differ from those found in the kidney.

MEASUREMENT OF PHARMACOKINETICS

Pharmacokinetics explores the changes in drug concentrations throughout the body with time as a result of ADME. The ability to measure changes in drug concentration over time

Cannot

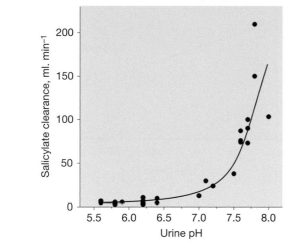

Fig. 5.6 Effects of urine pH on the excretion of a weak acid; aspirin.

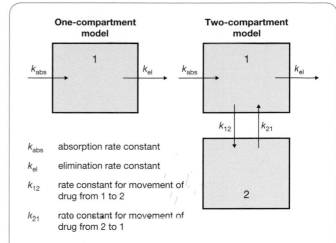

Fig. 5.7 One- and two-compartment models of drug distribution. In the simplest two-compartment model, absorption and elimination are to and from compartment 1, respectively.

is of vital importance to the process of drug discovery (where pharmacokinetics measured in animals is used to ascertain the likely 'therapeutic window' of a drug, and also for clinicians where patient variability in ADME requires dose adjustments to be made for a drug to remain effective and safety concerns manageable (therapeutic drug monitoring). There are two fundamental parameters, V_d (introduced above), and *clearance* (*Cl*) used to describe the interaction of a drug with ADME (readers are referred to the excellent book *Pharmacokinetics Made Easy* by DJ Birkett for depth of coverage). A third important parameter is the drug's half-life, often represented as the elimination rate constant (k_{el}), although this is determined by V_d and *Cl*. These parameters are determined by the rate of flux of a drug through different tissues, a concept known as 'compartments'. In practice, pharmacokinetics usually focuses on drug concentrations in plasma as these can be readily measured compared to tissue concentrations, and measurements such as the maximum plasma concentration (C_{max}), the time interval between drug administration and C_{max} (T_{max}) provide important characteristics, as does the area under curve (AUC) to measure total exposure.

Compartments

Whole body autoradiographs and chemical analysis of tissues show that drugs do not penetrate uniformly throughout the body. Particular tissues may well show higher or lower concentrations of drug than the plasma. Some tissues, however, may behave similarly (i.e. have similar drug concentration versus time profiles); it is then convenient to consider them as belonging to a common *compartment*. It is usual to adopt the minimum number of compartments (usually one or two) that can adequately describe the time course of drug disposition and predict the changes in concentrations that occur following administration. For many drugs, the volume of distribution (V_d, see above) appears to be a single entity and the situation is consistent with the *one-compartment model*. For other drugs, it is found that different tissues equilibrate with the drug at different rates. Where the tissues fall easily into two groups (e.g. well perfused and poorly perfused) a *two-compartment model* is sometimes applicable. Compartment 1 comprises the plasma and rapidly equilibrating tissues (e.g. lung and kidney). Compartment 2 represents the remaining more slowly equilibrating tissues (Fig. 5.7).

One-compartment distribution kinetics

Where passive diffusion is responsible for absorption or excretion, drug transport is often *first order*, i.e. the rate is proportional to the concentration gradient. First-order kinetics is exemplified by the exponentially declining plasma concentration of drug, c_p, which follows first-order elimination after intravenous administration (Fig. 5.8A):

$$c_p = c_p(0) e^{-k_{el}t}$$

where c_p is the drug concentration in plasma, $c_p(0)$ is initial plasma concentration at time $t = 0$ and k_{el} is the elimination rate constant.

The relationship may be linearized by taking logarithms (Fig. 5.8B). For natural logarithms (ln):

$$c_p = \ln c_p(0) - k_{el}t$$

A plot of $\ln c_p$ against t gives a straight line of slope $-k_{el}$.

The *plasma half-life*, ($t_{1/2}$ or $t_{0.5}$), applicable to drugs subject to first-order elimination, is the time taken for any given plasma concentration to decrease by 50% ($t_{1/2}$ is inversely related to k_{el}: $t_{1/2} = 0.693/k_{el}$).

Zero-order kinetics (Saturation kinetics)

This refers to the situation where the rate of the process (e.g. drug metabolism) is independent of the drug's concentration (Fig. 5.8C). Sometimes, drug elimination initially occurs as a result of saturation of a distinct mechanism (e.g. carrier-mediated transport or enzyme substrate). Examples include ethanol, phenytoin and salicylate.

Carrier-mediated transport

Drugs and enzymic biotransformations are saturable phenomena that, in the steady state, follow *Michaelis–Menten* kinetics, i.e. where the reaction rate is linear. Where such a process lowers c_p:

$$-\frac{dc_p}{dt} = \frac{v_{max} \cdot c_p}{c_p + K_m}$$

where V_{max} is the maximum rate of transport or biotransformation and K_m is the Michaelis constant. When the drug concentration is high (relative to K_m), this reduces to:

$$-\frac{dc_p}{dt} \approx v_{max}$$

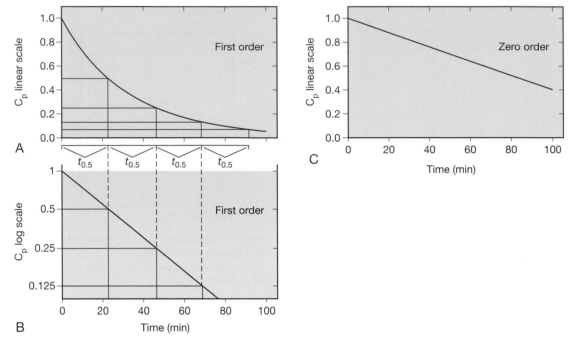

Fig. 5.8 Elimination of drugs. (A) First-order, linear concentration scale; (B) first-order, logarithmic scale. In a first-order situation, C_p decreases by half in successive half-lives (half-life here is 23 min). (C) shows the constant rate of elimination according to zero-order kinetics (here 0.006 units/min).

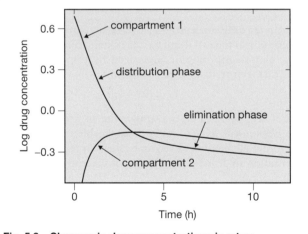

Fig. 5.9 Changes in drug concentrations in a two-compartment model of drug distribution following intravenous administration. Concentration falls quickly in compartment 1 as drug distributes into compartment 2. Note logarithmic concentration scale.

At this point the elimination process is saturated and, being independent of concentration, obeys zero-order kinetics (c_p declines at a fixed rate, Fig. 5.8C). Zero-order kinetics applies to many drugs at high concentrations and to some at 'low' concentrations (e.g. ethanol).

Two-compartment kinetics

The kinetics of the two-compartment model will obviously be more complicated and the plot of ln c_p versus time after intravenous administration will not yield a straight line. Figure 5.9 shows drug concentrations in compartments 1 and 2 following intravenous injection. For first-order distribution and elimination, the decay of the plasma concentration of the drug will follow a bi-exponential curve. The two components roughly represent the processes of transfer between plasma and tissues (α phase) and elimination from the plasma (β phase).

Drug clearance

Drug Cl is thus the parameter that describes the efficiency of elimination (whether it be urine, faeces, sweat, etc.) of a drug from the body (systemic circulation). Thus, uptake of drug into tissues is not clearance since the drug will eventually come back out. Cl is defined as the volume of plasma cleared of drug per unit time. (Usual units are mL/min.) Thus (assuming first-order, one-compartment behaviour)

$$\text{Clearance} = \frac{\text{elimination rate}}{\text{plasma concentration}}$$

The elimination rate is also given by the amount of drug in body ($c_p V_d$) multiplied by k_{el}. Therefore,

$$Cl = \frac{k_{el} c_p V_d}{c_p} = k_{el} V_d$$

as $k_{el} = 0.693/t_{1/2}$ $Cl = 0.693 v_d/t_{1/2}$

Total body clearance is the sum of the clearances occurring by whatever routes are applicable to the drug in question; often only renal and hepatic clearances are important.

Repeated drug administration

Drugs are commonly given as repeated doses using a fixed *dosing interval*. Since most drugs are eliminated exponentially, whenever a second dose is administered some of the preceding dose will still be in the body and the new peak concentration achieved will exceed that after the first dose, i.e. *accumulation* occurs (Fig. 5.10). With repeated doses c_p, and hence elimination, increases until a plateau is reached where the whole of the dose is eliminated

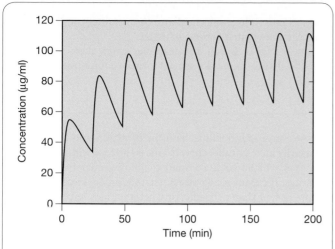

Fig. 5.10 **Drug accumulation.** Incomplete elimination of drug during the dosing interval results in a build-up of drug in the plasma.

during the dosing interval. Paradoxically, the rate of approach to the plateau is determined by the elimination rate constant rather than the absorption rate constant. A drug with a long half-life (e.g. digoxin) will thus approach the plateau concentration slowly. If this is undesirable, initial *loading doses* can be used.

The clearance concept can be usefully employed to determine the expected steady-state concentration of drug in the plasma, c_{ss}, during an infusion or regular intermittent dosing. In the steady state, the rate of drug administration (e.g. 500 mg per day) will equal the rate of loss (elimination rate, i.e. $Cl \times c_{ss}$). Therefore, c_{ss} is given by the dose rate divided by the Cl. Alternatively, by knowing the Cl of a drug and the desired target plasma concentration it is possible to calculate the required dose rate ($Cl \times c_{ss}$).

The action of drugs is usually measured by bioassay, which is the measurement of potency or activity of a drug using a biological response, using the principles of drug action and measurement provided in Chapter 3. It is used when it is necessary to:
- measure the activity of new/chemically unknown substances in research work or in new drug development,
- investigate endogenous mediators/transmitters, and
- measure unwanted actions of drugs.

A clinical trial in which, for example, a new drug is compared with one already in use is a special form of comparative bioassay.

PRINCIPLES OF BIOASSAY

Most bioassays involve measurements of the responses of isolated tissue or groups of animals. In the usual type of bioassay, the response to the unknown (or test) drug is compared with that of a standard (or control) drug. The response to a drug may be:
- graded, e.g. the contraction of a smooth muscle, the change in heart rate;
- all or none (quantal), e.g. the absence or presence of a pinch reflex, the success of maze-running in a stipulated time.

For accurate estimation, a parallel line assay is required (though in many cases this may not be feasible). Often, the effect of a drug (for which we have limited data) will be assessed (especially when compared with another drug or mediator) over several log order of magnitudes of concentration or dose (in vivo). This allows estimates of the equivalent concentrations of unknown and standard drugs to be compared for potency. Furthermore, an extensive assay can reveal unforeseen characteristics, for example synergism of receptor activation, selective functionalities at different doses, or polypharmacology. Sometimes pharmacologists will choose half-log (1, 3, 10, 30, 100, etc.) or third-log (1, 2, 5, 10, 20, 50, 100, etc.) intervals because these will provide recordings that are equally spaced on a graph (to improve accuracy of analysis). A more precise understanding of a compound's pharmacodynamic relationship might lead investigators to use concentrations with an arithmetic interval scaling.

The actions of drugs will be compared using familiar terms, for example the ED_{50} (or EC_{50}) or maximal responses (E_{max}). Other measurements are sometimes also used; for example the ratio ED_{75}/ED_{25} provides an assessment of the dose-response curve slope (otherwise measured exactly as h, the Hill coefficient: measured at the point of inflection for ED_{50}). It is used in a derivation of the Hill-Langmuir equation (see Chapter 3) of the dose-response relationship to quantify the degree of interaction between two ligand binding sites (taken from Page et al. *Integrated Pharmacology*, 2nd edition, Chapter 5):

$$E = E_{max} . [A]^h / [A]^h + (EC_{50})^h$$

Graded responses

Taking the contraction of an isolated strip of smooth muscle as an example, the log of the dose is plotted against the response expressed as the percentage of the maximal response (Fig. 6.1). When two agents act on the same receptor and have the same intrinsic activity (see Chapter 3), the log dose–response curves will be parallel and their relative potency (M) can be obtained from the separation of the two curves (log M in Fig. 6.1).

All-or-none responses (quantal responses)

In all-or-none situations (usually an *in vivo* response), the response is expressed as the percentage of individuals giving the all-or-none response. If a parallel log dose–response curve can be obtained, the potency ratio of unknown (or test) drug to control (standard) can be obtained as for a graded response. However, the two drugs may not have identical mechanisms of action and thus will not necessarily have parallel curves. This is the case with comparative bioassays, which seek to compare the biological activity of different drugs, for example to assess whether a new local anaesthetic is more potent than procaine, or whether a new antihypertensive vasodilator acting by a novel mechanism is more or less potent than the calcium antagonist nifedipine.

In comparative assays, a comparison of the ED_{50} (the dose which produces the particular outcome in 50% of the population) of each drug can be used to get a rough estimation of its relative potency. Note in this case the shape of the curve is determined by the statistical distribution of sensitivities of the individuals. A small standard deviation will produce a steep log dose–response curve and vice versa. Comparative assays are often used during the development of new drugs and in clinical trials (Fig. 6.2).

NEW DRUG DEVELOPMENT

Before a new drug can receive a product licence it must be tested for effectiveness and toxicity. Preclinical tests on isolated tissues and in intact animals* should ensure that the drug has the required

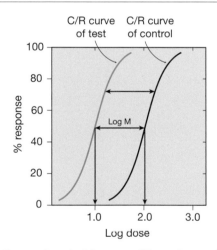

Fig. 6.1 Comparison by bioassay of the potency of the unknown (test) drug with standard (control). Since the concentration–response (C/R) curves are parallel, log M (the potency ratio) is the same at all points of the curve.

---

*Animal models. Initial tests of the potency of a drug such as a new vasodilator drug have necessarily to be done on animals. But there can be hazards in extrapolating such data to the use of the new agent as an antihypertensive drug in humans. Animal models can, however, be devised that attempt to mimic closely human conditions (such as anxiety, pain or hypertension) and which might provide valuable information on a drug's potential before exposure of human subjects. For example, animal models of hypertension have been established in which high blood pressure is induced by compromising renal function or by the selective breeding of strains that develop hypertension spontaneously.

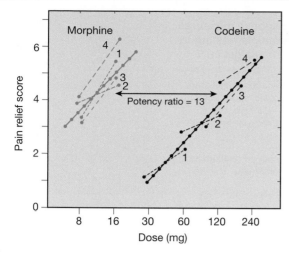

Fig. 6.2 Comparative assay of morphine versus codeine in humans. Each of four patients was given by intramuscular injection, on successive occasions, in random order, four different treatments (high and low doses of morphine and high and low doses of codeine). The subjective pain relief score was calculated for each treatment. The calculated regression line (solid line with dots) gave a potency ratio estimate of 13. (After Houde RW et al. In: *Analgesics*. New York: Academic Press, 1965.)

mechanism of action (e.g. β-adrenoceptor block) and at least in animals will produce appropriate system responses (e.g. analgesia). The characteristics of drug action can be made from the molecular, cellular, tissue, animal and population levels, and it is important to understand the qualitative nature of experiments conducted at each level (Fig. 6.3).

All bioassays should be designed to minimize variation and error through good experimental design. Bias can also be controlled through randomization of procedure allocation and blinding of an experimenter. Statistical tests need to be chosen at the time of experimental design to minimize erroneous conclusions. In particular, two types of error can be controlled:
- Type I error: Analysis shows a difference between A and B when none exists (false positive).
- Type II error: Analysis does not show a difference between A and B when it does exist (false negative).

The probability of avoiding these errors is influenced by the power of an experiment.

Animal models of disease are often required to assess the likelihood of efficacy in a human population. In this regard, animal models are fundamental to understanding the action of a drug in a physiological, integrated (whole) system. However, some important requirements for pharmacologists using animal models include understanding how these models resemble human disease:
- similar pathological phenotype (face validity)
- similar causation (construct validity)
- similar response to treatment (predictive validity)

At this stage the new drug will be tested against standard drugs in comparative assays. Toxicity tests in animals should in most cases allow some prediction of toxic/adverse effects in humans (see Chapters 7–9).

Clinical testing

In comparisons of drugs used clinically, potency does not necessarily relate directly to therapeutic usefulness; it is important to consider also the maximum achievable response and the incidence of unwanted effects.

Clinical testing in humans involves four phases:

Phase I
Measurement of pharmacological activity, pharmacokinetics and side effects in healthy volunteers (unless exposure of healthy individuals is unethical, e.g. trials of potentially toxic anticancer drugs can only be done in cancer patients).

Phase II
Pilot studies in small groups of patients to confirm that the drug works in the target condition and to establish the dosage regimen to be used in phase III.

Phase III
Formal clinical trials in a large number of patients to determine the drug's efficacy compared with existing treatment and to determine the incidence of unwanted effects.

Phase IV
Post-marketing surveillance to establish efficacy and toxicity in general use. The detection of rare, adverse effects is most likely to occur in this phase.

CLINICAL TRIALS

The object of a clinical trial is to obtain an objective assessment of two or more methods of treatment. This frequently involves comparing a new drug with a standard drug – as is necessary in phase III of clinical testing (see above).

Principles of clinical trials
Ideally the log dose–response curve of the new test drug is compared with the log dose–response curve of the standard control drug. This is rarely feasible. In practice, two points on the dose-response curves (chosen in a preliminary trial) of each may be used (see Fig. 6.2). More commonly still, single doses of each are compared. In essence, most clinical trials give information on the *comparative efficacy* and not the *comparative potency* of the two drugs. The starting dose during phase I will be determined based on doses of drugs that did not produce a safety or toxicity concern from preclinical safety testing in animals, after an appropriate safety margin has been added (see Chapters 7 and 8). Dose escalation will then occur gradually, via a single ascending dose (SAD) or multiple ascending dose (MAD).

Two important principles in the conduct of a clinical trial are:
- random allocation of patients to test and control groups, and
- a double-blind design.

Random allocation of patients to test and control groups
There is a real possibility that bias could affect the allocation of patients to test or control treatment. To minimize such bias, it is essential to allocate patients to new or old treatments on a random basis. For a large group of patients, randomization should ensure that each group has an equivalent spectrum of ages, males or females, severity of disease, etc. In some trials, with smaller numbers of participants, and where the patients' condition is stable, a *cross-over design* allows each patient to receive both treatments.

Double-blind design
If either the patient or doctor knows which treatment is being administered, the assessment may be subject to bias according to the expectations of either or both. This is usually countered by a double-blind design, i.e. neither the patient nor the investigator

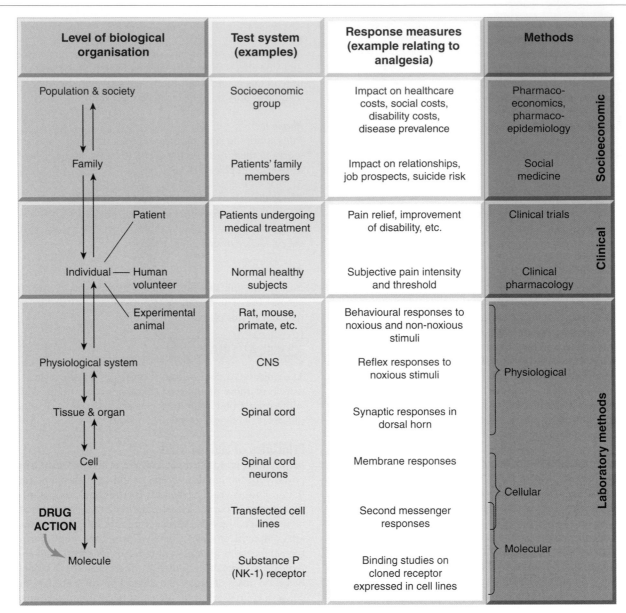

Level of biological organisation	Test system (examples)	Response measures (example relating to analgesia)	Methods	
Population & society	Socioeconomic group	Impact on healthcare costs, social costs, disability costs, disease prevalence	Pharmaco-economics, pharmaco-epidemiology	Socioeconomic
Family	Patients' family members	Impact on relationships, job prospects, suicide risk	Social medicine	Socioeconomic
Patient	Patients undergoing medical treatment	Pain relief, improvement of disability, etc.	Clinical trials	Clinical
Individual — Human volunteer	Normal healthy subjects	Subjective pain intensity and threshold	Clinical pharmacology	Clinical
Experimental animal	Rat, mouse, primate, etc.	Behavioural responses to noxious and non-noxious stimuli	Physiological	Laboratory methods
Physiological system	CNS	Reflex responses to noxious stimuli	Physiological	Laboratory methods
Tissue & organ	Spinal cord	Synaptic responses in dorsal horn	Physiological	Laboratory methods
Cell	Spinal cord neurons	Membrane responses	Cellular	Laboratory methods
DRUG ACTION	Transfected cell lines	Second messenger responses	Cellular	Laboratory methods
Molecule	Substance P (NK-1) receptor	Binding studies on cloned receptor expressed in cell lines	Molecular	Laboratory methods

Fig. 6.3 Levels of biological organization and types of pharmacological measurement. (From Rang HP, Ritter JM, Flower RJ, Henderson G. *Rang & Dale's Pharmacology*. 8th ed. Philadelphia: Elsevier; 2016.)

knows which treatment is being given. The importance of a patient's belief is emphasized by the *placebo* effect: an inert preparation may be found to have a demonstrable effect if the patient believes it to be pharmacologically effective.

Number of subjects required

The number of patients needed for a trial depends on the significance level sought and the power of the trial. These are influenced by consideration, respectively, of type I errors (proposing a difference when none exists) and type II errors (failure to detect a real difference). If it is thought to be worthwhile to detect a small improvement (such as a 1%–2% decrease in death rate) then a large number of patients will be required. Statisticians determine the detailed design of a trial, including the number of patients required to meet the declared aim.

A more recent and instructive means of expressing the benefits (or risks) of a treatment is based on an assessment of the absolute risk reduction (ARR) and the number needed to treat (NNT). The NNT is the number of patients who must be treated to produce one individual who has the given response, either desired or harmful. For example, if a treatment reduces the mortality of a disease from 5% to 2.5%, the ARR is 0.025 and, on average, the NNT (given by 1/ARR) is 40. For every 40 individuals treated, 1 life would be saved.

Meta-analysis

For some conditions it may be difficult to recruit many subjects, and the ensuing small trials may produce inconclusive results or opposing results. Meta-analysis is a procedure for combining the results of several independent trials to provide an unbiased conclusion on the likely potency (and safety) of a drug in the human population. It is therefore an objective assessment and is preferable to a subjective choice of clinical trial reports. (The constituent trials must of course have been properly designed.)

Ethical principles

Ethical principles are clearly a major issue in clinical trials. Independent ethics committees should always approve the design and conduct of clinical trials.

The therapeutic index, TD₅₀ and LD₅₀

A proper measure of a drug's value depends on a benefit–risk assessment. Very few drugs have no untoward effects; the amount of risk that is tolerated depends on the seriousness of the condition being treated. Greater risks will be accepted in the treatment of a life-threatening condition than for a trivial ailment (headache). A simple measure of benefit versus risk is the therapeutic index (TI), where:

$$TI = \frac{TD_{50}}{ED_{50}} \text{ or } \frac{LD_{50}}{ED_{50}}$$

The TD_{50} is the dose required to produce a toxic effect in 50% of the subjects (the median toxic dose) and the ED_{50} is the median effective dose. In animal studies, toxicity may be measured by death, in which case the median lethal dose (LD_{50}) replaces the TD_{50}. Clearly if the TD_{50}, or LD_{50}, is much greater than the ED_{50}, then the TI will be large and the drug might be considered to have a large safety margin. The LD_{50}, necessarily measured in animals, is a poor measure of human toxicity since:

- it measures only death, not other potentially serious sublethal effects, and it will almost certainly be different in experimental animals compared with humans;
- it is a measure of acute toxicity and neglects long-term adverse effects; and
- it takes no account of idiosyncratic responses, i.e. it will not allow for the rare individuals who are much more sensitive to the drug (often genetically determined).

Although it is almost impossible to quantify the TI in a satisfactory way, the concept is a valuable one. The concept is used throughout preclinical development to gauge the likelihood of a chemical entity in achieving efficacy and tolerability for a given condition, the accuracy increasing as more data is produced that can be directly compared. For example, directly comparing safety and efficacy data in same species, rather than from *in vitro* assays, will increase accuracy of predicting tolerability (Fig. 6.4). The simple therapeutic ratio might be misleading if the log (dose) response curves for efficacy and toxicity are not parallel, i.e. they do not have the same slope h (Fig. 6.5). Theoretically h is expected to be the integer 1 if the ligand binds competitively and reversibly. Drugs with an h higher than 1.0 have a steep increase in response that can be dangerous. Indeed, application of probabilistic derivations of the Hill equation allows estimations of the likelihood of an adverse event for a given dose. Therefore, one Hill equation can be used to describe the efficacious relationship, whilst a second Hill equation can be used to describe the toxicity. The therapeutic range will be between the two curves. Furthermore, information regarding the degree of parallelism (i.e. difference in slope, the h coefficient) informs pharmacologists as to whether the safety of a drug should be addressed with greater concern if dose escalation or accumulation occurs. Thus, non-parallel therapeutic versus toxicity curves

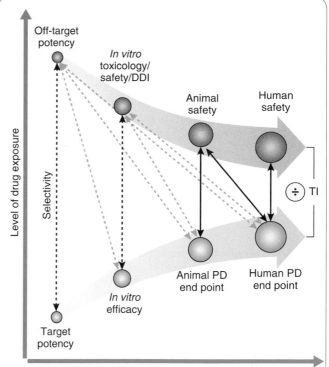

Fig. 6.4 An exposure-centric approach to therapeutic index determination. The extent of safety data (indicated by the size of the grey circles on the grey arrow) and extent of efficacy data (indicated by the size of the circles on the blue arrow) increase as a candidate drug progresses from *in vitro* to animal to human studies (indicated from left to right in the figure). Safety margins and therapeutic indices (TIs) are calculated by dividing the level of drug exposure (indicated by the position on the vertical axis) at which the safety end point occurs by the level of exposure at which the efficacy end point occurs. Dark grey vertical arrows indicate margins involving data of an analogous type. Light grey arrows indicate margins involving data of a different type. Solid arrows (light or dark grey) refer to margins of *in vivo* data involving both concentration-based (maximum (Cmax) or average (Cav)) and/or area (integral) under the concentration–time curve (AUC)-based data. Dashed arrows (light or dark grey) indicate margins that are restricted to concentration-based data as in vitro data are compared to *in vitro* or *in vivo* data. Often, the margins decrease as the candidate progresses from *in vitro* to animal to human studies. (Modified from Muller PY, Milton MN. The determination and interpretation of the therapeutic index in drug development. *Nat Rev Drug Discov.* 2012;11(10):751-761.)

can lead to misleading assumptions from simple TD_{50}/ED_{50} ratios, and more conservative estimates such as TD_{25}/ED_{75} or TD_{10}/ED_{90} can provide a better assessment of tolerability (as suggested by Ehrlich). Often, an *integrated risk assessment* of all collated data will be assessed (as described in Muller & Milton, 2012).

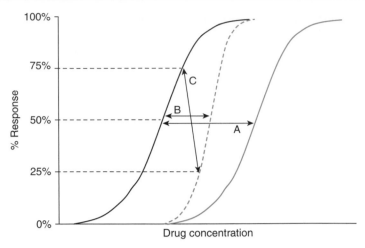

Fig. 6.5 Therapeutic versus toxicity curves. The therapeutic dose response curve (black) and toxicity dose response curve (blue) have parallel gradients at the point of inflexion (ED_{50} and TD_{50}), therefore assumptions can be made about the tolerability of the drug using the ratio A. If the gradient of the toxicity response curve (blue dotted line) is steeper, then the same ratio B clearly does not predict tolerability at different doses of a drug. Therefore, an improved therapeutic index can be calculated with a greater safety margin by comparing the ratio TD_{25}/ED_{75} C.

Drug discovery has evolved in the last 50–60 years from a purely phenotypic screening approach (compound libraries subjected to systems-based assays to identify compounds with biological effects) towards a target-based approach, whereby a rational hypothesis-based design of compounds is created through the use of technologies such as molecular biology understanding, structure-based drug design, combinatorial and parallel chemistry and human genome sequencing. Nevertheless, the discovery of first-in-class drugs is still dependent on these two differing approaches.

The stages of drug discovery and development of small molecules can be divided into three main phases and taking an idea to an approved medicine can take 10–15 years of research and development and cost up to a billion US dollars:

- *Drug discovery*: Pharmacological characterization of small molecules or larger molecules such as antibodies or peptides (see Chapter 8) to choose a lead drug candidate.

- *Preclinical development*: Regulatory safety and toxicological testing (see Chapter 9), along with development work to choose the appropriate route of administration and formulation to deliver the drug.
- *Clinical development:* Phase I studies to evaluate safety, followed by clinical trials in patients to select appropriate doses and to evaluate efficacy and safety.

For ease of understanding, the different phases of drug development are discussed in a linear way (Fig. 7.1). However, in reality the knowledge gained within each phase provides the basis of an iterative approach to optimize the development of a new medicine as often the first candidate selected for evaluation is not the drug finally approved, with many thousands of compounds often needing to be tested to ultimately find the best compound.

THE DRUG DISCOVERY PHASE

Target selection

The identification of a target occurs through the intelligence and knowledge of the research team building on evidence that a particular protein (e.g. receptor, enzyme, transport protein, signalling molecule) or mediator/neurotransmitter is involved in a pathophysiological process. Clearly, it is important to demonstrate that the target is expressed in humans, and better still that the target is differentially expressed in cells or tissue from patients with the disease that the drug is ultimately trying to target (e.g. the expression of an antigen on a cancer cell that is not found on healthy cells, or an enzyme found in bacteria or parasites that is not found in mammalian cells) to improve the likelihood of finding a drug with a wide therapeutic window. Various cell-based expression assays, *in vitro* functional assays, and *in vivo* disease modelling assays are used, or discerned from literature searches to better understand the apparent importance of the target. Given the high costs of developing new medicines, in most cases, the research group identifying new molecules that interact with the target will have some form of intellectual property protecting their intellectual investment in identifying new drugs to provide them with a period of exclusivity to market their new medicine and thus be able to both recoup their discovery and development costs and make a profit. Without this incentive new medicines would not be made.

Identification of a lead candidate

After a biochemical target has been decided, the research team will search for *lead compounds*. The human form of the target protein will be cloned and assays developed, so that the functional activity

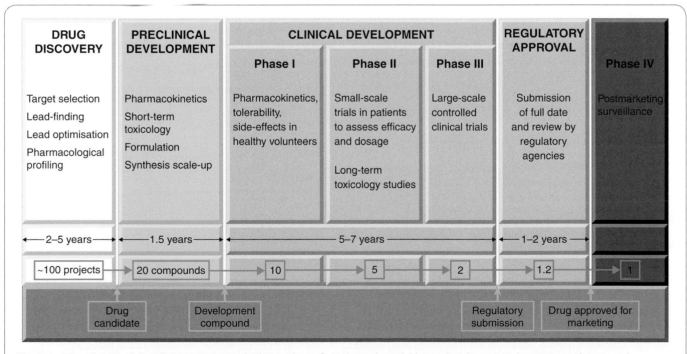

Fig. 7.1 The stages of development of a typical new drug. Only the main activities undertaken at each stage are shown, and the details vary greatly according to the drug and disease area. (From Rang HP, Ritter JM, Flower RJ, Henderson G. *Rang & Dale's Pharmacology*. 8th ed. Philadelphia: Elsevier; 2016.)

of the target can be measured in the presence of lead compounds for *potency* and *efficacy* and other basic pharmacological characteristics such as *affinity* and *selectivity* (see Chapter 3).

Several approaches might be undertaken to find or create lead compounds:

1. Compound screening of large libraries of chemical entities (>1 million compounds).
2. Structural knowledge of known ligands (endogenous or existing synthetic, plant/insect/marine organism-based chemicals, etc.).
3. The use of X-ray crystallography and other techniques to provide knowledge of the three-dimensional structure of the target that allows for rational computer-based modelling to identify novel lead compounds and to help with optimizing structure-activity relationships.

Lead optimization

Lead compounds that show desired actions *in vitro* are referred to as *hits*. Their chemical structures and physiochemical characteristics are then further explored to improve the features of the molecule such as affinity and selectivity for a target, metabolic stability, solubility and duration of action. Through an iterative process and testing of a limited number of compounds *in vivo* for bioavailability and acute toxicity, a small number of lead compounds are then tested in a range of different *in vitro* and *in vivo* functional assays, mimicking aspects of the human condition. Various *in vitro* safety and toxicology assays will also be employed to ascertain whether any of the lead compounds might have unwanted side effects that would lead to them being rejected as candidates before going into the next regulatory stage of development, which is a particularly expensive part of the process.

THE PRECLINICAL DEVELOPMENT PHASE

A lead compound will require tests to understand whether it produces unwanted effects on the major organ systems via regulatory safety and toxicology testing (see Chapter 9). Some safety and toxicological issues might be as a result of *exaggerated pharmacology* (i.e. hazardous events based on the *on-target* effect), or unpredictable pharmacology based on *off-target* effects. Clearly,

the more selective a lead compound is for a target, the less likely these unpredictable events will occur. Toxicology as a science has been said to be like fishing in a pond and never knowing what type of fish you may catch.

Pharmacokinetic testing will be undertaken, including absorption, distribution, metabolism and excretion (ADME) studies in the same laboratory animal species used for toxicity testing (usually rat and dog). This is required because exposure levels (blood plasma concentration) can then be related to pharmacological and toxicological effects. This will inform the dosing for the Phase I studies.

There is also a need for scale up chemistry to produce the larger amounts required for both the regulatory toxicology, which requires typically 28 days dosing with the drug at various doses until a safety signal is obtained, and for the larger amounts of drug required for clinical testing. There is also a need for pharmaceutical chemists to assess the stability and formulation of the new drug for these parts of the development.

Preclinical development studies required for regulatory purposes such as toxicology are required to be conducted under *good laboratory practice* (GLP), covering record keeping, instrument calibration, data analysis, staff training, material homogeneity, etc. GLP compliance therefore aims to reduce human error and reliability of data submitted to regulatory agencies such as the European Medicines Agency (EMA), the Medicines and Healthcare products Regulatory Agency (MHRA) or the US Food and Drug Administration (FDA).

All preclinical data is entered into an *Investigator's Brochure* (IB) to inform the regulatory agencies as to risk/benefit of a lead compound, now known as an investigational medicinal product (IMP). The IB is as an integrated risk assessment and reviewed for permission to proceed into human studies. An IB also informs clinicians working on a trial as to the starting dose; maximum dose; route and frequency of administration; assessment of pharmacodynamics (PD), pharmacokinetics (PK) and safety; and stopping and withdrawal criteria.

A starting dose is calculated based on findings from the toxicological studies. A dose of the IMP that provided a no observed adverse effect level (NOAEL) in the most clinically relevant species

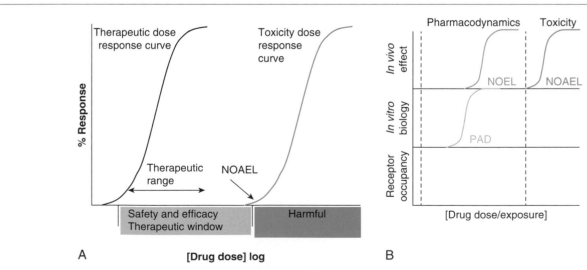

Fig. 7.2 Calculation of no observed adverse effect level (NOAEL). A, The maximum recommended starting dose (MRSD) is calculated several orders of magnitude below the NOAEL. Ideally the therapeutic window will be as wide as possible. **B,** Sometimes, knowledge of the NOAEL and pharmacologically active dose (PAD) is useful in providing an integrated risk assessment to determine the MRSD, if safety and toxicological concerns are evident with on-target effects below the no observed effect level (NOEL). (Courtesy Dr Roly Foulkes.)

is often used to determine a starting dose in humans (Fig. 7.2A), after conversion to the human equivalent dose (HED) based on the difference in body surface area between species. Finally, a safety factor is applied (usually 10-fold) to give a maximum recommended starting dose (MRSD). It should be noted that calculation of the MRSD might occur close to the NOAEL but above the pharmacologically active dose (PAD) from *in vitro* studies and knowledge of receptor occupancy (Fig. 7.2B).

THE CLINICAL DEVELOPMENT PERIOD

The four different phases of clinical studies, designated phases I, II, III and IV, are described in more detail in Chapter 6 and are carried under GCP. Clinical trials are designed to conservatively assess the safety and efficacy of the new drug, and the regulatory authorities who oversee these clinical studies are primarily involved to protect the public.

The use of biotechnology has led to the creation of novel classes of drugs that have transformed therapeutic approaches for various diseases that were otherwise difficult to obtain with traditional small molecule drug development. Monoclonal antibodies (mAbs), peptides and RNAi are therefore engineered and have required different approaches with their development (to determine efficacy, pharmacokinetics, safety) into the clinic. By far the greatest class of biologicals are mAbs (>50 having clinical acceptance, and hundreds more being developed).

PROTEINS AND POLYPEPTIDES AND GENE THERAPY

Proteins and endogenous molecules have been used for many years as therapies; some examples are insulin, factor VIII and human growth hormone. They include *first generation* proteins that are copies of endogenous proteins or antibodies, sometimes produced by recombinant DNA technology. However difficulties in extraction, the use of animal hormones to evoke an immune response and the danger of transmission of infectious agents (e.g. Creutzfeldt-Jakob disease) led to *second generation* technologies which were engineered to improve on these limitations (Table 8.1). *Third generation* agents are macromolecules where the structure is completely novel and the result of a biochemical design process. An example is **mipomersen,** an antisense RNA product that binds to mRNA coding for apolipoprotein B100, in the treatment of familial hypercholesterolemia.

Gene therapy involves the transfer of recombinant nucleic acid into cells to cause genetic modification to prevent, alleviate or cure disease. It has potential application and requires the use of vectors (e.g. viral or non-viral) to deliver DNA.

ANTIBODIES

Pharmacology of antibodies

The very nature of antibodies means that they will have exquisite *affinity* and *selectivity* for a target protein. Thus, *off-target* effects are rarely observed, which can make toxicology studies less demanding. However the predicted *on-target* effects have to be carefully considered. They may have multiple modes of action relating to the target that exhibits non-linear log dose-response curves (Fig. 8.1). MAbs often have a single optimal biological dose and this creates a biological response that is *quantal* rather than *graded* (i.e. a very steep dose-response relationship) due to mAb affinity for a target, instead of the proportional effects that are more accustomed to the small molecule drug-receptor relationships. Therefore traditional Scatchard plots that assume only a K_d variable have to be replaced by non-linear algorithms.

Consideration has to be made of the sheer size of antibodies (human IgG is 150,000 daltons) compared to small molecules (around 150 daltons). However the architecture of antibodies can be manipulated so that certain characteristics of the protein structure are modified. Therefore the size of these fragments can be varied (Fig. 8.2). Administration tends to be limited to intravenous or depot routes. Generally, whole antibodies do not internalize into cells, nor are they able to pass the blood–brain barrier. Therefore target selection for antibodies has to be made with these constraints in mind, although new technologies are being creating to engineer antibody fragments that can circumvent these constraints.

Furthermore, antibody technology has been most successful with targeting soluble mediators (e.g. **Infliximab** anti-tumour necrosis factor α (anti-TNF-α); **Omalizumab** anti-immunoglobulin E (anti-IgE)) and receptors and proteins expressed on the surface of cells that have a relatively stable conformation (e.g. **Trastuzumab** anti-epidermal growth factor receptor; **Ipilimumab** anti-CTLA4; **Nivolumab** anti-PD-1). The targeting of G-protein-coupled

Table 8.1 Some examples of second generation biopharmaceuticals

Type of change	Protein	Indication	Reason for Change
Altered amino acid sequence	Insulin	Diabetes	Faster-acting hormone
	Tissue plasminogen activator analogues	Thrombolysis	Longer circulating half-life
	Interferon analogue	Antiviral	Superior antiviral action
	Factor VIII analogue	Haemophilia	Smaller molecule, better activity
	Diphtheria toxin-interleukin-2 fusion protein	T-cell lymphoma	Targets toxin to appropriate cells
	Tumour necrosis factor receptor-human immunoglobulin G Fc fusion protein	Rheumatoid disease	Prolongs half-life
Altered carbohydrate residues	Glucocerebrosidase enzyme	Gaucher's disease	Promotes phagocyte uptake
	Erythropoietin analogue	Anaemia	Prolongs half-life
Covalent attachment to polyethylene glycol	Interferon	Hepatitis C	Prolongs half-life
	Human growth hormone	Acromegaly	Prolongs half-life

Modified from Walsh G. Second-generation biopharmaceuticals. *Eur J Pharm Biopharm*. 2004;58(2):185-196.

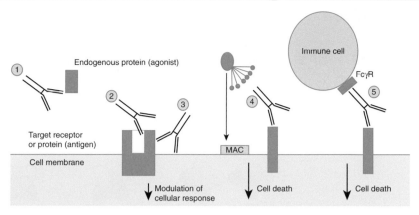

Fig. 8.1 Modes of action of antibodies. Whilst restricted to extracellular targets, antibodies can mediate their biological activities via multiple mechanisms: (1) to sequester soluble endogenous mediators (agonists), (2) to act in an agonistic or antagonistic manner at a receptor and (3) to sterically inhibit protein conformation required for signalling. Furthermore, antibodies can be used therapeutically to mediate immune functions, such as (4) complement-dependent cytotoxicity (CDC); or (5) antibody-dependent cell-mediated cytotoxicity (ADCC).

receptors (GPCRs) and ion channels provides a greater challenge, due to conformational energies of these proteins.

Lastly, mAbs tend to have long half-lives (days/weeks). Such a characteristic can be a positive attribute, depending on the disease and pathology. However this does mean that phase I and phase II metabolism cannot be used to predict how they are eliminated, but rather protein degradation kinetics are applicable.

Production and engineering of antibodies

Antibody production in the body of immunized animals will produce *polyclonal antibodies* (PAbs). These are a polyvalent mixture from all the plasma cell clones that reacted to the antigen that have different affinities and physical characteristics. In 1975 Milstein, Köhler and Jerne created a method of producing an abundance of mAbs *in vitro* from immunized mice using hybridomas (separation and fusion of particular lymphocyte clone creating one clone of antibody with immortalized tumour cells) (Fig. 8.3). However, on their own, such antibodies can raise immunogenicity against the host and have a short half-life in the circulation.

To bypass these problems, it is possible to produce *chimeric* or *humanized* mAbs (Fig. 8.4). *Chimeric* antibodies have been genetically engineered to replace the murine Fc region (constant domain) with its human equivalent by altering and splicing the gene. This greatly extends the plasma half-life and functionality of the antibody when administered into humans. Alternatively, *humanized* antibodies only contain the murine hypervariable region. The differences in architecture and naming of these antibodies is shown in Figure 8.5.

Fully human mAbs can also be made through the development of transgenic animals and from human antibody phage-display techniques.

During the development phase of antibodies, there are various properties of an antibody that can be modified (Table 8.2). These include immunogenicity, antigen-binding specificity and affinity; biological activity associated with variable domains; effector function associated with constant domains; pharmacokinetics; internalization; and chemical, proteolytic and thermolytic stability.

CONSIDERATIONS DURING ANTIBODY CHARACTERIZATION PHASE

The generation of a therapeutic antibody generally requires a company or research group to also produce a package of other materials in house to evaluate affinity, potency and selectivity:
- Target protein: specificity/affinity.
- Other related proteins: selectivity.
- Species cell lines/protein: assess cross-reactivity for efficacy measurement.
- Animal models that express human antigen: efficacy prediction in humans.
- Surrogate (murine) antibodies to demonstrate efficacy in animal models with no human antigen might be required.

SAFETY ASPECTS DURING PRECLINICAL DEVELOPMENT

Toxicological issues with antibodies tend to be minimized due to the lack of *off-target* effects. However, *on-target* effects may lead to an exaggerated pharmacology that is in itself dangerous to the patient. Therefore within the preclinical toxicology studies, attention needs to be made with the use of suitable species (e.g. non-human primates) to ensure on-target risks are understood.

In 2006 a phase I clinical trial for a new mAb (TGN1412, developed to activate T cells for the treatment of B-cell leukaemia) induced a cytokine storm in participants. One outcome of this disaster was to re-evaluate how preclinical safety screens should be used for biologicals with high target affinity and specificity. Thus, guidelines to find a safe starting dose in humans do not use the concept of assessing a no observed adverse effect level (NOAEL) (see Chapter 7), but rather a *minimal anticipated biological effect level* (MABEL) (Fig. 8.6). It is anticipated because an integrated risk assessment is conducted based on estimating where the human biological effect will occur, including animal data with human cell and animal cell *in vitro* data, calculated dose occupancy versus concentration and degree of species specificity.

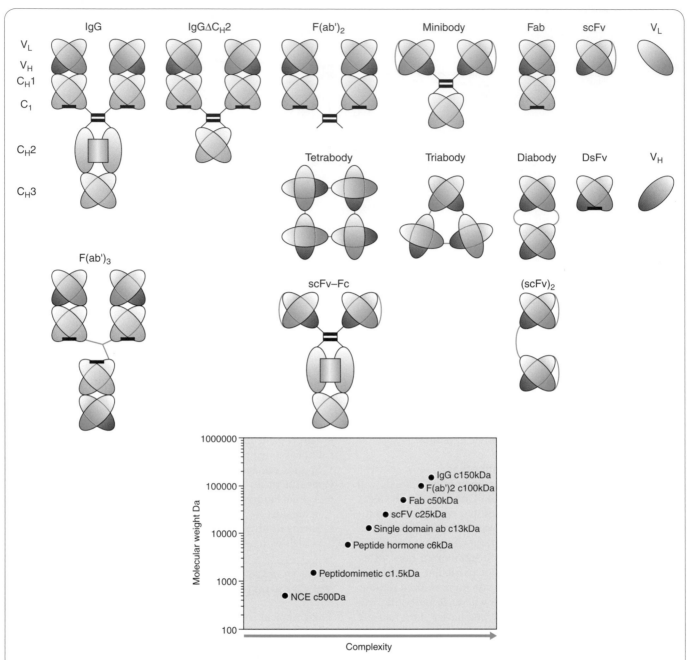

Fig. 8.2 Representative antibody formats. A, The modular domain architecture of immunoglobulins has been exploited to create a growing range of alternative antibody formats that spans a molecular-weight range of at least 12–150 kDa and a valency (n) range from monomeric, dimeric, trimeric to tetrameric. The building block that is most frequently used to create novel antibody formats is the single-chain variable (V)-domain antibody fragment (scFv), which comprises V domains from the heavy and light chain (VH and VL domain) joined by a peptide linker of up to ~15 amino-acid residues. Peptide and chemical linkers are shown as black and blue lines, respectively. *CH*, C domain of immunoglobulin heavy chain; *CL*, C domain of immunoglobulin light chain; *dsFv*, disulphide-stabilized variable (V)-domain antibody fragment. B, An appreciation of the size of antibodies compared to traditional small molecules used as drugs. (A, Modified from Carter PJ. Potent antibody therapeutics by design. *Nat Rev Immunol*. 2006;6(5):343-357. B, Courtesy Dr Roly Foulkes.)

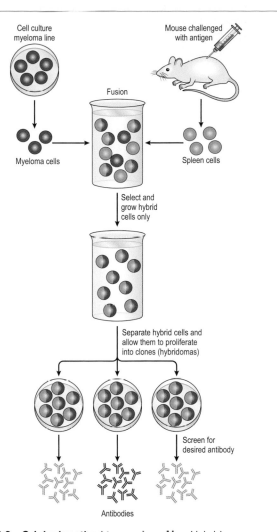

Fig. 8.3 **Original method to create mAbs.** Hybridoma technology was created to allow the production of monoclonal antibodies specific to a target antigen. Milstein, Köhler and Jerne won the Nobel Prize in Physiology or Medicine in 1984 "for theories concerning the specificity in development and control of the immune system and the discovery of the principle for production of monoclonal antibodies." (Modified from NobelPrize.org. Available at https://www.nobelprize.org/prizes/medicine/1984/press-release/.)

Immunogenicity of therapeutic antibodies occurs with all known marketed antibodies containing a xenogeneic protein sequence. Despite advances in humanization and the introduction of human antibodies, it is necessary during toxicology studies to measure the plasma concentrations of any host anti-antibody production, and to predict hypersensitivity reactions after repeat administration.

Dose escalation of antibodies in clinical trials will be conservative if the dose response curve is steep.

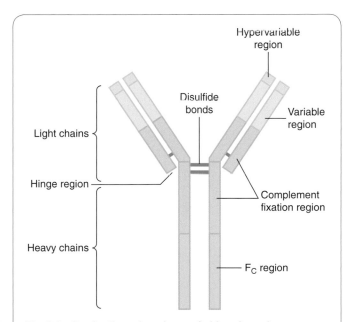

Fig. 8.4 **Production of engineered chimeric and humanized monoclonal antibodies.** (From Rang HP, Ritter JM, Flower RJ, Henderson G. *Rang & Dale's Pharmacology*. 8th ed. Philadelphia: Elsevier; 2016.)

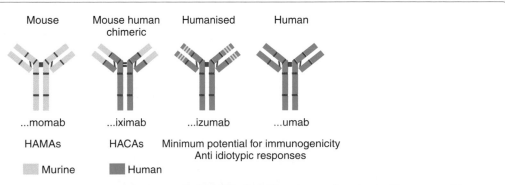

Fig. 8.5 **Structural differences of chimeric and humanized monoclonal antibodies.** The mixture of murine and human peptide sequencing is shown as differences between grey and blue segments. Naming strategies to identify different types of antibodies that sometimes make the clinic are provided. *HACA,* Human anti-chimeric antibody; *HAMA,* human anti-mouse antibody. (Courtesy Dr Roly Foulkes.)

Table 8.2 Adaptations to antibodies during development

Minimize risk of immunogenicity	Minimize non-human sequence via chimerization or humanization techniques	Improved efficacy due to more efficient effector function Improved safety Longer half-life
Increase antigen selectivity	Select from display libraries, structural-based design (Alter V_L region)	Target therapy
Increase species cross-reactivity	Select from display libraries, structural-based design (Alter V_L region)	Facilitates preclinical development (efficacy testing, toxicology)
Modulate antigen-binding affinity	Select from display libraries, structural-based design (Alter V_L region)	Increased efficacy; reduced dose or frequency of administration; increased potency of ADCC; control tissue localization
Reduce plasma half-life	Use antibody fragments; use IgG with impaired affinity for FcRn	Less whole-body exposure to antibody; improved target-to-non-target ratios
Increase plasma half-life	Use IgG with increased affinity for FcR; modify antibody fragments (binding to molecules with a long half-life)	Increased plasma concentrations might improve localization to target; increased efficacy; reduced dose or frequency of administration

Modified from Carter PJ. Potent antibody therapeutics by design. *Nat Rev Immunol.* 2006;6(5):343-357.
ADCC, Antibody-dependent cell-mediated cytotoxicity; *FcR,* fragment crystalline receptor of IgG; *FcRn,* neonatal form of FcR; *IgG,* immunoglobulin G; *VL,* V domain from light chain.

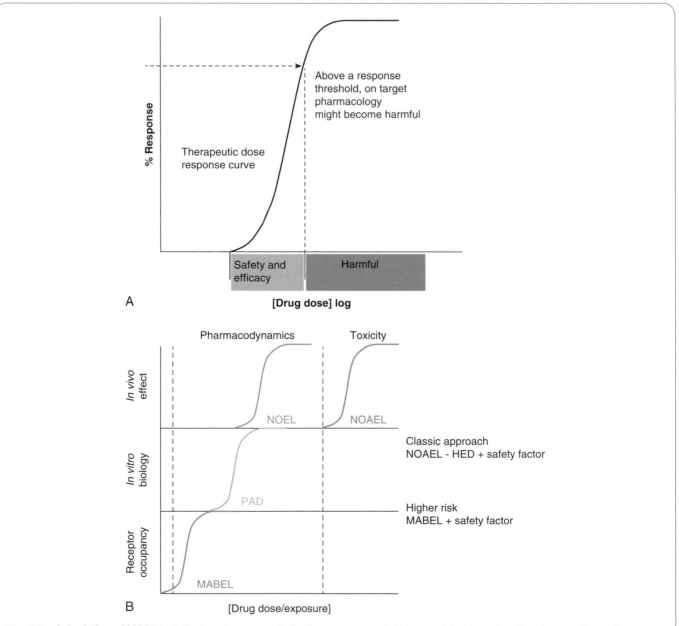

Fig. 8.6 Calculation of MABEL. A, On target, exaggerated safety concerns might be predicted based on the pharmacology of antibodies as opposed to a separate toxicological dose response. B, Given the exquisite nature of antibody binding to antigens, a biological effect can occur at very low concentrations. Therefore calculations for first human doses have to take into account potential *on-target exaggerated* pharmacology and provide a very conservative dose based on *in vitro* function and knowledge of receptor occupancy. *HED,* human equivalent dose; *MABEL,* minimum anticipated biological effect level; *NOAEL,* no observed adverse effect level; *NOEL,* no observed effect level; *PAD,* pharmacological active dose. (Courtesy Dr Roly Foulkes.)

A drug has to be demonstrated to be reasonably safe and effective before it can enter the clinic (see Chapter 10). An integrated risk assessment will be made on the efficacy and safety of the medicine to provide a risk-benefit analysis as an interpretation of the therapeutic index (see Chapter 6). To ensure medicinal products around the globe have been tested to the same degree of stringency, the International Council for Harmonisation of Technical Requirements for Pharmaceuticals for Human Use (ICH) brings together the governmental regulatory authorities and pharmaceutical industry to discuss scientific and technical aspects of drug registration, including guidelines to assess safety and toxicity issues. Below is a summary of the recommendations taken from the ICH guidelines (https://www.ICH.org). The scale and timing of these safety tests occur during various stages of the lifespan of the development of a drug (Fig. 9.1).

SAFETY PHARMACOLOGY

The purpose of safety pharmacology during *preclinical* drug development is to assess the potential undesirable effects of a medicinal product on essential physiological systems (cardiovascular, respiratory and central nervous system (CNS), known as the core battery). A selection of *in vitro* and *in vivo* tests are used (Table 9.1) with the following considerations:

- Time course and resolution, usually from a single dose.
- Evaluation of a wide range of doses to cover the anticipated therapeutic range and higher to determine at what doses adverse effects appear.
- Doses that might cause toxicity are not used, since these may hide an effect on the physiological system being investigated.
- Evaluation of safety is usually assessed using the proposed clinical route of administration, but other routes of administration (e.g. systemic) are sometimes also evaluated if warranted.
- Appropriate negative and positive control groups used.

Follow-up tests

Depending on the outcome of the initial core battery tests, it may be necessary to conduct further investigations to gain a meaningful understanding of a medicinal product's effects on a particular physiological system (Table 9.2).

Supplemental studies

Potential adverse effects on other organ systems (e.g. gastrointestinal, renal/urinary, autonomic nervous system, immune, endocrine) are also assessed when it is believed necessary.

TOXICOLOGY

Toxicity studies are carried out to identify any target organ(s) that may be damaged as a result of exposure to high doses of the new medicine, the dose level at which this occurs, the mechanism of action of any toxic effect and whether such effects are reversible. Toxicity studies are made up of *in vitro* and *in vivo* tests, and the aim is to identify and reject compounds whose toxicity would provide an unattractive *therapeutic index* as fast as possible during the development process.

Thus single/repeat dose toxicity, toxicokinetics, genetic toxicity, reproductive toxicity, teratogenicity (sometimes) and carcinogenicity studies are required. The various toxicity studies will be conducted at different time points along the developmental pathway of a compound, but this is also dependent on the drug characteristics and mechanism of action in terms of risk (Fig. 9.1).

Generally repeat dose toxicity studies are carried out in two species (rodent and non-rodent, usually rat and dog), and the length of time the animals are dosed is characterized by the expected

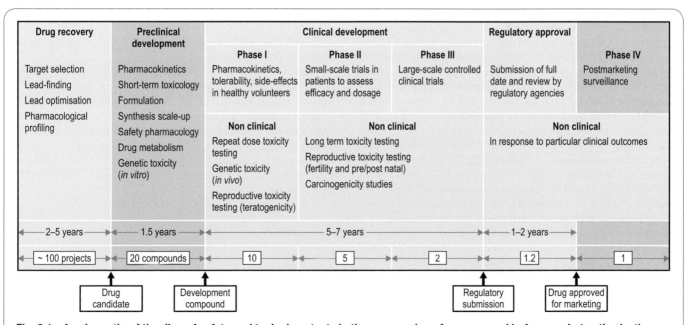

Fig. 9.1   A schematic of timeline of safety and toxicology tests in the progression of a compound before market authorization.
(Modified from Rang HP, Ritter JM, Flower RJ, Henderson G: *Rang & Dale's Pharmacology*. 8th ed. Philadelphia: Elsevier; 2016.)

Table 9.1   Core Battery Measurements

Central Nervous System: Motor activity, behavioural changes, coordination, sensory/motor reflex responses and body temperature. **Cardiovascular System:** Blood pressure, heart rate and the electrocardiogram. *In vivo, in vitro* and/or ex vivo evaluations, including methods (e.g. use of human ether-a-go-go-related gene (hERG) that codes for the Kv11.1 alpha subunit of a cardiac potassium channel) for repolarization and conductance abnormalities. **Respiratory System:** Respiratory rate and other measures of respiratory function (e.g. tidal volume or hemoglobin oxygen saturation).

Table 9.2   Follow-Up Measurements

Central Nervous System: Behavioural pharmacology, learning and memory, ligand-specific binding, neurochemistry, visual, auditory and/or electrophysiology examinations. **Cardiovascular System:** Cardiac output, ventricular contractility, vascular resistance, the effects of endogenous and/or exogenous substances on the cardiovascular responses. **Respiratory System:** Airway resistance, compliance, pulmonary arterial pressure, blood gases, blood pH, cough.

duration of future clinical trials. The frequency and route of administration will also reflect the intended human dosing regimen, but low, medium and high doses will be used all markedly higher than the estimated efficacy dose in humans. Studies are undertaken to investigate the effects of systemic exposure to high doses and exposure levels are assessed through toxicokinetic measurements. Biomarkers might be identified for subsequent use in clinical trials, and pivotal toxicological studies are a regulatory requirement to help select safe doses for use in clinical trials (see Chapters 7 and 8).

BIOLOGICALS

Due to the specificity of antibody target binding and target affinity, safety issues are often related to *on-target* exaggerated pharmacology, rather than inherent safety concerns related to the biologic. Therefore, genotoxicity; absorption, distribution, metabolism and excretion (ADME); and biodistribution measurements tend not to be conducted on biologicals. Safety pharmacology and toxicity studies are sometimes tailor-made, dependent on the mechanism of action of the biologic. However, being peptides or proteins, many biotechnology-derived pharmaceuticals can be immunogenic if they contain parts of a foreign protein, and therefore auto-antibodies against the biologic are often measured (e.g. titer, number of responding animals, neutralizing or non-neutralizing) as part of repeated dose toxicity studies of biologicals.

Whilst biologicals are considered to be neater options for drugs given their target specificity, species exclusivity (or lack of cross-reactivity) can create problems and often preclude standard toxicity testing designs in commonly used species (e.g. rats and dogs).

The following therefore have to be considered:
* The use of a relevant species in which the biological entity is pharmacologically active (affinity and cellular sensitivity) with a similar cross-reactivity profile to humans. This sometimes means higher primates need to be used in such evaluations.

* If no relevant species exists, the creation of transgenic animals expressing the human receptor or homologous protein is required.
* The use of disease models with similarity to human disease if the protein of interest has modulated expression and warrants investigation under these circumstances.

Increased number of biologicals are being approved for the treatment of a range of chronic diseases, rather than the initial use as acute therapy in life-threatening diseases which may lead to changes to guidelines for the development of such molecules:
* The use of chronic disease models to assess safety and toxicology.
* Timing of genotoxicity and carcinogenicity studies.
* The use of a relevant species (e.g. primates) rather than routine use of two species (rodent and non-rodent).
* Consideration that effects might be prolonged due to extended half-life of many biologics.

PHARMACOVIGILANCE

Despite the use of the extensive preclinical tests and clinical trials (see Chapter 7) to understand the safety of a drug and potential toxicity issues, it is still possible for adverse and unpredictable drug effects to occur in the wider population after clinical trials have ended. Therefore post-marketing surveillance (pharmacovigilance) is important for the centralized reporting of these reactions. These can be *hypothesis-generating* which is the voluntary reporting of an adverse events (yellow form in the United Kingdom), which provides information on the number of events (the numerator); or these can be *hypothesis-generating and testing* (green form in the United Kingdom), which provides information on the frequency of events as it monitors prescription events (data contains numerator and denominator). If events are frequent and adverse, then the drug can be removed from market or subjected to a hypothesis testing study, using cohorts of patients to prospectively test the hypothesis before a decision is made by the regulatory authorities.

Adverse drug reactions frequently mimic ordinary diseases and tend to affect:
* systems in which there is rapid cell multiplication (e.g. skin, haematopoietic system, gut lining);
* organs in which drugs are detoxified and/or excreted (e.g. liver, kidneys); or
* drug-drug interactions.

A recent example of a novel drug class being removed after approval because of unacceptable side effects occurred with the cyclooxygenase (COX)-2 inhibitors. These drugs were developed as novel analgesics for the treatment of patients with arthritis and were claimed to have less gastrointestinal side effects than older nonsteroidal anti-inflammatory drugs such as aspirin. However, this drug class was later found to elicit adverse effects on the cardiovascular system, including deaths in patients with underlying heart disease.

Drug regulation seeks to ensure the quality of the whole process of making and using a new medicine. Thus there are strict regulatory requirements to adhere to on the synthesis, scale up and purity of the active ingredient of any medicine, alongside strict requirements to assess efficacy and safety before a medicine can be granted a licence for use in people (and indeed for use in veterinary medicine). The various control and regulatory mechanisms that regulate drug approval are pan-national and internationally adhered to during the preclinical and clinical development of a drug (which are summarized in Chapters 6–9). These mechanisms aim to:

- Protect the public from the conflict of interest between the necessity of drug companies to make a profit on their investment in developing a new medicine and the need of patients for beneficial medication.
- Ensure standardized and agreed test panels for safety are used, and clinical efficacy testing is stringent.
- Ensure the agreed pharmacopeia is adhered to with regard to purity and physicochemical properties (and therefore manufacturing processes).
- Control access to drugs that require monitoring, and restrict access to drugs with abuse potential.

DRUG REGULATION FOR NEW DRUGS

There are some differences in the approval processes between different bodies, for example the US Food and Drug Administration (FDA), the EU European Medicines Agency (EMA) and the Japanese Ministry of Health and Welfare. However there is also a process of harmonization (promoted by the International Council for Harmonisation of Requirements for Pharmaceuticals of Human Use (ICH), Chapter 9) attempting to make the regulatory processes more uniform across the world. The regulation processes for new drugs is described in Page et al., *Integrated Pharmacology, 2nd edition* pp. 83–87, and is condensed below.

United States
In the United States, upon conclusion of a successful phase III clinical trial, the drug developer submits all preclinical and clinical data to the FDA in a New Drug Application (NDA) for review before a decision is made for approval for the drug to be used. The drug developer is required to create a 'label' that provides summarized details of the manufacturing process, pharmacokinetics, efficacy, toxicity and clinical trials and for which uses the drug is claimed to be of benefit. Once approved, the drug developer (company) is then given a licence for the drug to be marketed and used for the claimed indication(s). However, whilst the FDA has the power to approve the licencing and marketing of a drug for a particular indication, it cannot regulate use. Thus a physician may choose to use a drug on a patient for a non-approved disease indication which is termed 'off-label' use. If sufficient evidence is obtained from off-label use, this sometimes leads to the label being modified to reflect this broader use of the medicine.

Europe
In Europe, drug approval is currently regulated by both centralized and decentralized processes reporting to the EMA after clinical drug development is completed. A drug developer will summarize data in a 'Summary of Product Characteristics' (SmPC) file. Similar to the label in the United States, this will be reviewed before approval to market the drug is granted.

Centralized submissions in the EU are via the European Medicines Evaluation Agency (EMEA), with representatives from all member states, that appoints a rapporteur with a particular country's regulatory agency that has responsibility for initial review on behalf of the member states. The rapporteur then submits an opinion to the Committee for Proprietary Medicinal Products (CPMP) to decide drug approval. Decentralized submissions in the EU occur via a member state initially, and the report and decision is then circulated to other member states to decide whether to adopt the decision in their own territories. Off-label use of a drug is less prevalent in Europe compared to the United States.

Japan
In Japan, the approval process is carried out under the authority of the Ministry of Health and Welfare (MHW) and the Central Pharmaceutical Affairs Council (CPAC), which consists of medical and pharmaceutical science experts. CPAC recommends a decision that is then implemented by the MHW. It is usually a requirement to make decisions from clinical trials conducted on the Japanese population, due to the perception that genetic variations in ethnic groups (for example Japanese compared to European or American populations) and cultural differences (that might influence preferred dosing regimens) require such tailored studies.

Rest of the world
Drug acceptance and use is regulated in most countries by other national agencies. Some may accept the decisions made in the United States, Europe and Japan, which have experienced and large regulatory authorities as a result of being the largest drug markets.

DRUG INFORMATION TO PUBLIC

Drugs are packaged with a leaflet (Patient Information Leaflet (PIL)), that contains information from the SmPC (Europe). Public information in the United States is provided in the label. The patient is thus provided information on indications and use, contraindications, caution, adverse events and ingredients.

DRUG REGULATIONS RELATING TO ACCESS TO DRUGS

Countries have different regulations related to possessing and prescribing of drugs. Some drugs will be licensed by the above agencies to be sold 'over the counter' (OTC), whilst others will be sold only with a prescription from a physician. Regulation depends on safety concerns, the requirement for monitoring and abuse potential.

The nervous system controls conscious and subconscious (autonomic) activities, and the higher order processes memory, emotion and intelligence. It is composed of the following systems:
- The peripheral nervous system (PNS) that processes the external environment and sensations. The PNS is composed of afferent fibres that originate in peripheral tissues and pass to the spinal cord.
- The regulation of peripheral tissue activity by the autonomic nervous system (ANS). Efferent neurons originate from the spinal cord and pass to peripheral tissues.
- The central nervous system (CNS) (brain and spinal cord) connects the afferent and efferent neurons of the PNS with the brain to regulate and process bodily actions.

In this chapter we summarize the neurotransmitters in the CNS and ANS and how neurotransmission can be modified by drugs.

CENTRAL NERVOUS SYSTEM

Drug action

Drugs have important therapeutic effects in a variety of disorders of the nervous system. Normal CNS function can also be modified by general anaesthetics and by drugs taken for non-medical use (alcohol, nicotine, caffeine, cannabis, etc.). A full understanding of how drugs affect CNS function is currently hampered by our poor understanding of the ways in which the activity of particular neurons in the brain influence complex processes such as memory, mood and consciousness. Therefore, although the molecular targets and cellular actions of many centrally acting drugs are well established, the exact way in which the events at neuronal level are converted into therapeutically useful actions, as with antidepressants and anxiolytics, is usually much less clear. The action of drugs in Parkinson's disease (Chapter 12) provides perhaps the best example of how knowledge of the neuronal pathways and neurotransmitters involved, along with knowledge of the pathological deficit, provides a rational basis for drug use.

An important consideration in the design of drugs to have direct effects within the CNS is the requirement that they are able to traverse the blood–brain barrier. This barrier serves a valuable role in protecting the brain from many potentially neurotoxic agents which have gained entry into the systemic circulation, but it also impedes the uptake of most lipophobic drugs into the cerebrospinal fluid. Certain lipophobic drugs, however, can make use of active transport systems to enter the brain, e.g. **levodopa** in Parkinson's disease.

Chemical signalling in the CNS

The description of transmitter synthesis, storage and release is largely applicable to both CNS neurotransmission and the PNS. However, chemical transmitters in the CNS operate over quite different time scales.

Neurotransmitters

By convention these are the agents responsible for fast excitatory and inhibitory postsynaptic potentials. Typically they are released by terminal boutons and act on postsynaptic receptors concentrated in postsynaptic densities on a single neuron. Their action is normally rapidly terminated by reuptake or enzymatic degradation. Neurotransmitters commonly act on ionotropic receptors (e.g. N-methyl-D-aspartate (NMDA) acting on NMDAR) though mediators acting on some G-protein-coupled receptors (GPCRs) may produce quite rapid action and thus also be considered neurotransmitters (e.g. noradrenaline acting on α_1-adrenoceptors can qualify).

Neuromodulators

These are more slowly acting and their effects, both pre- and postsynaptically, may be more diffuse, spreading from the site of release to influence many surrounding neurons. Neuropeptides acting on GPCRs (e.g. somatostatin, substance P) are included in this category. Neuromodulators also include lipid mediators (e.g. prostaglandins, endocannabinoids) and nitric oxide, which are not released in the same way as conventional neurotransmitters. Neuromodulators may be released by the same terminals as neurotransmitters – co-transmission. Neuromodulators are involved in synaptic plasticity and modulate the effects of neurotransmitters on action potential firing rate. Steroids also have a role in synaptic plasticity.

Neurotrophic factors

These act over the longest time scale, regulating neuronal growth and morphology. Many are peptides acting on receptor tyrosine kinases to control gene expression (e.g. brain-derived neurotrophic factor).

A complication in understanding drug action is that, although a drug's action on its target receptor or enzyme may be manifest within minutes, the clinical effect may be delayed for some days (e.g. antidepressant activity or development of dependence on opioids). These delays are attributed to adaptive changes to drug-induced perturbations and may involve receptor up- or downregulation, modification of transmitter synthesis, etc.

Neurotransmitters in the CNS

Within the CNS, neurotransmitters can be amino acids, for example *glutamate* is the main fast excitatory transmitter and γ-aminobutyric acid (*GABA*) and *glycine* are the fast inhibitory amino acid transmitters. *Aspartate* may also serve as an excitatory transmitter acting at glutamate receptors. Other neurotransmitters include noradrenaline, 5-hydroxytryptamine (5-HT, serotonin), histamine, purines, peptides, dopamine, acetylcholine, eicosanoids and endogenous cannabinoids.

Glutamate

Glutamate is synthesized in neural tissues either by transamination of α-ketoglutarate (from the Krebs cycle) or from glutamine by the action of glutaminase. Like most transmitters it is stored in vesicles and released by exocytosis. Its action in the synaptic cleft is terminated mainly by active recapture into either the nerve ending or nearby astrocytes.

Glutamate receptors

There are four types of glutamate receptors: three ionotropic and one metabotropic receptors (Fig. 11.1).

The combination of subunits in ionotropic receptors varies widely so that the properties of the channels in different brain regions can also vary. NMDA receptors mediate a slow excitatory postsynaptic potential and have a greater calcium ion (Ca^{2+}) permeability. NMDA receptors will only open in response to released glutamate if glycine (or D-serine) occupies its binding sites on the NR1 subunits. (Variations in the local concentration of glycine may in some cases have an important regulatory role.) An important property of the NMDA receptor is that it is blocked by magnesium ions (Mg^{2+}) at the resting potential of neurons and the channel will only conduct ions (sodium ion (Na^+), Ca^{2+}) when the block is relieved by depolarization (produced by AMPA or kainate receptors). Entry of Ca^{2+} through NMDA receptors is involved in synaptic plasticity (e.g. long-term potentiation (LTP)) and also in cell damage (excitotoxicity)) (Fig. 11.2).

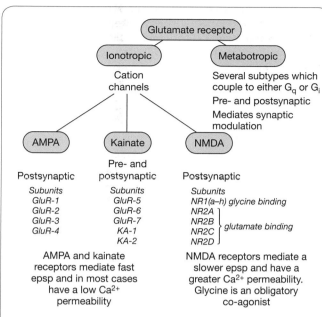

Fig. 11.1 Glutamate receptors. The ionotropic receptors are named after their selective agonists: NMDA, *N*-methyl-D-aspartate; AMPA, α-amino-3-hydroxy-5-methylisoxazole-4-propionic acid; and kainate. *epsp*, Excitatory postsynaptic potential; *IP₃*, inositol trisphosphate.

Drugs acting on glutamate receptors Only a few drugs are known to work by affecting glutamate receptors and include **ketamine** (which produces dissociative anaesthesia and works partly by blocking the NMDA receptor channel) and **memantine**, advocated for the treatment of Alzheimer's disease. Several other compounds with potent and selective actions on glutamate receptor subtypes have been identified; they are useful tools in the study of these receptors but do not have a recognized clinical value. One example is phencyclidine (angel-dust), a 'street' drug that, like ketamine, may act partially by blocking the NMDA receptor channel.

GABA

GABA is produced from glutamate by glutamic acid decarboxylase. The activity of released GABA is terminated mainly by reuptake into GABAergic neurons and astrocytes.

GABA receptors

There are two main kinds of GABA receptor: $GABA_A$ and $GABA_B$ (Fig. 11.3). $GABA_A$ is a ligand-gated Cl^- channel that occurs postsynaptically (Fig. 11.4).

Activation of $GABA_A$ receptors tends to clamp the membrane potential close to the chloride ion (Cl^-) equilibrium potential (which is usually near to, or more negative than, the membrane potential) and so decreases electrical excitability. Transmitter action at $GABA_A$ receptors typically produces fast inhibitory postsynaptic potentials.

$GABA_B$ is a GPCR that acts via G_i to:
- inhibit voltage-gated Ca^{2+} channels in nerve endings to reduce transmitter release;

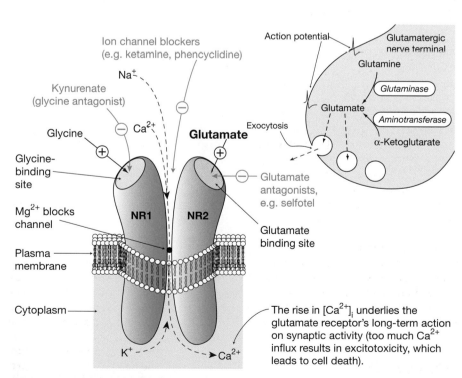

Fig. 11.2   A glutamate *N*-methyl-D-aspartate (NMDA) receptor in a postsynaptic cell membrane and the action potential-induced exocytosis of glutamate from a glutamatergic neuron. Only two of the four subunits are shown. The positions of the receptor sites for glycine and glutamate are purely diagrammatic.

- open potassium ion (K⁺) channels in nerves to reduce excitability.

Drugs acting on GABA receptors GABA_A receptors are important targets for the therapeutic actions of **benzodiazepines** and **barbiturates**. Useful experimental tools for GABA_A receptors are muscimol, an agonist, and **bicuculline**, a competitive antagonist. The convulsant picrotoxin blocks the ion channel

directly. **Benzodiazepines** modulate the binding and activity of GABA by binding to a modulatory site associated with the γ-subunit. Drugs may act as agonists (e.g. **diazepam**), antagonists (e.g. flumazenil) and inverse agonists (e.g. β-carbolines) at the benzodiazepine 'receptor'. Agonists enhance the activity of GABA whereas inverse agonists reduce the activity. Diazepam has anticonvulsant activity whereas flumazenil is proconvulsant. **Barbiturates** and **neurosteroids** such as **alphaxalone** bind to other modulatory sites on the GABA_A receptor to enhance GABA action.

Baclofen is an agonist at GABA_B receptors and has useful antispastic activity. Phaclofen, an antagonist, is a useful experimental agent.

Glycine

Glycine has two important actions; one direct on the inhibitory glycine receptors, the other as a co-agonist with glutamate on NMDA receptors. It is released particularly from inhibitory interneurons in the brainstem and spinal cord.

Glycine receptors

The glycine receptor is a pentameric ligand-gated Cl⁻ channel made up of glycine-binding α-subunits (α_1–α_4) and β-subunits. The convulsant action of strychnine results from antagonism at the glycine receptor. No clinically useful drugs are thought to act on these receptors.

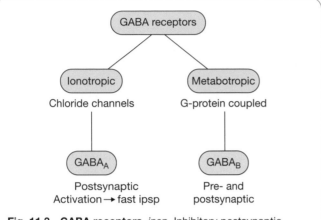

Fig. 11.3 GABA receptors. *ipsp*, Inhibitory postsynaptic potentials.

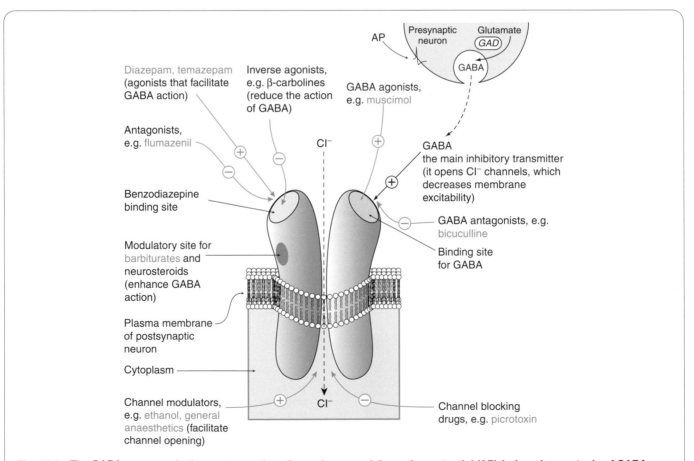

Fig. 11.4 The GABA_A receptor in the postsynaptic cell membrane and the action potential (AP)-induced exocytosis of GABA from a nerve ending. The positions of the receptor sites are purely speculative. Only two of the five subunits are shown. *GAD*, Glutamic acid decarboxylase.

Noradrenaline

Noradrenaline (NA) has both pre- and postsynaptic actions in the central nervous system (CNS). The bodies of noradrenergic neurons are found mainly in the pons (especially in the locus ceruleus), the medulla and brainstem (reticular formation) and project diffusely to the cortex, limbic system, hypothalamus, cerebellum and spinal cord. Synthesis, storage, release and reuptake of NA are essentially as described for peripheral sympathetic neurons (see below). The CNS effects of NA are mediated by both α- and β-adrenoceptors acting either pre- or postsynaptically.

α_2-Adrenoceptors can cause inhibition of calcium ion (Ca^{2+}) channels to inhibit transmitter release or activate potassium (K^+) channels to inhibit excitability. β-receptors may increase cell firing rate by inhibiting the hyperpolarizations that follow action potential discharge. Activation of noradrenergic pathways is thought to increase wakefulness and alertness, whereas reduced activity may contribute to depression (Chapter 12). Noradrenergic mechanisms are also involved in the central regulation of blood pressure and in the control of mood. (Some compounds previously thought to act on α_2-adrenoceptors, e.g. clonidine, are now thought to work at least partly through distinct G-protein-coupled imidazoline receptors.)

5-HT (serotonin) in the CNS

Serotonergic neurons are found in the raphe nuclei (in the pons and medulla) and project to many areas of the brain including the cortex, hippocampus, basal ganglia, limbic system and hypothalamus. Activity in 5-hydroxytryptamine (5-HT) pathways is known to modulate mood, emotion, sleep, appetite and vomiting, and to have some role in pain perception. The synthesis of 5-HT is dependent on the plasma concentration of its precursor tryptophan (itself dependent on dietary intake) and on the activity of tryptophan hydroxylase. There are seven classes of 5-HT receptor, all G-protein coupled except for the ionotropic $5-HT_3$ receptor. Most types of 5-HT receptors are found in the central nervous system (CNS) where they may act as either excitatory or inhibitory autoreceptors or act on heteroreceptors on the terminals of nerves utilizing other transmitters. Many will have postsynaptic actions. The different G-protein-coupled receptors may link to $G_q/11$, $G_{i/o}$ or to G_s.

5-HT released from dense core vesicles in serotonergic neurons is mainly inactivated by reuptake by specific carriers different to those for noradrenaline, but subject to inhibition by some of the same inhibitors (e.g. tricyclic antidepressants), as well as by selective serotonin reuptake inhibitors (SSRIs, Chapter 12). $5-HT_1$ receptors in the cortex and amygdala are targets for anxiolytic and antidepressant drugs. Actions on $5-HT_2$ receptors in the hippocampus and cortex may underlie the hallucinogenic effects of some drugs. $5-HT_3$ receptors are found mainly in the brainstem, especially the area postrema, which is concerned with vomiting.

Histamine

Histamine is synthesized from histidine by histidine decarboxylase. Four histamine receptors have been discovered and at least three of the subtypes (H_1, H_2 and H_3) are found in the CNS, although only a few histaminergic pathways have been identified. Nevertheless older H_1 antagonists that are able to cross the blood–brain barrier have useful sedative and anti-emetic actions. These include chlorpheniramine and diphenhydramine.

Purines

Adenosine triphosphate (ATP) is now well established as a neurotransmitter both in the CNS and periphery and has both ionotropic (P_{2X}) and G-protein-coupled (P_{2Y}) receptors. Adenosine receptors (A_1, A_{2A}, A_{2B}, A_3) are G-protein coupled. Caffeine and some other methylxanthines are adenosine receptor antagonists which certainly contribute to some of the side effects of this drug class. Adenosine receptor agonists have potential value as sedatives, anticonvulsants and neuroprotective agents.

Neuropeptides

Many peptides (e.g. somatostatin, enkephalins, substance P, neuropeptide Y) act as neuromodulators, influencing a wide range of CNS activity. In some cases they are released as co-transmitters with monoamines. Peptide receptors are most usually G-protein coupled; no examples of peptides gating ionotropic receptors are documented.

Dopamine

There are three main dopaminergic pathways in the central nervous system (CNS); the *nigrostriatal tract*, which contains most of the dopamine in the CNS, runs from the substantia nigra – where the cell bodies of the neurons lie – to the corpus striatum. Another dopaminergic pathway, the *mesolimbic system*, runs from the midbrain to the limbic system and the cortex. A third pathway, the *tuberohypophyseal system*, runs from the hypothalamus to the anterior pituitary. Dopamine is synthesised by the same pathway that produces noradrenaline (and is in fact a precursor of noradrenaline). Like noradrenaline, it is metabolized by monoamine oxidase and catechol-*O*-methyltransferase yielding dihydroxyphenylacetic acid (DOPAC) and homovanillic acid (HVA).

After release, dopamine can be recaptured by nerve endings using a selective dopamine transporter (T). Dopamine receptors belong to the G-protein-coupled receptor (GPCR) family and comprise five subtypes separated into D_1-like (D_1 and D_5) and D_2-like (D_2, D_3 and D4):

- D_1-like receptors couple to G_s-protein to stimulate adenylate cyclase.
- D_2-like receptors, acting via G_i/G_o, inhibit adenylate cyclase, reduce calcium ion (Ca^{2+}) currents and increase outward potassium ion (K^+) currents. The latter effect reduces electrical excitability and one action is to cause autoinhibition of dopamine release.

Functions of dopaminergic pathways: The *nigrostriatal pathway* is concerned with motor control and damage to these dopaminergic neurons leads to conditions manifesting motor incoordination, notably Parkinson's disease (Chapter 12). An increase in dopaminergic activity in the *mesolimbic/mesocortical* system induces stereotypic behaviour. An important role of dopaminergic neurones in schizophrenia is suggested by the valuable antischizophrenic action of D_2 receptor antagonists (Chapter 12). The *tuberohypophyseal pathway* regulates hormonal release from the pituitary, especially prolactin (reduced) and growth hormone (increased).

Acetylcholine

Cholinergic nerves are widely distributed in the central nervous system (CNS), the main pathways being from the magnocellular forebrain nucleus to the cortex, from the pons to the thalamus and cortex and the septohippocampal pathway. Cholinergic neurons also have an important role in the control of motion by the striatum (Chapter 17). Synthesis, storage, release and inactivation are the same as in the periphery (see below).

Brain acetylcholine (ACh) has mainly excitatory actions. Both nicotinic and muscarinic receptors are found, both occurring mainly presynaptically. The former are ionotropic, the latter G-protein coupled. Activation of the muscarinic receptors (which are mainly of the M_1 class) inhibits ACh release. Activation of the presynaptic nicotinic receptors (which are fewer) facilitates glutamate and dopamine release. Some postsynaptic nicotinic receptors mediate fast excitatory transmission. Inhibition of postsynaptic potassium ion (K^+) channels by muscarinic receptors can increase neuronal excitability.

Cholinergic pathways are important mainly in arousal, learning and memory and motor control; so that scopolamine for example has amnesic effects when used for premedication and anticholinesterases are advocated for use in Alzheimer's disease (Chapter 12). Scopolamine is also used to treat motion sickness. The cholinergic activity in the striatum provides a target for drug action in Parkinson's and Huntington's diseases (see Chapter 12). Cholinergic projections to the cortex influence electroencephalographic (EEG) activity; muscarinic antagonists increase slow wave activity which, paradoxically, causes excitement.

Arachidonic acid and its metabolites, including cannabinoids

Eicosanoids (leukotrienes, prostaglandins and HETES) as well as endogenous cannabinoids are synthesised from arachidonic acid within the brain. Arachidonic acid and the eicosanoids may act as intracellular messengers (for example, modifying ion channel activity) or interact with cell surface receptors. The neuromodulatory roles of eicosanoids are not well established but prostaglandins (PG) appear to be involved in temperature regulation (inhibition of PG production explains the antipyretic action of aspirin and other non-steroidal anti-inflammatory drugs (NSAIDs)) and perhaps in sleep.

G-protein-linked (G_i/G_0) cannabinoid (CB_1) receptors are found in the hippocampus (related perhaps to the memory-impairing action of cannabis) and in the cerebellum, substantia nigra, mesolimbic system and cortex. Metabolism of arachidonic acid yields the endogenous transmitters 2-arachidonyl glycerol and anandamide. CB_1 receptors act via inhibition of adenylate cyclase, inhibition of N- and P/Q-type calcium channels, stimulation of potassium channels and activation of mitogen-activated protein kinase. Synthetic cannabinoids (e.g. nabilone) have potential for use as anti-emetics and analgesics.

AUTONOMIC NERVOUS SYSTEM

The ANS regulates smooth muscle tone and cardiac function. It also has actions on exocrine and some endocrine secretions, and on intermediate metabolism. Efferent autonomic pathways usually consist of two neurons, a preganglionic fibre synapsing with a postganglionic fibre in the autonomic ganglion. There are also afferent nerves within the ANS but these are not targets of drug action and will not be considered further.

There are two major divisions of the ANS, the **parasympathetic** and **sympathetic** (Fig. 11.5). The **enteric nervous system** of the gut, a third division, is under the influence of the former two. Sympathetic and parasympathetic actions are often in opposite directions.

Pharmacologists who do not read dictionaries might find the term 'sympathetic' strange. To have sympathy is to have support of an idea or action, and thus the sympathetic nervous system prepares the body for physical activity, whilst the parasympathetic nervous system ('para' alteration, or distinct from) often has the opposite effect, relaxing the body and inhibiting physical activity, but in some tissues the action of one branch is unopposed (e.g. contraction of ciliary muscle by parasympathetic action).

The sympathetic nervous system

The cell bodies of sympathetic preganglionic neurons are found in the lumbar and thoracic spinal cord. The preganglionic nerve fibres synapse with postganglionic neurons either just outside the spinal cord, in the **paravertebral chains** or in the **midline (prevertebral) ganglia**. The preganglionic fibres branch and synapse with postganglionic neurons in several segments above and below their origin in the spinal cord – an anatomical basis for a diffuse response. Many of the postganglionic fibres from the sympathetic chain join the spinal nerves.

Widespread sympathetic effects also result from the release of catecholamines from the adrenal medulla.

The parasympathetic nervous system

Parasympathetic preganglionic fibres leave the CNS in the cranial nerves (III, VII, IX and X) and in spinal roots from the sacral region of the spinal cord. In contrast to their sympathetic counterparts, parasympathetic ganglia lie close to the target sites and the postganglionic fibres are often entirely within the tissue of the target organ. Most parasympathetic preganglionic fibres connect with only a few postganglionic fibres – an anatomical basis for discrete, localized responses.

The enteric nervous system

The enteric nervous system consists of neurons with cell bodies in the plexuses in the intestinal wall. Autonomic nerves terminate on these cells but the system can operate autonomously in the control of peristalsis and secretion.

NEUROTRANSMITTERS AND CO-TRANSMITTERS

The two main neurotransmitters in the ANS are **acetylcholine** (ACh) and **noradrenaline** (NA, or norepinephrine), released from postganglionic parasympathetic and sympathetic neurons, respectively (Fig. 11.6). An important exception is the autonomic innervation of sweat glands: although these are anatomically part of the sympathetic system, the postganglionic nerves utilize ACh as the neurotransmitter.

All preganglionic neurons in the ANS and somatic motor nerves innervating skeletal muscle release ACh. NANC (non-adrenergic, non-cholinergic) transmitters occur as primary transmitters in enteric neurons and sensory neurons and as co-transmitters with NA and ACh in autonomic nerves; examples include **ATP, GABA, 5-HT, dopamine, NO** (nitric oxide) and **peptides** (e.g. enkephalins, somatostatin, vasoactive intestinal peptide and neuropeptide Y). NO is also involved in the control of airway smooth muscle tone and partial relaxation of the corpus cavernous in the penis.

Co-transmitters are released together with neurotransmitters and commonly have a response speed that differs from that of NA or ACh (Fig. 11.7). The terminals of postganglionic nerves may carry several different kinds of presynaptic receptors that modulate the release of the neurotransmitter (e.g. NA acting on α_2-adrenoceptors inhibits ACh release from parasympathetic nerves in the gastrointestinal tract and stimulation of opioid receptors will inhibit NA release in various tissues).

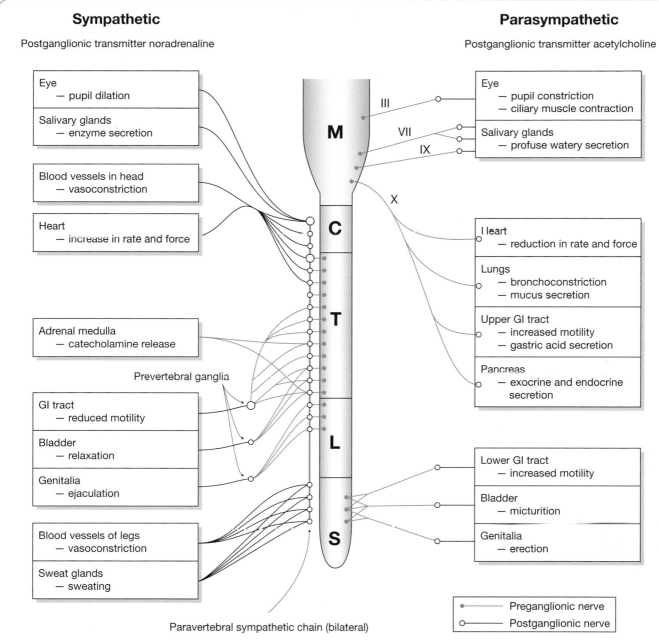

Sympathetic

Postganglionic transmitter noradrenaline

Eye
— pupil dilation

Salivary glands
— enzyme secretion

Blood vessels in head
— vasoconstriction

Heart
— increase in rate and force

Adrenal medulla
— catecholamine release

Prevertebral ganglia

GI tract
— reduced motility

Bladder
— relaxation

Genitalia
— ejaculation

Blood vessels of legs
— vasoconstriction

Sweat glands
— sweating

Paravertebral sympathetic chain (bilateral)

Parasympathetic

Postganglionic transmitter acetylcholine

Eye
— pupil constriction
— ciliary muscle contraction

Salivary glands
— profuse watery secretion

Heart
— reduction in rate and force

Lungs
— bronchoconstriction
— mucus secretion

Upper GI tract
— increased motility
— gastric acid secretion

Pancreas
— exocrine and endocrine secretion

Lower GI tract
— increased motility

Bladder
— micturition

Genitalia
— erection

• —— Preganglionic nerve
○ —— Postganglionic nerve

Fig. 11.5 The basic layout of the autonomic nervous system with illustrative actions. *C*, Cervical; *L*, lumbar; *M*, medullary; *S*, sacral; *T*, thoracic; *III*, *VII*, *IX* and *X*, cranial nerves.

Drugs modulation of neurotransmission

Drugs can be targeted to modulate:
• the central nervous system (CNS) control of autonomic nerve activity
• release of acetylcholine (ACh) and noradrenaline (NA), through an action on presynaptic receptors
• release of non-adrenergic, non-cholinergic (NANC) transmitters
• breakdown of ACh or NA
• postsynaptic action of autonomic nervous system (ANS) neurotransmitters/co-transmitters.

CHOLINERGIC TRANSMISSION

ACh is the transmitter at the neuromuscular junction (NMJ), autonomic ganglia, postganglionic parasympathetic nerve endings and various synapses in the CNS. It is produced in nerves and broken down by acetylcholinesterase (AChE found in the synapse with a pseudocholinesterase found in plasma). There are nicotinic (Fig. 11.8) and muscarinic (Fig. 11.9) receptors for ACh.

SYNTHESIS, STORAGE AND RELEASE OF ACETYLCHOLINE AND SUMMARY OF DRUG ACTION

ACh is an ester synthesised from choline and acetic acid (as acetyl-CoA) by choline acetyltransferase (CAT). It is stored in vesicles and released by Ca^{2+}-mediated exocytosis triggered by a nerve action potential. Uptake of choline into the nerve endings, and the storage and release of ACh, can each be inhibited though not in a clinically useful way (Fig. 11.10). Modulation of ACh release by presynaptic receptors is probably an important physiological mechanism and may, for example, contribute to the effects of opioids on gut motility.

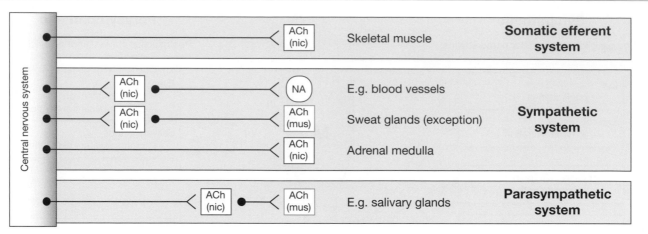

Fig. 11.6   Acetylcholine (ACh) and noradrenaline (NA) as transmitters in the peripheral nervous system. The location of nicotinic (nic) and muscarinic (mus) receptors are indicated.

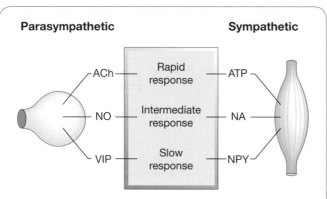

Fig. 11.7   The main co-transmitters at postganglionic parasympathetic and sympathetic neurons give rise to fast, intermediate and slow responses of the target tissue. *ACh,* Acetylcholine; *NA,* noradrenaline; *NPY,* neuropeptide Y; *NO,* nitric oxide; *VIP,* vasoactive intestinal peptide.

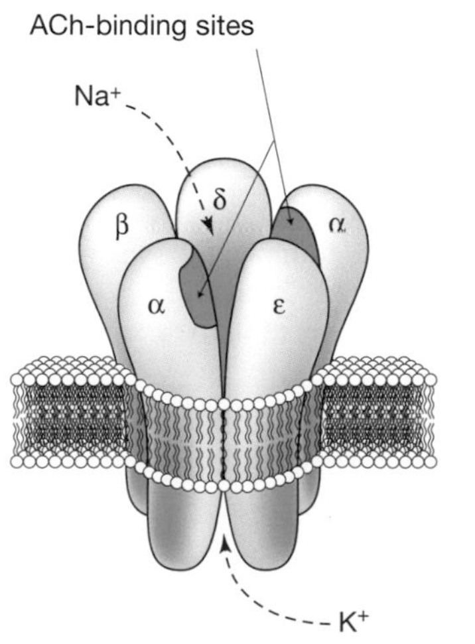

ACh-binding sites

Na⁺

β   δ   α

α   ε

K⁺

A nicotinic receptor is shown embedded in the cell membrane. It is a cation channel-forming protein comprising five subunits:

• NMJ: 2α, β, δ and ϵ

• neurons: 2α and 3β

To date, ten different α- and four different β-subunits have been cloned. Some drugs have selective actions on either neuronal or muscle type receptors. Channel opening allows Na⁺ influx leading to membrane depolarization and action potential initiation.

Ca²⁺ permeation is important in neurons.

Fig. 11.8   The structure of the nicotinic receptor. *ACh,* Acetylcholine; *NMJ,* neuromuscular junction.

NICOTINIC RECEPTORS

Drugs acting on nicotinic receptors (Fig. 11.11 and Table 11.1)

The main peripheral sites at which ACh acts on nicotinic receptors are:

• the NMJ in skeletal muscle;
• autonomic (ANS) ganglia.

At both sites the receptors are mainly postsynaptic.

Neuromuscular-blocking agents

Both agonists and antagonists can produce neuromuscular block.

• *Non-depolarizing blocking agents*: all those used clinically are competitive antagonists. Agents such as **vecuronium** reduce the size of the end-plate potential and so block transmission. Their effect can be reversed by anticholinesterases (see below), which increase the concentration of ACh at the receptor.
• *Depolarizing blocking agents*: these activate the receptor and so, at least initially, cause some contraction of muscle fibres (e.g. **succinylcholine**). However, the maintained depolarization which they produce causes the Na⁺ channels in the skeletal muscle membrane adjacent to the end-plate to enter the inactivated state and thus prevents the end-plate potential from producing a propagated action potential. Anticholinesterases will not reverse depolarization block since any increase in ACh concentration only serves to enhance the depolarization of the skeletal muscle fibres.

Pharmacokinetic aspects

All the neuromuscular blockers are quaternary ammonium compounds, which penetrate cell membranes poorly. They are given intravenously. Durations of action are pancuronium, 1–2 h; vecuronium, 30–40 min; atracurium, <30 min; succinylcholine, 10 min. Pancuronium and vecuronium undergo both renal excretion and hepatic metabolism. Atracurium was designed to be largely broken down by a simple chemical reaction in the blood stream, so its duration of action is less dependent on renal or hepatic function and is of particular use in the presence of kidney or liver disease. The short half-life of succinylcholine, a choline ester, results from its rapid hydrolysis in the plasma. (A genetic variant – occurring in 1 in 2000 people – which reduces the activity of plasma cholinesterase can result in a duration of up to 2 h.)

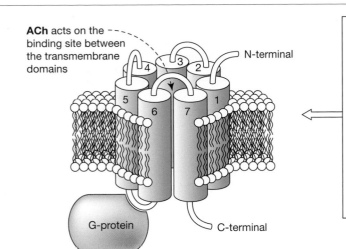

ACh acts on the binding site between the transmembrane domains

N-terminal

G-protein

C-terminal

A muscarinic receptor is shown embedded in the cell membrane. Muscarinic receptors are members of the G-protein-coupled receptor family, having 7 transmembrane segments in their amino acid sequence. Five muscarinic receptor subtypes (M_1–M_5) have been cloned, though only 3 (M_1–M_3) are well characterised.

M_1 (neural) and M_3 (glandular) couple to G_q and increase cellular inositol trisphosphate and diacylglycerol concentrations. M_2 (cardiac) couple to G_i and inhibit adenylate cyclase and open K^+ channels. M_1 receptors can also inhibit K^+ channel opening. The cellular events triggered by G-protein activation are discussed in detail in Chapter 2.

Fig. 11.9   The structure of the muscarinic receptor.

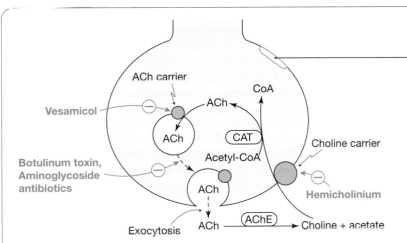

ACh carrier

Vesamicol

CoA

ACh

CAT

Acetyl-CoA

Choline carrier

Botulinum toxin, Aminoglycoside antibiotics

Hemicholinium

Exocytosis   ACh ⟶ (AChE) ⟶ Choline + acetate

Presynaptic receptors modulate ACh release

Some *inhibit* release: α_2-adrenoceptors, muscarinic and opioid receptors do so at parasympathetic post-ganglionic nerve endings.

Some *facilitate* release: e.g. β-adrenoceptors do so at parasympathetic nerve endings; nicotinic receptors do so at the NMJ.

Fig. 11.10   Diagram of the terminal of a cholinergic nerve including drugs that can modify acetylcholine uptake into and release from the terminal. *AChE*, Acetylcholinesterase; *NMJ*, neuromuscular junction.

Unwanted effects

Tubocurarine causes hypotension, mainly by ganglion block. It also releases histamine from mast cells, which adds to the hypotension and may cause bronchoconstriction. Pancuronium, vecuronium and atracurium are less prone to induce these effects. Pancuronium has some antimuscarinic activity, which may cause tachycardia. Succinylcholine produces bradycardia (agonist action at muscarinic receptors) and a rise in intraocular pressure (contraction of extraocular muscles). In patients with severe trauma or burns, the K^+ efflux from skeletal muscle mediated by succinylcholine may increase plasma K^+ levels sufficiently to cause cardiac dysrhythmias.

Ganglion-blocking agents

Ganglion blockers have widespread and predictable actions consequent on blocking both sympathetic and parasympathetic transmission (e.g. hypotension from blocking sympathetic vaso-constriction, a dry mouth from blocking parasympathetic saliva-tion, tachycardia by vagal block). Ganglion block is caused either by receptor antagonism (trimetaphan) or by direct channel block (hexamethonium). An excess of nicotine may cause depolarizing block of ganglion.

Clinical uses of drugs acting on nicotinic receptors

- **Neuromuscular-blocking drugs**, such as **succinylcholine, atracurium**, pancuronium and **vecuronium**, are used to produce muscle relaxation in anaesthetized patients during surgery. They also prevent injuries during electroconvulsive therapy.
- **Ganglion-blocking drugs**, such as trimetaphan, are occasionally used to lower blood pressure during surgery.

MUSCARINIC RECEPTORS

Drugs acting on muscarinic receptors

Muscarinic agonists and antagonists are listed in Table 11.2.

Pharmacological actions

Muscarinic agonists cause:

- smooth muscle contraction (e.g. gut, bladder) (M_3),
- pupillary constriction, ciliary muscle contraction,
- decreased rate and force of heart beat (M_2),

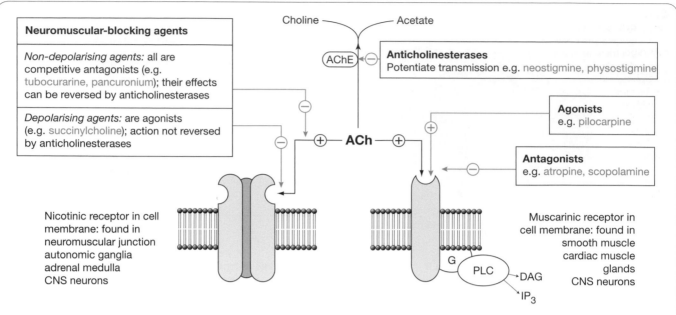

Fig. 11.11 **Summary of drug action at cholinergic receptors.** *DAG*, Diacylglycerol; *G*, G-protein; *IP₃*, inositol trisphosphate; *PLC*, phospholipase C; note that PLC activation is only one of several transduction systems that can be activated by muscarinic receptor stimulation.

Table 11.1 **Examples of Drugs Acting on Nicotinic Receptors**

	NMJ	ANS ganglia
Agonists	ACh*	ACh*
	Nicotine*	Nicotine*
	Succinylcholine (suxamethonium)	
	Decamethonium	
Antagonists	Tubocurarine	Trimetaphan
	Pancuronium	Mecamylamine
	Vecuronium	
	Atracurium	
	Rocuronium	
	Mivacurium	
	α-Bungarotoxin*	

*No clinical use, of historical or experimental interest.
ACh, Acetylcholine; *ANS*, autonomic nervous system; *NMJ*, neuro-muscular junction.

- glandular secretion (salivary, sweat, exocrine pancreas) (M₃),
- gastric acid secretion (M₁),
- vasodilatation via release of endothelial NO (M₃),
- inhibition of neurotransmitter release (M₂; M₁ may *facilitate* release),
- slow excitation of ganglia (M₁).

Muscarinic antagonists (those in regular use) all act in a reversible competitive fashion. Most show no selectivity between the receptor subtypes. They cause:

- inhibition of secretions (e.g. dry mouth),
- tachycardia,
- pupillary dilatation and paralysis of accommodation,
- relaxation of smooth muscle,
- inhibition of gastric acid secretion,

Table 11.2 **Examples of Drugs Acting on Muscarinic Receptors**

Agonists	Antagonists
ACh	**Atropine**
Carbachol	**Scopolamine** (hyoscine)
Pilocarpine	Pirenzepine (M₁ selective)
	Benzatropine
	Ipratropium
	Tiotropium
	Oxybutynin
	Tropicamide
	Cyclopentolate

ACh, Acetylcholine.

- CNS excitation (atropine) or depression (scopolamine),
- antiemetic action,
- antiparkinsonian action.

Pharmacokinetics

Atropine and **scopolamine** (tertiary amines) are well absorbed from the gastrointestinal (GI) tract and have half-lives of ~3 h. **Oxybutynin** has a half-life of 12 h. **Tropicamide** and cyclopentolate are used topically for effects on the eye and have a shorter duration of action than atropine.

Ipratropium and tiotropium (both quaternary ammonium) are administered by inhalation and, given this way, have no systemic actions. Both are used for the treatment of asthma and chronic obstructive pulmonary disease (COPD), with the effects of ipratropium on the airways lasting for ~4 h. Tiotropium is much longer acting drug providing beneficial effects for up to 24 h. **Benztropine** is usually given orally but can be given intravenously or intramuscularly; it penetrates the brain well. **Pilocarpine** (tertiary amine) given as eyedrops can cross the conjunctival membrane to produce effects which last for a day.

Clinical uses of drugs acting on muscarinic receptors

- **Antagonists:**
  - Cardiovascular: to treat sinus bradycardia (**atropine**).
  - Ophthalmic: to dilate the pupils (**tropicamide**, cyclopentolate).
  - Respiratory: to reduce cholinergic bronchospasm in patients with asthma or chronic obstructive pulmonary disease (COPD) (**ipratropium**, tiotropium; (see Chapter 20) for anaesthetic premedication to reduce airway secretions.
  - During anaesthesia for surgery (**atropine, scopolamine**).
  - Gastrointestinal: as an antispasmodic (**dicyclomine**), to reduce acid secretion as part of the treatment of peptic ulcer (**pirenzepine**; M_1 selective).
  - Urinary incontinence (**oxybutynin**).
  - Neurological: to prevent motion sickness (**scopolamine**), for Parkinson's disease (**benztropine**).
- **Agonists:**
  - Ophthalmic: to lower intraocular pressure in glaucoma (**pilocarpine**).
  - Gastrointestinal: to increase motility (bethanechol).

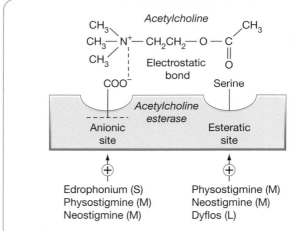

Fig. 11.12 Acetylcholine binding to AChE. As shown, anticholinesterases may bind to either or both sites. The duration of drug action is indicated: short (S), medium (M) or long (L).

Unwanted effects

Muscarinic antagonists can cause a wide range of unwanted effects. Some occur through parasympathetic block: constipation, urinary retention, blurred vision and raised intraocular pressure (problem in narrow-angle glaucoma). Some result from CNS actions, e.g. sedation (scopolamine) or excitement (atropine) and mental confusion.

CHOLINESTERASES AND ANTICHOLINESTERASES

Cholinesterases

There are two forms of cholinesterase: AChE and plasma or butyrylcholinesterase (BuChE). Both are serine hydrolases which hydrolyse ACh and other esters but have differing locations and specificities (Table 11.3). AChE is the enzyme that terminates the action of ACh released from nerves.

Enzyme action

Hydrolysis of ACh occurs in three steps:
1. ACh binds to the enzyme (Fig. 11.12).
2. The acetyl group is transferred to a serine OH in the esteratic site of the enzyme, resulting in a transiently acetylated enzyme plus free choline.
3. Hydrolytic cleavage of the serine-acetyl bond releases the acetyl group.

At fast synapses, such as those at the NMJ and in ganglia, but not at slow ones (cardiac muscle, smooth muscle, glands), AChE hydrolyses the released ACh in about 1 ms.

Table 11.3 Differences Between AChE and BuChE

	AChE	BuChE
Location	Basement membrane at cholinergic synapses; erythrocytes	Soluble form in plasma; also in liver and elsewhere
Substrate specificity	ACh and closely related compounds	Less specific: butyryl-choline, other esters (e.g. succinylcholine and procaine)

ACh, Acetylcholine; *AChE*, acetylcholinesterase; *BuChE*, butyrylcholinesterase.

Anticholinesterases

Anticholinesterases inhibit cholinesterase. There are three main groups, the differences in their duration of action depending on how they interact with AChE (see Fig. 11.12).
- Short acting: simple reversible association with the anionic site of the enzyme (e.g. edrophonium).
- Medium duration of action: interact with the serine hydroxyl at the active site to give a carbamylated product, which is only slowly hydrolysed (e.g. neostigmine, physostigmine, pyridostigmine).
- Irreversible (long acting): irreversibly phosphorylate the serine hydroxyl group. Most are organophosphate compounds with generalized toxic effects. Ecothiopate has a more or less selective action at postganglionic parasympathetic receptors and has been used in glaucoma.

Organophosphates are also used as insecticides (parathion) and chemical weapons (sarin and novichok) and poisoning with these agents is clearly serious. At an early stage their action can be reversed by the cholinesterase reactivator **pralidoxime**, which has such a high affinity for the phosphate group that it can effectively remove it from the esteratic site.

Pharmacological actions and unwanted effects

Enhancement of cholinergic transmission results in the following:
- **Autonomic effects**, including bradycardia, hypotension, excessive secretions, bronchoconstriction, GI tract hypermotility and decreased intraocular pressure.
- **Action at the neuromuscular junction**, causing muscle fasciculation and increased twitch tension; an excessive rise in ACh concentration may produce depolarization block.
- Action in CNS: drugs crossing blood–brain barrier can activate muscarinic receptors; they can cause respiratory failure and loss of consciousness (antagonized by atropine).

Clinical uses of the anticholinesterases

- **Ophthalmic:** eyedrops to treat glaucoma (**ecothiopate**, but now largely superseded by β-adrenoceptor blockers).
- **Musculoskeletal**
  - myasthenia gravis: neostigmine, pyridostigmine.
  - reversal of non-depolarizing neuromuscular block: neostigmine.
- **Alzheimer's disease:** donepezil (Chapter 18).

ADRENERGIC TRANSMISSION

Noradrenergic neurons in the periphery are postganglionic sympathetic neurons. The cell bodies lie in sympathetic ganglia and most have long axons with a series of varicosities strung like beads along the branching terminal network. The varicosities are the sites where synthesis and release of NA occurs. After release, NA acts on adrenoceptors in various target organs, including vascular smooth muscle, gland cells and cardiac cells.

TRANSMISSION AT THE NORADRENERGIC VARICOSITY WITH SUMMARY OF DRUG ACTION

High concentrations of NA are present in the varicosities, the NA being held in dense-cored storage vesicles from which it is released by Ca^{2+}-mediated exocytosis triggered by a nerve action potential. (The vesicles are produced in the cell body and pass down to the varicosities.) Fig. 11.13 depicts the events at the junction of the noradrenergic varicosity with vascular smooth muscle.

The action of the released NA is short lived because there is rapid reuptake into the varicosity and then into the storage vesicles; any NA not taken up is metabolized. Termination of the action of NA, therefore, differs from that of acetylcholine, which is hydrolysed after release.

NA is a catecholamine, as are adrenaline and isoprenaline. Differences in the responses to these three drugs in different tissues led to the understanding that there were different types of adrenoceptors: α and β, and several subtypes. The relative potencies of the three catecholamines on these are:

- α_1 and α_2 subtype: adrenaline = NA >> isoprenaline,
- β_1 subtype: isoprenaline > adrenaline = NA,
- β_2 subtype: isoprenaline = adrenaline > NA.

Subtypes of the α_1 and α_2 receptors have been identified, as has a β_3 subtype.

The term 'sympathomimetic' refers to the action of agents that mimic – to a greater or lesser degree – the actions of NA or adrenaline. Many clinically important drugs act by modifying noradrenergic transmission, notably those that act as agonists and antagonists on β-adrenoceptors. (The recommended international drug name for adrenaline is epinephrine and for noradrenaline is norepinephrine.)

THE ACTION OF DRUGS ON ADRENOCEPTORS

Many drugs that act on adrenoceptors have selective effects on the various receptor subtypes. Fig. 11.14 summarizes these. More details on α- and β-adrenoceptors follow below.

α-Adrenoceptor agonists and antagonists

Fig. 11.15 shows the lower part of a varicosity and the events and drugs modifying α-adrenoceptor action.

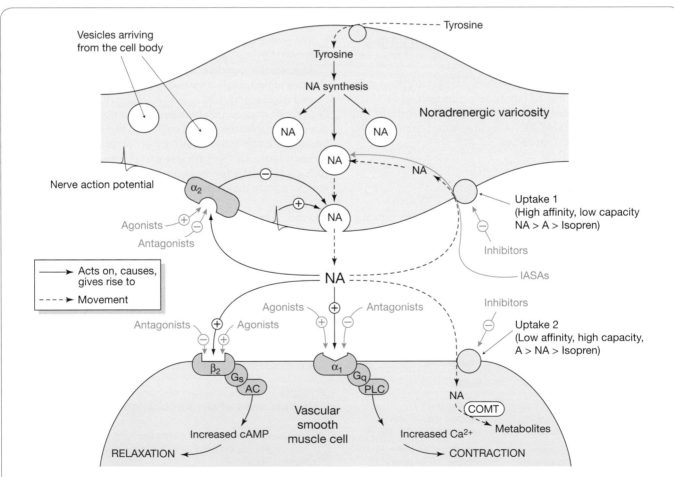

Fig. 11.13 The noradrenergic varicosity, emphasizing the action of NA on receptors and the events in a postsynaptic cell.
A, Adrenaline; *AC*, adenylate cyclase; *COMT*, catechol-*O*-methyltransferase; *G*, G-protein; *IASAs*, indirectly acting sympathomimetic amines; *Isopren*, isoprenaline; *PLC*, phospholipase C.

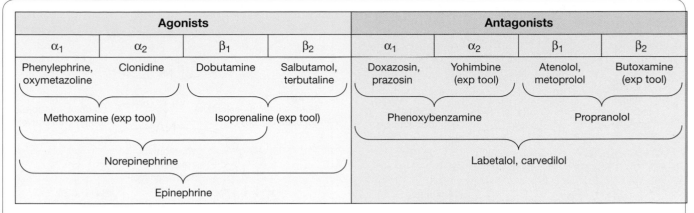

Agonists				Antagonists			
α_1	α_2	β_1	β_2	α_1	α_2	β_1	β_2
Phenylephrine, oxymetazoline	Clonidine	Dobutamine	Salbutamol, terbutaline	Doxazosin, prazosin	Yohimbine (exp tool)	Atenolol, metoprolol	Butoxamine (exp tool)
Methoxamine (exp tool)		Isoprenaline (exp tool)		Phenoxybenzamine		Propranolol	
Norepinephrine				Labetalol, carvedilol			
Epinephrine							

Fig. 11.14 Some examples of drugs that act mainly on particular subtypes of adrenoceptors. Note: the names norepinephrine and epinephrine are now used for the *drug* forms of NA and adrenaline, respectively.

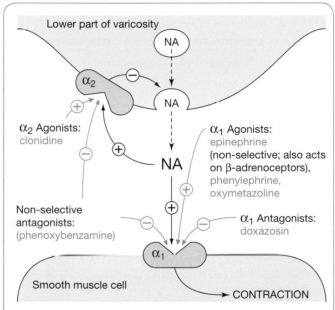

Fig. 11.15 The α-adrenoceptors modifying NA action at a noradrenergic varicosity. The main clinically useful agonist and antagonist drugs are shown, with drugs that are rarely used given in parentheses. NA release is modulated by autoinhibitory feedback of NA on α_2-adrenoceptors. Note: epinephrine is the name now used for the drug form of adrenaline.

α Agonists

The main α agonists that are of value clinically are epinephrine (adrenaline) and norepinephrine (noradrenaline); others are shown in Figs 11.14 and 11.15.

Pharmacological actions
- At α_1-adrenoceptors:
  - contraction of the smooth muscle of blood vessels (causing increase in blood pressure), uterus, the sphincters of the GI tract, the bladder sphincter and the radial muscle of the iris;
  - glycogenolysis in liver cells.
- At α_2-adrenoceptors:
  - inhibition of NA release,
  - inhibition of lipolysis.

Mechanism of action
Stimulation of α_1-adrenoceptors results in G-protein-mediated activation of phospholipase C (PLC) with generation of the second messengers inositol trisphosphate (IP$_3$) and diacylglycerol (DAG). IP$_3$ increases intracellular Ca^{2+}, which activates the contractile mechanism in smooth muscle cells. DAG activates protein kinase C (PKC), which phosphorylates various proteins; there are various isoforms of PKC with multiple intracellular actions. The α_2-adrenoceptors inhibit adenylate cyclase: this leads to reduction in cyclic adenosine monophosphate (cAMP), which would otherwise enhance Ca^{2+} influx with the passage of the nerve action potential. They also inhibit opening of Ca^{2+} channels directly and promote opening of K$^+$ channels.

Unwanted effects
The main adverse effects with the various α_1 agonists are:
- **epinephrine**: hypertension, increased heart rate (a β-adrenoceptor effect) with possibility of dysrhythmias (though reflex bradycardia can occur);
- **phenylephrine**: increased blood pressure, reflex bradycardia.

α Antagonists
The main α antagonists used clinically are the α_1-selective agents, **doxazosin**, prazosin and terazosin. Others are the non-selective α-antagonists **phenoxybenzamine** (which is irreversible and binds covalently to the receptor) and phentolamine. Labetalol blocks both α- and β-adrenoceptors. Ergot alkaloids are antagonists/ partial agonists at α-adrenoceptors.

Pharmacological actions
The main actions are:
- a fall in blood pressure,
- a rise in heart rate owing to reflex cardiac β-adrenoceptor response to the fall in blood pressure,
- decreased tone of the smooth muscle at the bladder neck.

Mechanism of action
α Antagonists act by blocking the effect of endogenous mediators (and exogenous agonists) on the relevant receptors by competitive inhibition.

Unwanted effects
Most unwanted effects are extensions of the pharmacological actions: increased heart rate, postural hypotension, congestion of the nasal blood vessels. Some agents can cause impotence.

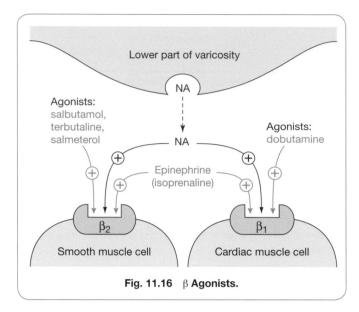

Fig. 11.16 β Agonists.

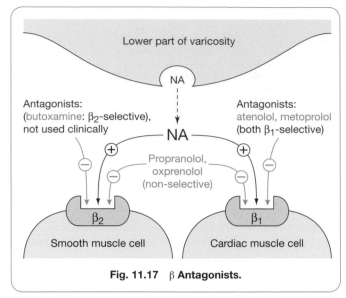

Fig. 11.17 β Antagonists.

β-adrenoceptor agonists and antagonists

β Agonists

The main β agonists that are used clinically include the β_2-selective agents **salbutamol**, terbutaline, **salmeterol** and the β_1-selective agent **dobutamine**. Isoprenaline and **epinephrine** stimulate both β_1- and β_2-adrenoceptors (Fig. 11.16).

Pharmacological actions

- At β_2-adrenoceptors:
  - dilatation of bronchioles and arterioles,
  - relaxation of the bladder detrusor muscle and of the ciliary muscle of the eye,
  - glycogenolysis.
- At β_1-adrenoceptors: increase in the rate and force of the heart.
- At β_3-adrenoceptors: lipolysis.

Agents with actions on β_1-, β_2- and β_3-adrenoceptors will have a mixture of the effects given above.

Mechanism of action

The cellular action depends on the signal transduction mechanism. β-adrenoceptor activation results mainly in G-protein-mediated activation of adenylate cyclase with increase of cyclic adenosine monophosphate (AMP), which in turn activates protein kinase A (PKA). In smooth muscle, PKA phosphorylates and inactivates myosin light chain kinase and thus reduces the contractile action. In the heart, PKA phosphorylates Ca^{2+} channels, increasing the inward Ca^{2+} current and thus the force of contraction (see Chapter 14). The cardiac effects of dobutamine are less potent than those of the other β_1 agonists.

Unwanted effects

The main unwanted effects are extensions of the pharmacological effects, mainly cardiac dysrhythmias with the β_1 agonists and tremor and peripheral vasodilatation with the β_2 agonists.

β Antagonists

The main β antagonists used clinically are **atenolol** (β_1 selective), **propranolol, alprenolol** (non-selective, partial agonist), labetalol (non-selective, also acts on α-adrenoceptors) (Fig. 11.17).

Table 11.4 Cardiovascular Effects of the Catecholamines

	Norepinephrine	Epinephrine	Isoprenaline
Diastolic BP	↑	↓	↓
Systolic BP	↑	↑ (moderate)	↓
Heart rate	↓ (reflex)	↑	↑

BP, blood pressure.

Pharmacological actions

The β antagonists have limited action in normal individuals at rest; the main actions are seen in pathological conditions. These include the following:

- An antihypertensive effect, which is caused by reduced cardiac output, decreased release of renin, central decrease of sympathetic action.
- An antianginal effect, which is caused by slowing of the heart rate and thus decreased metabolic demand.

Mechanism of action

The β antagonists act by blocking the effect of endogenous mediators (and exogenous agonists) on the relevant receptors, most acting as competitive antagonists.

Unwanted effects

The main unwanted effects are extensions of the pharmacological actions. Some are unpleasant but not critical for the patient:

- cold extremities,
- fatigue.

Some are particularly important in the presence of other diseases:

- Bronchoconstriction: this is potentially life-threatening in subjects with asthma.
- Slowing of heart rate: this can cause heart block in patients with coronary disease.
- Cardiac failure can occur in patients with heart disease.
- Decrease of the warning sympathetic response to hypoglycaemia in diabetic patients.

Table 11.4 summarizes the cardiovascular effects of the catecholamines.

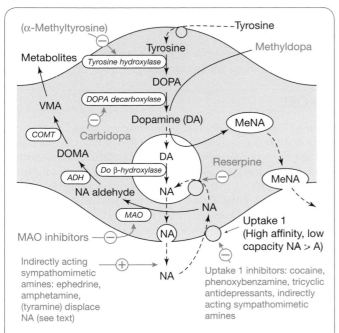

Fig. 11.18 Diagram of a varicosity. The sites of action of drugs are shown; those agents that are not used clinically are given in parentheses. *ADH*, Aldehyde dehydrogenase; *COMT*, catechol-O-methyltransferase; *DOMA*, dihydroxymandelic acid; *MAO*, monoamine oxidase; *MeNA*, methylnoradrenaline; *VMA*, vanillylmandelic acid; some of the later steps in NA metabolism take place outside the neuron.

EVENTS IN THE VARICOSITY AND THE ACTION OF DRUGS

Fig. 11.18 summarizes events in the varicosity and action of drugs thereon.

Pharmacological actions

Uptake 1 inhibitors cause an increase in the effects of NA because they interfere with the main method for terminating NA action, namely the uptake mechanism. For most of the drugs specified in Fig. 11.18, this action is subsidiary to their main pharmacological effect. Thus **cocaine** is a local anaesthetic, while **phenoxybenzamine** is mainly an α antagonist. The main actions of the other inhibitors are clear from their names.

Indirectly acting sympathomimetic amines (IASA, e.g. ephedrine) have similar (but weaker) actions to NA on receptors. They are taken up by Uptake 1 then into the vesicle by exchange with NA, which in turn is released from the varicosity by exchange with IASAs at Uptake 1. Actions in the CNS include increased alertness and decreased appetite.

Carbidopa reduces peripheral sympathetic activity when used as an adjunct to levodopa in the treatment of parkinsonism. It does not cross the blood–brain barrier.

Methyldopa is taken up by an amino acid transporter and acted on by the NA-producing enzymes to give, within the vesicle, methylnoradrenaline, which is released as a false transmitter. It acts mainly on α2-adrenoceptors, thus reducing further the release of NA. It has antihypertensive action by this effect and also by postsynaptic action on central neurons.

Clinical use and pharmacokinetic aspects of drugs affecting adrenoceptors

Agonists
- **Epinephrine** (adrenaline) is given subcutaneous (SC) or intravenous (IV) for anaphylactic shock and IV in cardiac arrest; it can be included in local anaesthetic preparations to delay absorption by inducing local vasoconstriction.
- **Salbutamol** and terbutaline (β2-selective agonists) are given by inhalation to treat bronchoconstriction in subjects with asthma. Both have a <30 min onset and are short acting (4–6 h) and can also be given SC for severe attacks. Salmeterol is longer acting (12 h) with vilanterol and olodaterol providing maintenance bronchodilation for up to 24 h following inhalation.
- **Ritodrine** or salbutamol may be used to inhibit preterm labour.
- **Dobutamine** (β1-selective) may be given for cardiogenic shock.
- **Phenylephrine** and oxymetazoline are given intranasally to reduce nasal congestion.
- Unwanted effects of β2 agonists are skeletal muscle tremor, tachycardia (at higher doses) and hypokalemia (which can lead to cardiac arrhythmias).

Antagonists
- **Doxazosin** (α1 antagonist; half-life 4 h) is used orally to treat resistant hypertension; it is metabolized in the liver.
- **Phenoxybenzamine** (non-selective antagonist, also inhibits Uptake 1; half-life 12 h) is given orally and is used to treat pheochromocytoma.
- **Atenolol** (half-life 6 h) and metoprolol, alprenolol, propranolol (half-lives 3–4 h) are β-adrenoceptor antagonists used for hypertension, angina and cardiac dysrhythmias.
- **Timolol** (β antagonist) decreases aqueous humour production; used in eyedrops to treat glaucoma.
- **Labetalol** (α and β antagonist) is used to treat hypertension in pregnancy; it is given orally and has a half-life of 4 h.
- α-Methyltyrosine (experimental tool) inhibits the rate-limiting enzyme in NA synthesis, tyrosine hydroxylase.
- Guanethidine (experimental tool; not shown) also depletes NA in the vesicle.
- 6-Hydroxydopamine (experimental tool; not shown) is taken up into the varicosity and destroys it.
- Reserpine inhibits uptake of NA into the vesicle; it is used mainly as an experimental tool.

Clinical use of drugs affecting varicosal events

- **Carbidopa**, given orally, is used as an adjunct to decrease the peripheral sympathetic activity of levodopa.
- **Ephedrine**, an indirectly acting sympathomimetic, is used as a nasal decongestant.

Drugs are used to treat neurodegenerative disorders, anxiety, psychosis, depression, epilepsy and pain.

NEURODEGENERATIVE DISORDERS

The very limited capacity of neurons to divide and re-establish synaptic contacts means that neuronal death in the central nervous system (CNS) produces largely irreversible changes in brain function. The main neurodegenerative disorders are Alzheimer's disease and Parkinson's disease (PD); less common are Huntington's chorea and motor neuron diseases (amyotrophic lateral sclerosis); prion diseases, such as variant Creutzfeldt-Jakob disease, are less common still. Another major cause of neuronal death is the acute brain ischaemia resulting from a stroke.

Many neurodegenerative diseases are associated with protein misfolding and aggregation, believed to be the first step leading to neurodegeneration. Mechanisms are not clear, but misfolded proteins can be toxic and lead to neuronal cell death. Examples are provided in Table 12.1.

Mechanisms of neurodegeneration

Excitotoxicity This is neuronal damage produced by disproportionate action of the excitatory neurotransmitter glutamate. High concentrations of glutamate cause an excessive elevation of calcium ions $[Ca^{2+}]_i$ which leads to membrane damage and cell death (Fig.12.1).

Oxidative stress This results from the generation of reactive oxygen species following inflammatory insults or ischaemia (reactive oxygen species (ROS): oxygen and hydroxyl free radicals) which can damage proteins, membrane lipids and nucleic acids. Elevations of ROS are normally prevented by antioxidants such as glutathione and vitamins C and E and the activities of superoxide dismutase (SOD) and catalase. However, it seems that, in neurodegenerative diseases, these defence mechanisms can be overwhelmed.

Apoptosis Programmed cell death is frequently associated with excitotoxicity. Neural apoptosis is normally prevented by neuronal growth factors such as nerve growth factor and brain-derived neurotrophic factor.

Potential drug targets to reverse neurodegeneration

These might include elements of the excitotoxic glutamate cascade: Ca^{2+} entry, intracellular protease activation, free radical damage, the inflammatory response and membrane repair. Furthermore, neuroprotective strategies to induce neuro-regeneration (i.e. reverse apoptosis) might be employed.

STROKE

Brain ischaemia, usually due to thrombosis, leads to rapid cell death in the hypoxic area followed by a slower neurodegeneration in adjacent areas. The ischaemia causes depolarization of neurons, which leads to release of glutamate and the consequences shown in Fig. 12.1. At present, there are few effective drugs available. If given soon after the vascular occlusion, fibrinolytics (tissue plasminogen activators; e.g. **alteplase** (see Ch. 15)) can improve blood flow and reduce further damage; however, they can make matters worse if the stroke is due to haemorrhage rather than clot formation.

PARKINSON'S DISEASE

Patients with PD have tremor at rest, muscle rigidity and difficulty in performing voluntary movements (hypokinesia).

Pathogenesis

The motor symptoms of PD are due to a specific loss of dopaminergic neurons in the nigrostriatal pathway, which forms an essential link in the extrapyramidal motor system involved in fine motor control. Excessive activity of the intrinsic cholinergic fibres of the striatum (unchecked by dopamine) is probably implicated in the tremor. An imbalance between the two systems is thought to be a key factor in PD. The damage to the dopaminergic neurons is caused by excitotoxicity, oxidative stress and apoptosis. Mitochondrial abnormalities have been detected in PD. (Mitochondrial effects of 1-methyl-4-phenyl-1,2,3,6-tetrahydropyridine (MPTP), a contaminant of meperidine, are responsible for a PD-like condition induced in a number of abusers of this drug.) PD-like symptoms may be produced, as one might expect, by dopamine receptor antagonists. The pathways that are affected in PD are shown in Fig. 12.2.

In PD, the destruction of dopaminergic fibres projecting from the substantia nigra to the corpus striatum impairs the fine control of movement exerted by the basal ganglia. This is exacerbated by a resulting enhancement in the action of striatal cholinergic neurons.

Table 12.1 Examples of Neurodegenerative Diseases Associated With Protein Misfolding and Aggregation*

Disease	Protein	Characteristic pathology	Notes
Alzheimer's disease	β-Amyloid (Aβ)	Amyloid plaques	Aβ mutations occur in rare familial forms of Alzheimer's disease
	Tau	Neurofibrillary tangles	Implicated in other pathologies ('tauopathies') as well as Alzheimer's disease
Parkinson's disease	α-Synuclein	Lewy bodies	α-Synuclein mutations occur in some types of familial Parkinson's disease
Creutzfeldt-Jakob disease	Prion protein	Insoluble aggregates of prion protein	Transmitted by infection with prion protein in its misfolded state
Huntington's disease	Huntingtin	No gross lesions	One of several genetic 'polyglutamine repeat' disorders
Amyotrophic lateral sclerosis (motor neuron disease)	Superoxide dismutase	Loss of motor neurons	Mutated superoxide dismutase tends to form aggregates; loss of enzyme function increases susceptibility to oxidative stress

*Protein aggregation disorders are often collectively known as amyloidosis and commonly affect organs other than the brain.
(From *Rang HP* et al. *Rang & Dale's Pharmacology*. 8th ed. Philadelphia: Elsevier; 2016.)

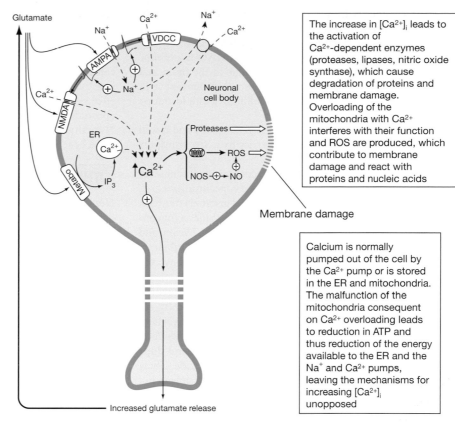

Glutamate-induced excitotoxicity is a major factor in ischaemic brain damage

↓

Glutamate activates receptors that lead to a sustained rise in [Ca²⁺]ᵢ

- Stimulation of AMPA receptors depolarises the plasma membrane which leads to the opening of voltage-dependent Ca²⁺ channels and also unblocks NMDA channels; this latter action plus...
- Stimulation of NMDA receptors allows Ca²⁺ influx (see Ch. 34)
- Stimulation of metabotropic (Metabo) receptors activates phopholipase C and leads to generation of IP₃, which releases Ca²⁺ from the endoplasmic reticulum (ER)
- Cell membrane Na⁺/Ca²⁺ exchange further increases [Ca²⁺]ᵢ

In glutamatergic neurons the increased [Ca²⁺]ᵢ leads to increased glutamate release and a positive feedback is initiated

The increase in [Ca²⁺]ᵢ leads to the activation of Ca²⁺-dependent enzymes (proteases, lipases, nitric oxide synthase), which cause degradation of proteins and membrane damage. Overloading of the mitochondria with Ca²⁺ interferes with their function and ROS are produced, which contribute to membrane damage and react with proteins and nucleic acids

Calcium is normally pumped out of the cell by the Ca²⁺ pump or is stored in the ER and mitochondria. The malfunction of the mitochondria consequent on Ca²⁺ overloading leads to reduction in ATP and thus reduction of the energy available to the ER and the Na⁺ and Ca²⁺ pumps, leaving the mechanisms for increasing [Ca²⁺]ᵢ unopposed

Fig. 12.1 The main mechanisms of excitotoxicity. *AMPA*, α-amino-3-hydroxy-5-methyl-methylisoxazole-4-propionic acid; *ER*, endoplasmic reticulum; *NMDA*, N-methyl-D-aspartate; *NO*, nitric oxide; *NOS*, nitric oxide synthase; *ROS*, reactive oxygen species; *VDCC*, voltage-dependent Ca²⁺ channel.

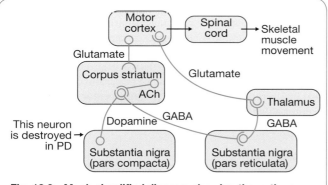

Fig. 12.2 Much simplified diagram showing the pathways between the cortex and the basal ganglia involved in motor control and the specific loss of dopaminergic fibres in Parkinson's disease (PD). *ACh*, Acetylcholine; *GABA*, γ-aminobutyric acid.

Treatment of PD

Drugs used to treat PD act by:
- redressing the loss of dopamine (**levodopa** or dopamine receptor agonists, e.g. **bromocriptine**);
- reducing the unbalanced action of acetylcholine in the striatum (muscarinic receptor antagonists, e.g. benztropine);
- inhibiting the breakdown of dopamine in CNS neurons with monoamine oxidase-B (MAO-B) inhibitors (**selegiline**);
- releasing dopamine (**amantadine**).

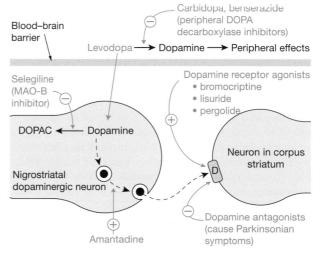

Fig. 12.3 Drug action on dopaminergic transmission in the treatment of Parkinson's disease. *D*, Dopamine receptor; *DOPAC*, dihydroxyphenylacetic acid.

None of the above actions halt the progression of the disease. Drugs affecting the dopaminergic system are shown in Fig. 12.3.

Levodopa (L-dopa)

Levodopa is the main treatment for PD.

Actions and mechanism of action Levodopa is decarboxylated to dopamine either within surviving nigrostriatal fibres or in other monoaminergic neurons and provides some restoration of nigrostriatal pathway activity. It is more effective against the akinesia and rigidity than against the tremor. The MAO-B inhibitor selegiline reduces the breakdown of dopamine in the brain and may enhance the action of levodopa. Combining **entacapone** (a catechol-*O*-methyltransferase (COMT) inhibitor) with levodopa can improve the response.

Pharmacokinetic aspects Levodopa is given orally and is well absorbed. It crosses the blood–brain barrier by active transport and has a half-life of approximately 2 h.

Unwanted effects These include an acute schizophrenia-like syndrome related to an increase in dopamine concentrations and, more commonly, confusion, disorientation and insomnia or nightmares. More slowly developing effects include dyskinesia (uncontrolled movements, which occur in most patients after 2 years) and 'on-off' effects, which are rapid fluctuations between dyskinesia and hypokinesia/rigidity. Outside the CNS, levodopa is converted to dopamine, which causes the unwanted peripheral side effects: postural hypotension and nausea. The latter is due to stimulation of the chemoreceptor trigger zone and can be reduced by co-administration of the dopamine antagonist domperidone, whose action is confined to the periphery. These peripheral side effects can be reduced by combining levodopa with a peripheral dopa decarboxylase inhibitor such as **carbidopa** or benserazide. These not only decrease the production of dopamine in the periphery but also substantially reduce the required dose of levodopa.

Dopamine receptor agonists

The dopamine receptor agonists **bromocriptine**, lisuride and pergolide have varying agonist activities on D_1, D_2 and D_3 receptors and can be used in place of, or as adjuncts to, levodopa. (Both D_1 and D_2 receptors are involved in the regulation of motor activity by the striatum.) They have similar side effects to levodopa.

Amantadine

Amantadine, an antiviral agent, also has a useful action in PD, possibly attributable to an increase in neuronal release of dopamine. It is less effective than levodopa or bromocriptine.

MAO-B inhibitors

Inhibition of MAO-B protects dopamine from extra neuronal degradation and MAO-B inhibitors may therefore be used with levodopa. However, **Selegiline** is metabolized to amphetamine, and may cause excitement, anxiety and insomnia. **Rasagiline** does not have this side effect and it is thought it might be neuroprotective, slowing disease progression. **Safinamide** inhibits both MAO-B and dopamine reuptake.

Muscarinic receptor antagonists

Muscarinic antagonists decrease the tremor of PD. The drugs used (e.g. **benztropine** and trihexyphenidyl (benzhexol)) show some CNS selectivity. Apart from the predictable effects due to antagonizing acetylcholine (ACh) in peripheral parasympathetic nerves, this drug class can have troublesome side effects in elderly patients such as sedation and confusion.

ALZHEIMER'S DISEASE

This age-related dementia is associated with a loss of neurons and shrinkage of brain tissue, particularly in the hippocampus and basal forebrain. Amyloid plaques and neurofibrillary tangles characterize the condition, leading to the selective loss of cholinergic fibres (in basal forebrain nuclei) that is thought to be a key factor.

Anticholinesterase drugs have a modest efficacy with predictable parasympathomimetic side effects, but do not retard or reverse disease progression. The drugs used are **tacrine** (short acting and can be hepatotoxic), **donepezil** (rather more effective and causes less liver damage), **rivastigmine** (fewer parasympathomimetic effects and longer lasting), and **galantamine** (may work partly by allosteric activation of CNS nicotinic receptors). **Memantine**, an N-methyl-D-aspartate (NMDA) receptor antagonist, provides some benefit probably by reducing excitotoxicity.

OTHER NEURODEGENERATIVE DISEASES

Huntington's disease is inherited (autosomal dominant) resulting in progressive brain degeneration and death in adults through protein misfolding of Huntington protein. Prion diseases such as Creutzfeldt-Jakob disease are transmissible through an infective agent (a prion) that causes protein misfolding (see Table 12.1).

ANXIETY AND HYPNOSIS

Anxiolytics are used to treat acute anxiety states. *Hypnotics* are drugs used to treat insomnia.

Anxiety is characterized by psychological symptoms such as nervousness and feelings of foreboding, accompanied by a variety of physical symptoms such as agitation, palpitations, sweating, sleeplessness and gastrointestinal (GI) tract disturbances. It can be a normal appropriate reaction to disturbing events but can in some circumstances be pathological and disabling, particularly if associated with panic attacks, phobic states or obsessive-compulsive disorders (OCDs). Many anxiety states, especially in the long term, may be better treated with antidepressants (e.g. the selective serotonin reuptake inhibitors (SSRIs) such as paroxetine).

Insomnia is difficulty in sleeping and may result from anxiety.

Both anxiety states and insomnia can be treated with CNS depressant drugs, which have effects that range from anxiolytic at low concentrations, to sedation and sleep at higher concentrations, to anaesthesia and, in toxic doses, coma and respiratory depression. However, some sedative and hypnotic drugs are ineffective in anxiety states.

The main drugs used are benzodiazepines, 5-hydroxytryptamine $(5\text{-HT})_{1A}$ receptor agonists and β-adrenoceptor antagonists. H_1 receptor antagonists (e.g. promethazine) may sometimes be used as hypnotics.

Benzodiazepines

Benzodiazepines have related chemical structures (e.g. **clonazepam, diazepam, lorazepam**) and are the most important and widely used anxiolytics and hypnotics.

Pharmacological actions
Benzodiazepines cause:
- a decrease in anxiety (less effective in obsessional states),
- a sedative effect,
- the induction of sleep,
- a reduction in muscle tone,
- an anticonvulsant effect.

The onset of their action is generally rapid. In general, most benzodiazepines exhibit similar pharmacological actions and choice is made mainly on the basis of duration of action. Shorter-acting agents are preferred as hypnotics to avoid sedative actions throughout the day. Table 12.2 gives a selection from the large number of benzodiazepines available.

Table 12.2 Commonly Used Benzodiazepines and Related Drugs Showing Their Main Clinical Uses and Half-Lives

Drug	Half-life	Main uses
Midazolam	Short (<10 h)	Premedication, induction
Zolpidem[a]	Short	Hypnotic (not anxiolytic)
Oxazepam	Short	Anxiolytic
Nitrazepam	Medium (10–24 h)	Hypnotic
Temazepam	Medium	Hypnotic
Flunitrazepam	Medium	Hypnotic, jet lag
Lorazepam	Medium	Anxiolytic, premedication
Alprazolam	Medium	Anxiolytic, panic disorder
Clonazepam	Long (>24 h)	Epilepsy
Diazepam	Long[b]	Anxiolytic, pre-medication, status epilepticus
Chlordiazepoxide	Long[b]	Anxiolytic

[a]Not a benzodiazepine.

[b]Long action due to slowly metabolized active metabolite. The drugs are also used in the treatment of spasticity and withdrawal from alcohol dependence.

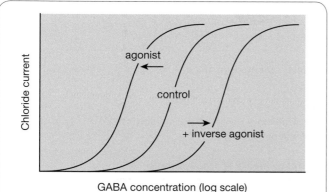

Fig. 12.4 Graph showing that agonists and inverse agonists at the benzodiazepine site have opposite effects on the opening of the GABA$_A$ receptor ion channel.

Mechanism of action
Benzodiazepines act by binding to distinct 'benzodiazepine regulatory sites' on γ-aminobutyric acid (GABA)$_A$ receptors to enhance the action of GABA, effectively increasing its affinity for its site on GABA-activated chloride (Cl$^-$) channels (Fig. 12.4; see Chapter 11). The increase in affinity is manifest as a shift of the GABA log dose–response curve to lower concentrations. The overall action of the benzodiazepines on the CNS is to produce a general enhancement of the neuroinhibitory actions of GABA. The actions at the GABA$_A$ receptor of benzodiazepines, competitive antagonists, such as flumazenil, and inverse agonists are shown in Fig. 12.5. Flumazenil can be used to treat an overdose of benzodiazepine.

Pharmacokinetic aspects
Benzodiazepines are lipid soluble and generally well absorbed from the gut and readily distributed into the brain. Most bind strongly to plasma proteins (up to 90% bound). Some benzodiazepines are metabolized to active agents with longer plasma half-lives. The final excretory product of most benzodiazepines is the glucuronide. Slower metabolism and increased half-life in elderly people necessitate lower doses.

Unwanted effects
These include drowsiness, confusion, forgetfulness and some loss of motor control. Together these actions impair complex tasks such as driving. In general, benzodiazepines are very safe on their own, although they can produce severe respiratory depression in combination with alcohol. *Tolerance* (not marked for the hypnotic action) and *dependence* can develop. Stopping the drug can, therefore, cause a withdrawal syndrome with both physical and psychological features: rebound anxiety, insomnia, photophobia, feelings of unsteadiness and even seizures. This is more likely to happen with short-acting agents. About a third of long-term users show withdrawal effects when they cease taking the drugs.

5-HT$_{1A}$ agonists
5-HT$_{1A}$ receptors occur extensively in the cerebral cortex and the amygdala. They are autoinhibitory presynaptic receptors and their activation results in decreased firing of the serotonergic neurons on which they occur. 5-HT$_{1A}$ receptor agonists will thus have mainly inhibitory effects. The important drug of this type is **buspirone**.

Pharmacological actions
5-HT$_{1A}$ agonists reduce anxiety but do not cause the sedation and motor incoordination seen with benzodiazepines. Buspirone is effective in generalized anxiety disorder but less active against OCD or posttraumatic stress disorder.

Mechanism of action
The drugs are believed to work by activating the presynaptic 5-HT$_{1A}$ autoreceptors, particularly in the dorsal raphe nucleus of the midbrain. The drugs also reduce the activity of some noradrenergic neurons (Chapter 11) and thus decrease arousal reactions (but do not induce sleep). However, there is a delay of several days before clinical effects are seen, which suggests a more complex mechanism of action.

Unwanted effects
These are less of a problem than with the benzodiazepines. They include nausea, nervousness, giddiness, restlessness, headache and light-headedness. The possibility of developing dependence and withdrawal is low.

β-Adrenoceptor antagonists
β-Adrenoceptor antagonists (e.g. **propranolol**) can reduce some of the peripheral manifestations of anxiety, notably tremor, sweating, tachycardia and diarrhoea. They have no effect on the central CNS affective component. They find use (abuse) in some sports and the performing arts.

Antihistamines
Antihistamines (H$_1$ receptor antagonists) with sedative action (see Chapter 16) have a useful hypnotic action that is made use of in some cold remedies and for wakeful children. However, many authorities feel that the use of drugs to help children sleep is rarely justified.

Barbiturates
Barbiturates, once used widely as both anxiolytics and hypnotics prior to the introduction of benzodiazepines, are no longer

1. The GABA$_A$ receptor on CNS neurons has binding sites for GABA and for benzodiazepine (BZD) anxiolytic drugs

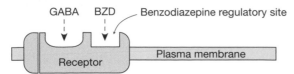

2. The receptor isomerises between a form that can bind the endogenous agonist GABA, which causes the Cl$^-$ channel to open...

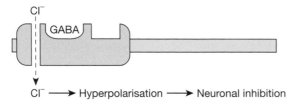

3. ...and an 'inactive' form, i.e. one that has much lower affinity for GABA

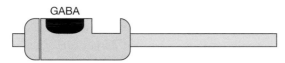

Normally there is equilibrium between the two conformations, with submaximal sensitivity to GABA

4. BZD agonists, such as diazepam, bind preferentially to the active form of the receptor and increase affinity for GABA

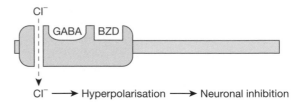

5. Inverse agonists such as the β-carbolines (βcar) bind preferentially to the 'inactive' form of the receptor, thus decreasing the proportion of receptors that bind GABA and reducing its effects

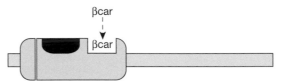

6. Competitive antagonists such as flumazenil (Flu) have equal affinity for the active and inactive configuration and, therefore, on their own, do not disturb the normal equilibrium. But their binding prevents the binding both of conventional agonists and of inverse agonists

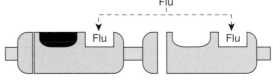

Fig. 12.5   Schematic diagram of the interaction of benzodiazepine agonists, antagonists and inverse agonists with the GABA$_A$ receptor.

recommended for these clinical uses in view of their low therapeutic index and dependence-producing properties. Barbiturates resemble benzodiazepines in increasing the activity of GABA$_A$ receptors but bind to a different site on the receptor and increase channel opening beyond that seen with GABA itself (Chapter 11). This is responsible for their severe depressant effect on the CNS. They retain useful roles in anaesthesia (Chapter 27) and epilepsy (see below).

PSYCHOSIS

Antipsychotic drugs, also known as *neuroleptics*, are used mainly in the treatment of schizophrenia, an important disabling mental illness that affects 1% of the population. The *positive symptoms* are delusions, hallucinations and thought disorders. The *negative symptoms* include social withdrawal, emotional flattening, reduced drive, inability to feel pleasure and poverty of speech. Schizophrenia often becomes overt in adolescence or early adulthood (though signs may be present earlier). Antipsychotic drugs may also be used for agitated depression and severe anxiety (see below).

Pathophysiology of schizophrenia
The cause of schizophrenia is not clear. Environmental factors play a part and there is a significant genetic component in that 10%–15% of first-degree relatives share the condition. Much evidence now indicates that it is associated with abnormalities of the cerebral cortex – often detectable before birth – and

alterations in various neurotransmitter systems (e.g. the dopaminergic pathways).

Dopamine theory of schizophrenia
Clear evidence for a malfunction of dopaminergic transmission comes from the well-established correlation between the potency of dopamine D$_2$ receptor antagonism and antipsychotic effect (Fig. 12.6). Abnormalities in the mesolimbic and mesocortical dopaminergic pathways are most likely since psychotic symptoms develop after injury or lesions in these areas. The involvement of dopamine is supported by the antipsychotic action of reserpine, which depletes monoamines, and by the action of the amine releaser amphetamine, which can generate psychotic symptoms (e.g. hallucinations). Positron emission tomography also shows increased D$_2$ receptors in the nucleus accumbens of schizophrenics (but in general the neurochemical evidence for an increase in dopamine receptors is not strong). The positive symptoms seem to be better correlated with changes in dopaminergic pathways than the negative symptoms.

Role of other transmitters
The production of schizophrenic-like symptoms by lysergic acid diethylamide (LSD) and NMDA antagonists (phencyclidine) suggests some malfunction of 5-HT and glutamate transmitter systems. Both 5-HT$_{2A}$ and 5-HT$_{1A}$ receptors may be involved, the latter showing some increase in the prefrontal cortex of schizophrenics. Recently a greater emphasis has been placed on alterations of glutamatergic pathways.

Antipsychotic drugs

Antipsychotic drugs can alleviate the positive symptoms of schizophrenia but have little effect on the negative symptoms; in fact, they can produce apathy and decreased initiative. The overall action of the drugs on the CNS is shown schematically in Fig. 12.7.

Mechanism of action

All currently used antipsychotics are dopamine D_2 receptor antagonists and have varying activity on the other dopamine receptor subtypes; antagonism of D_2 receptors seems to be most relevant. The drugs have a range of actions on other receptors (α_1-adrenoceptors, histamine H_1 receptors, muscarinic receptors,

5-HT receptors) that modifies their effectiveness or side effects (Table 12.3). Effects take some days to develop, suggesting that the antipsychotic effect is not simply due to receptor block, which will closely follow the rise in the concentration of the drug in cerebrospinal fluid.

The early antipsychotic drugs (examples in Table 12.3) are now referred to as 'typical' (or first generation) and share a strong tendency to produce extrapyramidal motor symptoms (see below). The typical neuroleptics are often referred to by their chemical structure: **chlorpromazine** and fluphenazine are *phenothiazines*; **haloperidol** is a *butyrophenone* and **flupentixol** is a *thioxanthene*.

Newer (second generation) agents (e.g. **clozapine**) are deemed 'atypical' in the sense that they produce fewer extrapyramidal

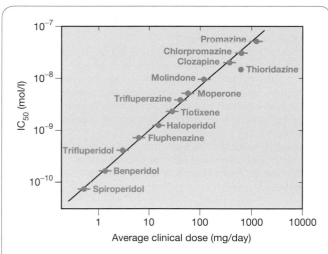

Fig. 12.6 The correlation between the clinical potency of antipsychotic drugs and their affinity for dopamine D_2 receptors. Binding is expressed as the concentration needed to give 50% inhibition of haloperidol binding.

Table 12.3 Unwanted Effects of Some Antipsychotic Drugs

Drug	EPS	Sedation	Antimusc	BP↓
Typical				
Chlorpromazine	++	++	+++	++
Fluphenazine	+++	+	++	+
Haloperidol	+++	+	0	++
Flupentixol	++	+	0	+
Atypical				
Clozapine	0	++	+++	++
Olanzapine	+	++	++	+
Risperidone	+	++	0	++
Amisulpride	+	+	+	0
Aripiprazole	+	+	0	+
Quetiapine	+	++	+	++

Antimusc, Antimuscarinic; *BP*, blood pressure; *EPS*, extrapyramidal symptoms. Number of '+' signs indicates intensity of effect.

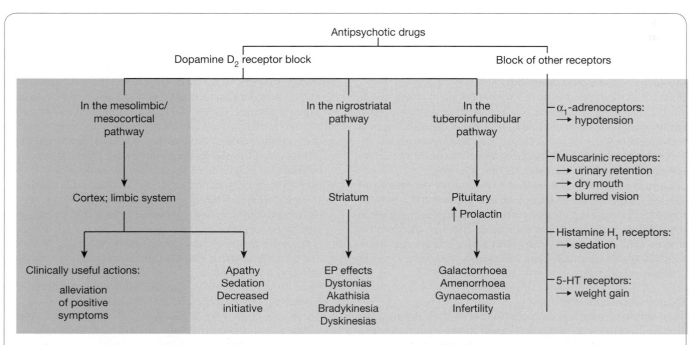

Fig. 12.7 Schematic diagram showing the main effects of antipsychotic drugs. The blue area shows the wanted actions of the drugs; the grey area shows the unwanted actions. The unwanted actions of some individual drugs are shown in Table 12.3. *EP*, Extrapyramidal; *HT*, hydroxytryptamine.

actions and may be effective in cases where the typical agents are not. They are also more effective against the negative symptoms. The improved profile of the atypical agents may reflect reduced activity on D_2 receptors and increased antagonism of 5-HT$_{2A}$ receptors (implying an alternative mechanism for the antipsychotic action). A role for agonist activity on 5-HT$_{1A}$ receptors, which increase dopamine release in the prefrontal cortex, has been suggested.

Some second generation antipsychotic drugs also possess muscarinic antagonist properties (e.g. **olanzapine**). This poly-pharmacology might help reduce extrapyramidal side effects observed in first generation antipsychotic drugs, because there is interplay in the striatum between D_2 receptor activation and muscarinic activation, where dopaminergic nerve terminals innervate cholinergic interneurons that express inhibitory D_2 receptors. Thus antagonizing D_2 receptors alone can result in the release of acetylcholine acting on the muscarinic receptors to produce extrapyramidal side effects.

Dopamine receptor antagonists have some other useful actions: a central anti-emetic action (Chapter 22), a prominent sedative effect (in some cases aided by antihistamine action) and potentiation of analgesics and general anaesthetics.

Unwanted neurological effects

Adverse neurological effects comprise extrapyramidal motor symptoms (parkinsonian effects) caused by D_2 receptor antagonism in the striatum:

- Rigidity, a mask-like face and bradykinesia (slowness in movement and in initiating movement).
- Dystonias (spasms of the face and neck muscles, which can be relieved with antimuscarinics).
- Akathisia (motor restlessness: an uncontrolled drive to move about, countered by β-blockers or benzodiazepines).
- Tardive dyskinesias (stereotyped repetitive 'tic'-like movements or worm-like twisting movements; these appear very late in treatment).

Atypical agents (e.g. clozapine and risperidone) have much reduced extrapyramidal effects. Agents with intrinsic anticholinergic action are also less likely to produce the extrapyramidal effects.

Antipsychotic malignant syndrome is a rare but potentially fatal effect of haloperidol, flupentixol or chlorpromazine.

Unwanted non-neurological effects

Blockade of the dopaminergic tuberoinfundibular pathway results in increased prolactin secretion (usually insignificant with atypical agents such as clozapine but does occur with risperidone), with consequent breast swelling, galactorrhoea and amenorrhoea.

A range of other effects follow from the actions on other receptor systems (see Fig. 12.7 and Table 12.3).

Chlorpromazine potentiates the respiratory depression of opiates. Clozapine causes serious agranulocytosis in 1% of those treated and is reserved for those resistant to other antipsychotics (risperidone and olanzapine may be as effective as clozapine without causing agranulocytosis). Obstructive jaundice may occur with chlorpromazine and related phenothiazines. Several agents produce weight gain.

Pharmacokinetic aspects

Most antipsychotic drugs have a half-life of 15–30 h and are given orally or intramuscularly (IM). There is, however, considerable individual variation, both in the plasma concentration achieved for a given dose and the response to a given plasma concentration. This means that doses need to be determined on an individual basis. Elderly people require reduction in dosage. Several neuroleptics

have been esterified with long-chain fatty acids to yield depot formulations that are only slowly absorbed from the IM injection site (e.g. **fluphenazine decanoate**). These are effective for up to 28 days. Depot formulations can help to ensure effective treatment in the high percentage of schizophrenic patients who do not take the drugs reliably. There is an increased risk of extrapyramidal motor symptoms with depot formulations. Binding to plasma proteins is commonly high (e.g. >90% for chlorpromazine, haloperidol and olanzapine).

Therapy with antipsychotic drugs

- Antipsychotic agents provide effective long-term treatment of schizophrenia in up to 70% of patients, allowing many to lead normal lives in the community.
- The older 'typical' first generation agents are more effective against the positive than the negative symptoms.
- The newer 'atypical' second generation agents, especially clozapine, may be effective in some patients resistant to the typical agents (e.g. a proportion of patients with chronic schizophrenia) and are better able to control the negative symptoms.
- The extrapyramidal effects and the effects due to increased prolactin are less marked with the atypical agents.
- Intramuscular depot preparations may be used for long-term therapy.

AFFECTIVE DISORDERS

Affective disorders are characterized by disturbances in mood and the main types are *depression* and *mania*.

Depression is the most common mental illness. It may be *unipolar* (the mood is always low) or *bipolar* (low mood alternates with mania – manic-depressive illness). It may be *reactive* (i.e. a response to traumatic life events), or *endogenous* (i.e. with no obvious cause). Severe endogenous depression may border on the psychotic and can carry a high risk of suicide.

Pathophysiology

The neurological basis of depression is poorly understood. The monoamine theory, which currently provides the best explanation, states that in depression there is a functional deficit of the transmitters noradrenaline (NA) and 5-HT in the forebrain and in mania there is a functional excess. Evidence for this theory comes from the antidepressant action of drugs acting at NA/5-HT nerve endings.

In support of this theory are the following observations:
- Inhibition of NA or 5-HT reuptake improves mood.
- Inhibition of monoamine oxidase (MAO, which metabolizes NA and 5-HT; see below) has an antidepressant effect.
- Reserpine, which depletes monoamine stores in the nerve endings, causes depression.

Against this theory are the following observations:
- The sympathomimetic drugs cocaine and amphetamine lack an antidepressant action.
- Some drugs (e.g. **iprindole**) have an antidepressant effect in the absence of clear effects on NA/5-HT transmission.
- There is a 2- to 4-week delay in the onset of the clinical action of antidepressant drugs despite immediate effects on neurotransmission.
- There are inconsistent changes in NA and 5-HT receptor densities and in the turnover of amine transmitters in depressed patients.

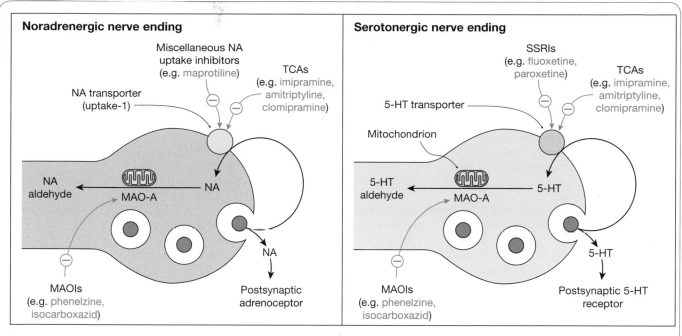

Fig. 12.8   Schematic diagram showing the probable sites of action of antidepressant drugs. *MAOIs*, Monoamine oxidase inhibitors; *SSRIs*, selective serotonin reuptake inhibitors; *TCAs*, tricyclic antidepressants.

Drugs used in affective disorders

The main categories of drugs used in affective disorders are:

- those used to treat unipolar depression, namely the antidepressants,
- those used to treat bipolar depression.

Antidepressant drugs

The main classes of antidepressant are:

- inhibitors of the reuptake of monoamine transmitters:
  - tricyclic antidepressants (TCAs), e.g. **imipramine**, amitriptyline, clomipramine
  - SSRIs, e.g. **fluoxetine**, paroxetine, citalopram
  - miscellaneous reuptake inhibitors, e.g. **maprotiline**, venlafaxine
- MAO inhibitors (MAOIs), e.g. phenelzine, isocarboxazid
- atypical antidepressants, e.g. trazodone, bupropion.

Mechanisms of action

Monoamine reuptake inhibitors   The explanation of how these drugs act is given by their names. Inhibition of reuptake raises the concentration of transmitter in the synaptic cleft and increases stimulation of postsynaptic receptors (Fig. 12.8). The selectivity for NA and 5-HT reuptake varies between the three main groups and between compounds in the same group. The relative potencies in inhibiting 5-HT or NA reuptake are indicated in Fig. 12.9.

MAOIs   These inhibit MAO within nerve endings. The cytosolic NA/5-HT concentration thus increases and more leaks out into the synaptic cleft. There are two MAO isoenzymes (A and B). The selectivity of MAOIs for the isoenzymes is shown in Table 12.4. Selective inhibitors of MAO-A are more effective antidepressants with fewer side effects. The older MAOIs bind covalently to the enzyme and consequently have a long duration of action; some newer drugs bind reversibly (e.g. **moclobemide**) and are safer.

Atypical antidepressants   These have less well characterized mechanisms of action; some combine actions on monoamine transporters and on receptors. Trazodone has weak 5-HT uptake

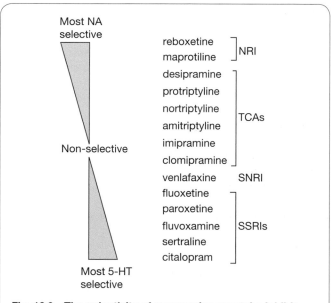

Fig. 12.9   The selectivity of monoamine reuptake inhibitors for 5-HT or noradrenaline (NA), based on the ratio of inhibitory constant values for 5-HT and NA reuptake inhibition. *NRI*, Noradrenaline reuptake inhibitor; *SNRI*, serotonin and noradrenaline reuptake inhibitor.

Table 12.4   The Selectivity of Drugs for MAOIs

Selectivity	Drugs
Non-selective	Iproniazid, isocarboxazid, tranylcypromine, phenelzine
MAO-A selective	Clorgyline, moclobemide
MAO-B selective	Selegiline

MAO; Monoamine oxidase; *MAOI*, monoamine oxidase inhibitors.

inhibition and antagonism of 5-HT receptors; bupropion has dopamine and NA reuptake inhibition; mianserin and mirtazapine have α_2-adrenoceptor antagonism (the latter also has NA reuptake inhibition) and iprindole has dopamine reuptake inhibition.

Time course of action It is important to note that for both the reuptake inhibitors and MAOIs, effects on neurotransmission can be expected fairly rapidly. However, the antidepressant effect is not apparent for 2–6 weeks which may be due to slower changes in receptor density (β_1, α_2-adrenoceptors, 5-HT$_{1A}$ and 5-HT$_2$-receptors), desensitization of monoamine receptors or increased neurogenesis in the hippocampus.

Pharmacokinetics aspects

SSRIs These are given orally and are well absorbed. The half-lives are: fluoxetine 24–96 h; citalopram 24–36 h and paroxetine 18–24 h.

TCAs These are very lipid soluble and are well absorbed by mouth. They bind strongly to plasma and tissue components, which results in a large volume of distribution. Many TCAs are tertiary amines with two methyl groups attached to the side chain nitrogen. Removal of one of these methyl groups (e.g. imipramine to desmethylimipramine (desipramine) or amitriptyline to nortriptyline) yields active drugs. The desmethyl metabolites show a greater ratio of NA/5-HT reuptake inhibition. Many TCAs are subsequently conjugated with glucuronic acid. TCAs have long half-lives and dosage can often be once daily.

Unwanted effects

TCAs Dangerous in overdose. They are chemically related to the antipsychotic phenothiazines and many have a similar spectrum of side effects due to receptor block:
- Antimuscarinic actions: dry mouth, constipation, blurred vision, urinary retention.
- Antihistamine effect: sedation.
- α-Adrenoceptor block: hypotension.

SSRIs Generally safer and have fewer side effects than TCAs; those that occur include:
- nausea and vomiting,
- sexual dysfunction.

Serious adverse effects can occur if SSRIs are given concurrently with MAOIs.

Miscellaneous monoamine reuptake inhibitors These have fewer adverse actions than the TCAs.

Atypical antidepressants Fewer adverse effects than the TCAs. Trazodone causes marked sedation, which leads to low compliance. Mirtazapine can cause weight gain. All antidepressants can cause hyponatraemia, especially in the elderly.

MAOIs These drugs potentiate amine transmitters and indirectly acting amines, e.g. those used as decongestants. They can cause serious unwanted effects if given with tyramine-containing foods (e.g. cheese, red wine). This is referred to as the 'cheese reaction'. Because tyramine is normally rapidly metabolized by MAO in the gut and liver, therapy with MAOIs will lead to high concentrations of this amine in the plasma. The tyramine will then release NA from sympathetic nerve endings which can result in dangerous hypertension. Selective MAO-A inhibitors do not produce such a strong cheese-reaction. MAOIs cause hypotension.

Clinical use of antidepressants

- **SSRIs** and **TCAs** are used primarily to treat depression but are also used effectively in some anxiety disorders: panic disorder (citalopram), obsessive-compulsive disorder, and bulimia.
- The combination of an atypical agent with an SSRI may be beneficial in antidepressant-resistant patients.
- TCAs produce varying degrees of sedation: sedative agents being used for anxious patients; less-sedative agents for withdrawn patients.
- **MAOIs** are less effective and subject to more drug interactions than the reuptake inhibitors and are considered second line.

Drugs used for bipolar depression
Lithium

Lithium is an important drug for the prophylaxis of bipolar disorder. Its actions may be attributable to inhibition of the formation of inositol trisphosphate (as a result of protein kinase C activation), inhibition of kinases and/or by mimicking sodium ion (Na$^+$), thus modifying cell membrane potential and ionic balance. Lithium causes CNS toxicity and, in large concentrations, renal damage; its low therapeutic index makes it essential to monitor its plasma concentration.

EPILEPSY

Epilepsy is a condition in which intermittent abnormal high-frequency firing of a localized group of cerebral neurons results in seizures. The discharge may remain localized or may spread to other regions of the brain. The seizures may be *partial* or *general*.

Types of seizure

Partial seizures involve repeated jerking of a limb or complex behavioural changes (psychomotor epilepsy) but no loss of consciousness. In these cases, the abnormal discharge is localized to the relevant area of the cortex.

Generalized seizures can take several forms:
- An initial generalized tonic convulsion followed by jerking of the whole body (clonic convulsion) accompanied by sudden loss of consciousness; this is tonic-clonic epilepsy or *grand mal*.
- Episodic transient loss of consciousness (absence seizures); this is termed *petit mal* and is seen mostly in children.

In generalized seizures, the abnormal electrical activity involves the whole brain.

A state in which generalized convulsions follow each other without consciousness being regained is termed *status epilepticus* and is a medical emergency. About 75% of those with epilepsy respond well to treatment.

Antiepileptic drugs

Antiepileptic drugs (AEDs) may need to be taken life-long so the fewer adverse effects the better.

The main commonly used antiepileptic drugs are **carbamazepine, phenytoin, valproate, ethosuximide** and benzodiazepines such as **diazepam** and **clonazepam**. Other newer drugs are vigabatrin, gabapentin, lamotrigine, felbamate, tiagabine, topiramate, levetiracetam and zonisamide.

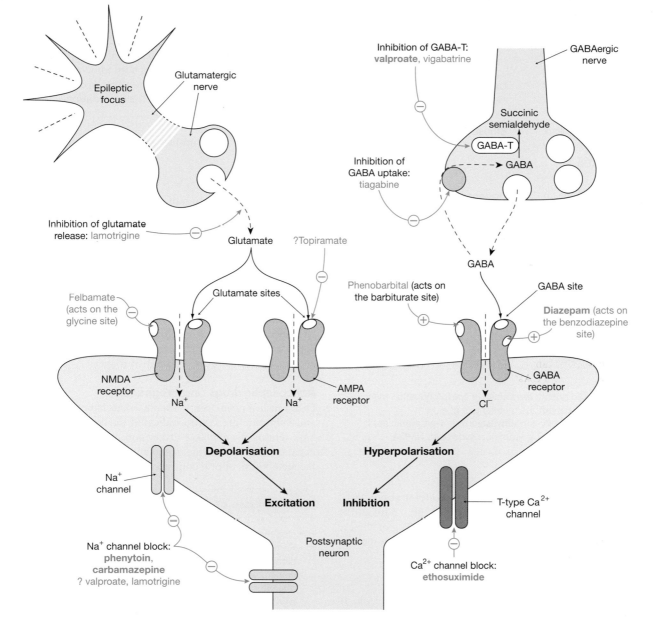

Fig. 12.10 Sites of action of antiepileptic drugs. The neurons undergoing abnormal high-frequency discharge release the excitatory transmitter glutamate; the postsynaptic neuron is depolarized and the discharge propagates. The main drugs used are shown in bold, less frequently used drugs or drugs still being assessed in smaller type. Vigabatrin and tiagabine also block uptake of GABA into, and metabolism in, glial cells. *GABA-T*, GABA transaminase.

Mechanisms of action of antiepileptic drugs
Drugs inhibit seizures by three main mechanisms (Fig. 12.10).

Table 12.5 gives examples of drugs that act by one or more of these means.

Carbamazepine and phenytoin

These agents inhibit the high-frequency discharge by binding preferentially to inactivated Na$^+$ channels. This prevents the return of the channel to the resting state which is necessary for the generation of action potentials (Chapters 11 and 27). Both drugs are effective in most types of epilepsy except absence seizures, carbamazepine (the most widely used AED) being preferred because it has fewer adverse effects.

Pharmacokinetic aspects They are both given orally. Carbamazepine's half-life is 30 h but is shorter with repeated administration. Phenytoin is subject to zero-order metabolism (see Chapter 5), which can lead to disproportionate increases in plasma concentration as the dose is increased. There is significant variation between individuals and a given dose can result in considerable differences in the plasma concentrations. Consequently monitoring of the plasma concentration is necessary.

Unwanted effects Both interact with other drugs because they induce the P450 liver enzymes. With phenytoin, the effective plasma concentration and the concentration causing adverse effects are uncomfortably close. It can cause dose-related vertigo, confusion, insomnia and ataxia. Non-dose-related effects include rashes, megaloblastic anaemia, teratogenesis, thickening of the gums and an increase in body hair. Carbamazepine can cause unsteadiness, sedation, mental disorientation and water retention.

Table 12.5 Sites and Mechanisms of Action of Antiepileptic Drugs

Mechanism of action	Drugs
Inhibition of action potential generation/conduction	
Use-dependent Na⁺ channel block	**Carbamazepine, phenytoin, valproate**, lamotrigine, topiramate, zonisamide
T-type Ca²⁺ channel block	**Ethosuximide**, gabapentin
Enhancement of GABAergic (GABA_A) transmission	
Agonist at the BZD site on the GABA_A receptor	**Diazepam, clonazepam**, clobazam
Ligand at the barbiturate site on the GABA_A receptor	Phenobarbital
Inhibiting GABA reuptake or metabolism	**Valproate**, vigabatrin, tiagabine
Reduction of glutamatergic transmission	
NMDA receptor antagonist	Felbamate
AMPA receptor antagonist	?Topiramate
Inhibition of glutamate release	Lamotrigine, ?levetiracetam

The commonly used agents are shown in bold. A question mark indicates uncertainty about the mechanism of action.
AMPA, α-amino-3-hydroxy-5-methylisoxazole-4-propionic acid; *BZD*, benzodiazepine; *GABA*, γ-aminobutyric acid; *NMDA*, N-methyl-D-aspartate.

Ethosuximide

Ethosuximide is given orally and has a half-life of about 48 h. It acts by inhibiting T-type Ca²⁺ channels (see Fig. 12.10) and is used only for absence seizures, for which it is the drug of choice. It can *precipitate* tonic-clonic epilepsy. *Unwanted effects* include GI tract disturbances, sedation and skin rashes.

Valproate

Valproate is given orally and has a half-life of about 15 h. It increases the GABA concentration in the brain and affects several processes involved in seizure generation (see Fig. 12.10), but its exact mechanism of action is not clear.

Unwanted effects These are fewer than with other antiepileptics and include alteration in hair thickness, GI disturbance and, rarely,

liver failure. It is teratogenic. It is effective in both tonic–clonic and absence seizures.

Benzodiazepines

Benzodiazepines (see above) also have a role in the treatment of epilepsy. **Clonazepam** is effective in both tonic-clonic and absence seizures. **Diazepam** is given intravenously (IV) or rectally for status epilepticus. The main unwanted effect is sedation.

Phenobarbital

Phenobarbital is a second-line antiepileptic drug; see Fig. 12.10 for site of action.

Newer antiepileptics

The mechanisms of action of **vigabatrin** (irreversible inhibitor of GABA transaminase, thus increasing releasable pool of GABA) and **lamotrigine** (similar to phenytoin and carbamazepine in mechanism of action) are shown in Fig. 12.10. Both are given orally. Both affect all types of epilepsy; vigabatrin can, in addition, be effective in epilepsy resistant to other agents; whilst lamotrigine has a broad therapeutic profile with efficacy against absence seizures.

Antiepileptics still being assessed include gabapentin, felbamate, topiramate and tiagabine, levetiracetam and zonisamide.

Unwanted effects Vigabatrin can cause giddiness, sedation, depression and hallucinations. Lamotrigine can cause giddiness, ataxia, skin rashes and GI tract disturbances.

Antiepileptic drugs and pregnancy

Drugs such as phenytoin, carbamazepine, lamotrigine, topiramate and valproate are contra-indicated during pregnancy, as they have teratogenic effects. Furthermore, through induction of the hepatic CYP3A4 enzyme, some antiepileptic drugs can increase the metabolism of oral contraceptives.

Clinical use of antiepileptic drugs

- Commonly used drugs are shown in bold.
- Partial seizures: carbamazepine, valproate, phenytoin, clonazepam, gabapentin, lamotrigine.
- Generalized tonic-clonic seizures: carbamazepine, valproate, phenytoin, gabapentin, lamotrigine, topiramate. Treatment with a single drug is recommended.
- Generalized absence seizures: ethosuximide, valproate, clonazepam, lamotrigine.
- Status epilepticus: diazepam IV, phenytoin.
- Antiepileptic drugs also find use for neuropathic pain (Chapter 13) and bipolar disorder (see above).

Pain (nociception) is a subjective experience with both sensory and emotional components arising from actual or potential tissue damage. It is frequently a traumatic feature of many diseases and the relief of pain is an important clinical priority. The main pain pathways are shown in Fig. 13.1. Acute pain is a normal physiological response to an excessively noxious stimulus associated with actual or potential tissue damage. In contrast, chronic pain might elicit *hyperalgesia* increased pain associated with a mild noxious stimulus), *allodynia* (pain evoked by a non-noxious stimulus) and *spontaneous pain* (no stimulus).

The sensation of pain arises from the activation of the peripheral terminals of nociceptive C and Aδ afferent fibres by thermal, mechanical and chemical stimuli. C fibres are non-myelinated and polymodal and give rise to slow burning pain; Aδ fibres are myelinated, activated by mechanical stimuli and give rise to acute localised pain.

When tissue is damaged, chemical mediators such as bradykinin (see Chapter 16), 5-HT (Chapter 12) and protons depolarise the C fibres (see below) and locally released prostaglandins sensitise the neurons to the action of these mediators (see below). At their central terminals in the DH of the spinal cord, the nociceptive fibres release peptides such as substance P (slow transmitters) and glutamate (a fast transmitter) that activate spinothalamic tract neurons; these carry the pain signals to the contralateral thalamus. From the thalamus, pain signals pass to the cortex and other CNS centres to elicit the conscious sensation of pain and the emotional response.

Pain transmission by the DHN is regulated by a 'gating' mechanism, which consists of (i) inhibitory input from GABAergic and enkephalinergic (enkeph) INs in the spinal cord (which are inhibited by the incoming C/Aδ fibres), see projection box, and (ii) descending inhibitory pathways from the midbrain and brainstem, the input of which is coordinated through the PAG.

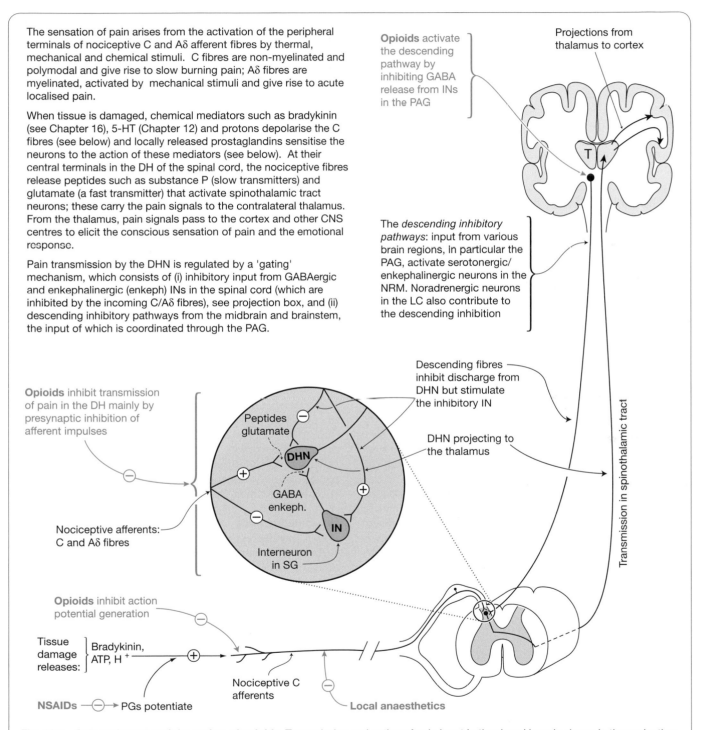

Opioids activate the descending pathway by inhibiting GABA release from INs in the PAG

Projections from thalamus to cortex

The *descending inhibitory pathways*: input from various brain regions, in particular the PAG, activate serotonergic/enkephalinergic neurons in the NRM. Noradrenergic neurons in the LC also contribute to the descending inhibition

Descending fibres inhibit discharge from DHN but stimulate the inhibitory IN

DHN projecting to the thalamus

Transmission in spinothalamic tract

Opioids inhibit transmission of pain in the DH mainly by presynaptic inhibition of afferent impulses

Peptides glutamate

DHN

GABA enkeph.

IN

Interneuron in SG

Nociceptive afferents: C and Aδ fibres

Opioids inhibit action potential generation

Tissue damage releases: Bradykinin, ATP, H⁺

Nociceptive C afferents

NSAIDs ⊖→ PGs potentiate

Local anaesthetics

Fig. 13.1   Pain pathways and the action of opioids. Transmission and gating of pain input in the dorsal horn is shown in the projection circle. *DH*, Dorsal horn; *DHN*, dorsal horn neuron; *enkeph*, enkephalin; *IN*, interneuron; *LC*, locus ceruleus; *NRM*, nucleus raphe magnus; *PAG*, periaqueductal grey matter; *PG*, prostaglandin; *SG*, substantia gelatinosa; *T*, thalamus.

ANALGESIA (THE RELIEF OF PAIN)

The main pain-relieving drugs are the *opioids*, which modify both the transmission of pain signals to the brain and the subjective perception of the painful stimulus, but other drugs can be helpful in alleviating some types of pain. Mild/moderate musculoskeletal pain can be alleviated by reducing the nociceptive stimulus through decreasing the formation of chemical mediators in areas of tissue damage (Fig. 13.1). *Nonsteroidal anti-inflammatory drugs* (*NSAIDs*) treat pain by inhibiting the enzyme cyclooxygenase leading to a reduction in the formation of prostaglandins (Chapter 16). (Note: **paracetamol,** which similarly inhibits cyclooxygenase, is also widely used for mild pain, but lacks anti-inflammatory action.) Certain types of pain can be controlled by *local anaesthetics* (Chapter 27) or **nitrous oxide** inhalation (Chapter 27). The pain of trigeminal neuralgia is susceptible to **carbamazepine** (an antiepileptic drug) and the pain of migraine to treatment with 5-HT$_1$ agonists (e.g. **sumatriptan**) or **ergotamine** (Chapter 12). Pain associated with damage to nerves (neuropathic pain) is often resistant to opioids and better treated with tricyclic antidepressants (e.g. amitriptyline) (Chapter 12) or selected antiepileptic drugs (e.g. gabapentin).

OPIOID ANALGESICS

There are two categories of opioid drugs:
- Morphine and related compounds such as diamorphine (heroin) and **codeine.**
- Synthetic analogues of morphine such as **pethidine, fentanyl, methadone,** pentazocine and buprenorphine.

Mechanism of action

Opioids act on opioid receptors, of which there are three main types: μ, δ and κ. A fourth receptor, the opioid-receptor-like (ORL) or nociception receptor, is now included in the same family, although it is insensitive to morphine-like drugs and a role in nociception is still uncertain.

Opioid analgesics act as agonists on opioid receptors. Some compounds structurally related to morphine act as partial agonists (nalorphine, levallorphan and buprenorphine) and can also have antagonist activity. Some are full antagonists (**naloxone, naltrexone**); these can inhibit/reverse the action of the agonists and can be used as antidotes in case of opioid overdose.

Many endogenous peptide agonists are essential components of an endogenous analgesia system which underlies the reduced pain sensations that occur under conditions of stress. These include β-*endorphin, met-enkephalin, leu-enkephalin, dynorphin* and the *endomorphins.* They are derived from the gene products *preproopiomelanocortin, preproenkephalin,* and *preprodynorphin.* Recent work suggests that endomorphins are the normal ligands

for the μ-receptor. Table 13.1 gives details of the actions of these various substances on the opioid receptors.

The opioid receptors are coupled to G-proteins, which:
- inhibit the action of adenylate cyclase, thus decreasing intracellular cAMP;
- couple directly to K$^+$ and Ca^{2+} channels increasing or decreasing their opening, respectively; this can inhibit presynaptic transmitter release and reduce postsynaptic excitability.

More than 75% of opioid receptors in the dorsal horn are found presynaptically and most of those are μ-receptors.

Pharmacological actions

Morphine will be taken as the reference drug. **Codeine** and dextropropoxyphene are relatively weak analgesics. **Tramadol** is a weak agonist at opioid receptors and its analgesic action is due in part to inhibition of 5-hydroxytryptamine (5-HT) and noradrenaline reuptake. It has less-marked unwanted action (i.e. less respiratory depressant and addictive effect; see below). The actions of the opioids are as follows.

Analgesia

Morphine relieves most types of pain, reducing both the sensory and the emotional components. It produces analgesia mainly by (1) inhibition of pain transmission in the dorsal horn, (2) activation of the descending pathways that inhibit pain transmission in the dorsal horn and (3) inhibition of activation of the nociceptive afferents in the tissues. The sites of analgesic action are shown in Fig. 13.1. Analgesia is mainly due to an action on μ-receptors.

Euphoria

A feeling of well-being mediated by μ-receptors is helpful in severe/terminal pain (κ receptors can cause dysphoria).

Sedation
Cough suppression

Opioids inhibit the cough reflex pathways in the brainstem. This can be therapeutically useful; codeine and pholcodine are able to exert this action selectively (Chapter 20).

Antidiarrhoeal action

Opioids have inhibitory actions on enteric nerves, which leads to reduced motility and constipation. This is usually an unwanted effect but is useful in the treatment of diarrhoea.

Unwanted actions
Respiratory depression

Activation of μ-receptors reduces the sensitivity of the respiratory centre to carbon dioxide (CO_2). This occurs even with therapeutic doses of morphine and is the main cause of death in overdose. The

Table 13.1 Agents Acting at the Various Opioid Receptors

	Receptor		
	μ	δ	κ
Endogenous agonists	β-Endorphin, endomorphins, leu-enkephalin, met-enkephalin	Enkephalins, β-endorphin	Dynorphins
Exogenous agonists	**Morphine**, heroin, codeine, fentanyl, pethidine, methadone, dextropropoxyphene, sufentanil, remifentanil	Experimental compounds	Pentazocine
Antagonists	Naloxone, naltrexone	Naloxone, naltrexone	Naloxone, naltrexone

reversible competitive antagonists **naloxone** and **naltrexone** can reverse opioid-induced respiratory depression, but may induce withdrawal reactions in addicts.

Nausea and vomiting
Stimulation of the chemoreceptor trigger zone in the medulla by opioids causes troublesome effects in 40% of patients.

Pupillary constriction
Stimulation of the oculomotor nucleus mediates parasympathetic constriction of the pupil; this is diagnostic of opioid abuse.

Psychological and physical dependence
This is very marked with the street use of morphine and other strong agonists but is less troublesome with their use as analgesics (Ch. 37). Withdrawal symptoms may be severe and can be reduced by methadone.

Histamine release
Morphine causes release of histamine from mast cells, other opioids having a lesser effect. The released histamine can cause bronchospasm and hypotension; therefore, an alternative should be used for pain relief in patients with asthma.

Pharmacokinetic aspects
Morphine and heroin can be given orally (sustained release preparations are available) but are commonly given by injection (intravenous (IV), intramuscular (IM), subcutaneous (SC)). Codeine, dextropropoxyphene and tramadol are given orally. Fentanyl can be given by injection or as a transdermal patch that provides analgesia for up to 3 days. A selective spinal action, with reduced central effects, can be achieved with intrathecal or epidural injection. Buprenorphine is longer acting than morphine and can be given sublingually. Heroin is faster acting than morphine because it is more lipid soluble and penetrates the blood–brain barrier more rapidly. Most opioids are metabolized in the liver, commonly by oxidation or, as with morphine, by production of the glucuronide. A newer opioid, **remifentanil** is very short acting (half-life 3–4 min) due to rapid metabolism by plasma and tissue esterases and is less dependent on hepatic and renal function. Some metabolites (e.g. morphine 6-glucuronide) retain analgesic activity. The analgesic action of codeine and heroin is due in large part to their conversion to morphine (by demethylation and deacetylation, respectively).

PARACETAMOL AND NSAIDS

NSAIDs are used to treat pain induced by inflammation and to reduce fever. The mechanism of action is discussed elsewhere (Chapter 16). Aspirin, ibuprofen and all other NSAIDs also have anti-inflammatory effects; however, paracetamol (acetaminophen) only has analgesic and antipyretic effects. It has been shown that paracetamol is a weak inhibitor of COX enzyme but shows selectivity for COX located in the brain. It remains contentious whether paracetamol relieves pain centrally via the COX-1 splice variant COX-3, or other mechanisms of action. For example, the active metabolites of paracetamol have been shown to activate TRPA1 to reduce voltage-gated calcium and sodium currents in sensory neurons.

Paracetamol is administered orally, with a plasma half-life of 3 h. It is metabolized by hydroxylation and excreted in the urine. Paracetamol can induce severe and fatal liver damage if over-dosed.

Opioids (codeine) and paracetamol are sometimes given in combination, since the different mechanisms of action appear to provide a synergistic analgesic effect (rather than additive).

TREATMENT OF NEUROPATHIC PAIN

Neuropathic pain is a severe chronic pain associated with various conditions and is sometimes suggested as being opioid resistant. Tricyclic antidepressants (amitriptyline, nortriptyline), certain antiepileptic drugs (gabapentin, carbamazepine, valproic acid, lamotrigine) and local anaesthetics (lidocaine) can relieve neuropathic pain.

OTHER PAIN-RELIEVING DRUGS

Cannabinoids acting on the CB_1 receptors reduce nociception in animal models of acute, inflammatory and neuropathic pain. Whilst the effects in these models are not particularly potent, **Sativex** (an extract of the cannabis plant containing Δ9-tetrahydrocannabinol (THC) and cannabidiol) at least provides benefit for neuropathic pain in patients with multiple sclerosis. CB_2 receptor agonists are also being evaluated for analgesic properties.

CARDIAC RHYTHM AND DYSRHYTHMIAS

Antidysrhythmic drugs are agents that are used to treat disorders of heart rate and rhythm termed dysrhythmias. The normal regular contractions of the heart are initiated and controlled by a specialized conducting system; dysrhythmias occur when the function of this is deranged. To understand the action of the antidysrhythmic drugs it is necessary to understand the actions of this conducting system.

The specialized conducting system in the heart

A heart beat is initiated in the sinoatrial (SA) node by the pacemaker potential. This triggers an impulse, the action potential, which passes across the atrial muscle to the atrioventricular (AV) node and then, via the Purkinje fibres, through the ventricles – coordinating the contraction of the cardiac muscle. The cardiac action potential has a long duration and long refractory period (Fig. 14.1) and differs from one part of the heart to another. The prolonged activation of calcium ion (Ca^{2+}) channels during the action potential plateau in the ventricles maintains Ca^{2+} entry, which is essential for the prolonged contraction required for the effective ejection of blood during systole.

The action of the SA node is controlled by autonomic activity.

Pathophysiology

Clinically important dysrhythmias include:

* *Tachycardia (rapid heart beat)*
  - In the atria ('supraventricular' tachycardias): paroxysmal tachycardia, flutter and fibrillation. In atrial fibrillation (the commonest dysrhythmia), the contraction of the muscle is fast, uncoordinated and ineffective; not all impulses get through to the ventricles, resulting in a very irregular heart rate.
  - In the ventricles: tachycardia, torsades de pointes (a particular type of tachycardia) and fibrillation (the last frequently fatal).
* *Bradycardia (slow heart beat) and heart block*
  - The latter is due to damage to the AV node or conducting tissue, causing the ventricles to beat at a slower, and often irregular, rate driven by pacemaker activity in the ventricular conducting tissue; an external pacemaker rather than drug therapy is usually required.

Myocardial ischaemia is a common cause of dysrhythmias, which can also be precipitated by reperfusion after an infarction.

The causes of dysrhythmias can be:

* *Abnormal pacemaker activity*: ischaemia-induced depolarization or increased sympathetic activity can cause pacemaker activity to be initiated at an ectopic focus in atria or ventricles.
* *Early or delayed after-depolarization (EAD, DAD)*: these can act as triggers for the generation of abnormal impulses or extra beats.
  - DADs: the action potential in non-pacemaker cells does not have a phase 4 depolarization (see Fig. 14.1), but these cells can become ectopic foci of action potential generation if a phase 4-like after-depolarization occurs. This is associated with increased $[Ca^{2+}]_i$ which can be produced by some drugs (cardiac glycosides, norepinephrine).
  - EADs: these can arise during phases 2 and 3 of the action potential and can themselves trigger propagated action potentials. They occur when repolarization is delayed and the action potential is abnormally long, as occurs during bradycardia. EADs can also be produced by class III antidysrhythmic drugs.
* *Re-entry*: under normal circumstances, the refractory period of the muscle prevents the action potential re-invading the tissue it has just traversed. If, however, there is damage that allows unidirectional propagation, a continuous cycling of the action potential may occur (circus rhythm) (Fig. 14.2). This is more

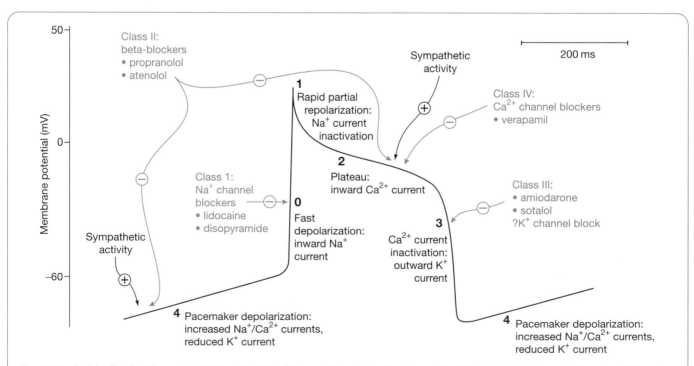

Fig. 14.1   An idealized action potential in a Purkinje fibre and the sites of actions of antidysrhythmic drugs. In the sinoatrial node, an action potential is triggered when the pacemaker potential reaches a critical threshold (approximately –60 mV).

likely in depolarized tissue where Ca^{2+} channels rather than Na^+ channels produce slowly propagated action potentials with a longer refractory period. Re-entry provides an abnormal site for cardiac excitation.

Antidysrhythmic drugs

Actions and mechanisms of action

Most drugs act on the ion channels involved in the various stages of action potential generation and propagation; some act on the sympathetic control of the heart (see Fig. 14.1 and Table 14.1).

All class I drugs show use-dependence, binding preferentially to sodium ion (Na^+) channels in their activated (open) or inactivated states. The block is thus more pronounced at rates above normal (when the channels spend more time in these states) or in depolarized tissues, where recovery from inactivation is delayed. Class I drugs dissociate at different rates from the channel, resulting in different degrees of use-dependence and leading to subdivision of the class into Ia, Ib and Ic; Ib drugs dissociate rapidly, Ia drugs less rapidly and Ic drugs most slowly. Ic drugs (e.g. flecainide) have been found to cause fatal dysrhythmias and so their use is restricted.

Amiodarone has class III actions and also blocks Na^+ channels and β-adrenoceptors. These multiple actions may explain its particular efficacy. **Sotalol** has actions in classes II and III. **Adenosine** activates adenosine (A_1) receptors in the heart to exert the same cardiac effects as acetylcholine interacting with muscarinic receptors. Its short duration of action reduces the likelihood of side effects. Digoxin has direct effects on myocardial contraction due to its inhibition of the sodium/potassium adenosine triphosphatase pump ($Na^+/K^+ATPase$), which include increased excitability; this may, in fact, cause the conversion of atrial flutter to fibrillation. However, by increasing vagal action on the heart, it blocks AV conduction and usefully reduces ventricular rate.

Pharmacokinetic aspects

Lidocaine is given intravenously (IV) following myocardial infarction. It is rapidly metabolized by the liver and so is ineffective orally owing to first-pass metabolism; by the same token it has a short half-life (2 h). **Propranolol** has a half-life of about 4 h with significant first-pass metabolism: its antidysrhythmic activity is maintained by an active metabolite. **Amiodarone** is extensively bound in tissues and only slowly eliminated; its half-life is 10–100 days. **Verapamil** is orally active and has a half-life of 6–8 h. **Adenosine** is given IV to terminate supraventricular tachycardia and acts for only 20–30 s due to rapid uptake into erythrocytes and subsequent metabolism.

Unwanted effects

Antidysrhythmics generally have a narrow therapeutic index. As most antidysrhythmics are metabolized by the cytochrome P450

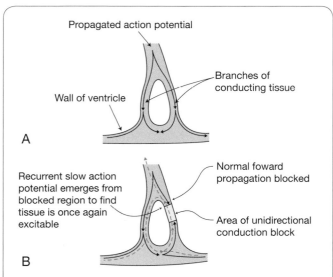

Fig. 14.2 Example of the production of circus rhythm. A: The normal conduction pattern. B: Unidirectional block and re-entry.

Labels in figure:
- Propagated action potential
- Branches of conducting tissue
- Wall of ventricle
- A
- Recurrent slow action potential emerges from blocked region to find tissue is once again excitable
- Normal foward propagation blocked
- Area of unidirectional conduction block
- B

Table 14.1 The Mechanism of Action, the Electrophysiological Actions and Clinical Uses of Selected Antidysrhythmic Drugs

		Example	Mechanism of action	Electrophysiological actions	Clinical use
Vaughan Williams classification	Class Ia Class Ib	Disopyramide Lidocaine	Na^+ channel block	Reduced rate of depolarization of action potential, increased ERP, decreased AV conduction	Ventricular fibrillation, especially associated with myocardial infarction
	Class II	Propranolol, atenolol	β-Adrenoceptor antagonism	Slowed pacemaker activity, increased AV refractory period	Dysrhythmia prevention in myocardial infarction; paroxysmal atrial fibrillation due to sympathetic activity
	Class III	Amiodarone, sotalol	K^+ channel block	Increased action potential duration and increased ERP	Atrial fibrillation; ventricular fibrillation
	Class IV	Verapamil	Ca^{2+} channel block	Decreased APD, slowed AV conduction	Supraventricular tachycardias; atrial fibrillation
Not classified by system		Adenosine	K^+ channel activation	Slowed pacemaker activity, slowed AV conduction	Given IV for supraventricular tachycardias
		Digoxin	K^+ channel activation (vagal action)	Slowed AV conduction (block)	Atrial fibrillation
		Magnesium sulfate	? Ca^{2+} channel block		Ventricular fibrillation; digoxin toxicity

APD, Action potential duration; *AV*, atrioventricular; *ERP*, effective refractory period; *IV*, intravenous.

system, pharmacokinetic interactions involving enzyme induction or inhibition may be clinically significant. Ca²⁺ channel blockers should be avoided in heart failure because of reduction in contractility. Class II drugs should not be used in subjects with asthma as they can precipitate bronchoconstriction. Amiodarone has important adverse effects, not only triggering torsades de pointes (shared with other class III drugs), but also exhibiting thyroid and pulmonary toxicity.

Vernakalant is a recently introduced anti-arrhythmic drug which is used IV to treat atrial fibrillation. It acts by delaying atrial repolarization by blocking atrial selective potassium and sodium channels.

BLOOD PRESSURE CONTROL AND HYPERTENSION

The cardiovascular system is regulated by complex mechanisms, the main variable under control being the arterial blood pressure, which is the driving force for the flow of blood through the systemic circulation. Fig. 14.3 gives a rough outline of the principal *homeostatic factors* controlling the arterial pressure. The arterioles play the major role in determining the *peripheral resistance* and also regulate the relative blood flow through individual organs. The *cardiac output* depends on the stroke volume (SV) and the *heart rate*. The main factors affecting the SV are the *plasma volume* and the *venous return*; the heart rate is controlled primarily by the

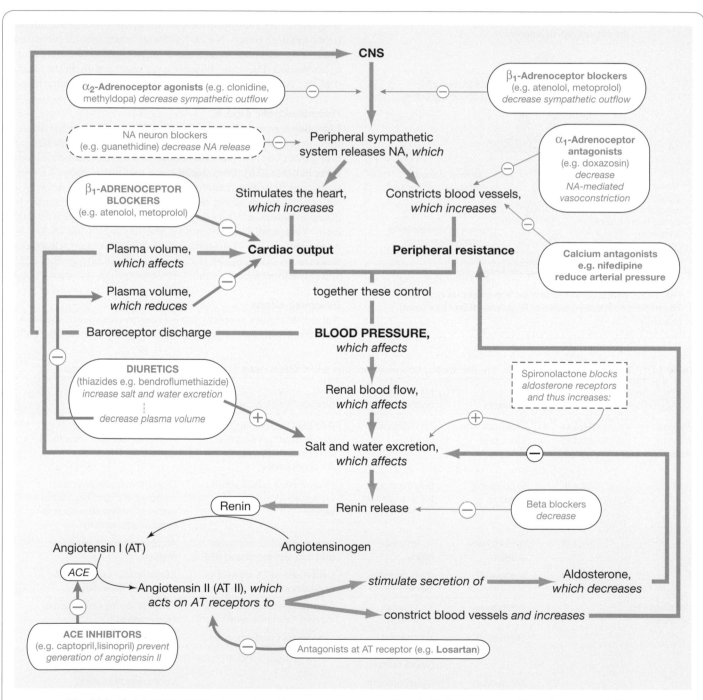

Fig. 14.3 Calcium ion (Ca2⁺) channel blockers such as verapamil and nifedipine are used to induce vasodilation.

sympathetic nerves (which increase the rate) and the parasympathetic nerves (which decrease the rate). Note that the kidney plays a vital part in blood pressure control as do some paracrine factors including nitric oxide and prostacyclin (PGI_2) released by vascular endothelial cells (which increases cyclic guanosine monophosphate, cGMP), adenosine and prostaglandins and bradykinin generated during inflammatory responses.

The boxes give the main antihypertensive drugs.

Vasodilatation involves an increase in cyclic adenosine monophosphate (cAMP) in vascular smooth muscle and is brought about partly by adrenaline acting on β_2-adrenoceptors. (A decrease in sympathetic tone can also produce vasodilatation.)

Vasoconstriction involves an increase in intracellular Ca^{2+} and is brought about primarily by noradrenaline (NA) released from sympathetic nerves acting on α_1-adrenoceptors (for more detail, see Chapter 11). Vasoconstriction can also be regulated by angiotensin II and local release of endothelin from endothelial cells.

Pathophysiology of hypertension

The main pathological condition affecting the vascular system is hypertension (high blood pressure). This can be caused by renal disease, endocrine disorders or phaeochromocytoma (a catecholamine-secreting tumour; rare), but in most patients the cause is unknown and the hypertension is termed 'essential' (for archaic and mistaken reasons). From Fig. 14.3, it is clear that a multitude of factors influence arterial blood pressure, all of which could be implicated in the pathogenesis of hypertension, although this is mainly caused by the kidney and/or the sympathetic nervous system. If hypertension is not treated, coronary thrombosis, stroke or kidney failure may result.

Antihypertensive drugs

The main drugs are:
- agents affecting the renin–angiotensin system (angiotensin-converting enzyme (ACE) inhibitors, angiotensin (AT) I receptor antagonists, see below);
- the thiazide diuretics (Chapter 18);
- calcium antagonists (see below);
- β-Adrenoceptor antagonists (see below and Chapter 11).

In young patients, initial treatment is with agents affecting the renin–angiotensin system; older patients are started on thiazides or a calcium antagonist.

Other drugs that can be used include:
- drugs acting centrally or peripherally on noradrenergic transmission: doxazosin, clonidine, methyldopa; these are dealt with in Chapters 11 and 12;
- vasodilators (covered briefly below).

Thiazide diuretics

Examples: bendroflumethiazide, hydrochlorothiazide.

Actions relevant to hypertension:
- Increase in salt and water excretion and thus reduction of extracellular fluid volume.
- Decrease in cardiac output through reduced plasma volume.
- Reduction in peripheral resistance (an as yet unexplained effect).
- Increase in renin release (which may counteract some of the above effects on the blood pressure).

Thiazides have antihypertensive actions when used alone and also potentiate the action of other antihypertensive drugs.

Drugs acting on the renin–angiotensin system

The sequence of events is outlined in Fig. 14.3. (AT III, a breakdown product of AT II, also stimulates aldosterone secretion; not shown.)

The release of renin, a proteolytic enzyme, is stimulated by:
- decreased blood flow through the kidney,
- reduced Na^+ concentration in the distal tubule,
- β-adrenoceptor agonists.

The renin–angiotensin system tends to increase blood pressure by:
- the vasoconstrictor action of AT II (partly through augmentation of NA release);
- the aldosterone-mediated retention of salt and water, which leads to increased extracellular fluid volume. The raised plasma volume increases cardiac output.

These effects can be decreased by ACE inhibitors and by AT_1 receptor antagonists, the sartans. In addition to their action as antihypertensives, these two groups of drugs are also used in heart failure and diabetic nephropathy.

ACE inhibitors

Examples include: captopril, lisinopril and enalapril.

Actions relevant to hypertension   ACE inhibitors cause a fall in blood pressure affecting particularly the vasculature of the brain, kidney and heart. The drop is more marked in hypertensive individuals, especially if diuretics are also being given. They are given orally, lisinopril once a day and captopril twice a day and are excreted in the urine.

Main unwanted effects
- A dry cough.
- Hypotension (initially; particularly in the presence of diuretics).
- Recent work suggests that chronic use of this drug class may have an increased risk of lung cancer.

Contraindications
- Renovascular disease.
- Pregnancy.

Sartans

Actions relevant to hypertension   These drugs antagonize the action of AT II on the AT_1 receptors thus decreasing the effects of AT II (see above).

Calcium antagonists

Examples are: nifedipine, amlodipine.

The calcium antagonists block Ca^{2+} entry through Ca^{2+} channels. Action relevant to hypertension is the inhibition of depolarization-induced Ca^{2+} entry into cardiac and vascular smooth muscle. The vasodilator effect reduces arterial pressure. They cause flushing and ankle oedema; the absence of more serious unwanted actions is a recommendation for their use as antihypertensives.

β_1-Adrenoceptor antagonists (sometimes referred to as cardioselective)

Examples: atenolol, metoprolol.

Actions relevant to hypertension
- Decrease in cardiac output.
- Decrease in sympathetic activity by an action in the CNS.
- Decrease of renin release, which reduces the generation of AT I and II and thus decreases AT II-induced vasoconstrictor activity and aldosterone-induced salt and water reabsorption.

Vasodilators

Various vasodilator agents have been used as antihypertensives (and are sometimes still so used in special circumstances).

Minoxidil is a K^+ channel activator which relaxes vascular smooth muscle by hyperpolarizing the plasma membrane, thus preventing Ca^{2+} entry through voltage-dependent Ca^{2+} channels. It is used with a β-adrenoceptor antagonist and a diuretic for very severe hypertension.

CARDIAC BLOOD FLOW, ANGINA AND MYOCARDIAL INFARCTION

The coronary arteries supply blood to the heart muscle. Blood flow only occurs during diastole and is markedly affected by adenosine being the main vasodilator. Other factors less important in the control of the coronary vessels are the sympathetic nerves, circulating catecholamines, and mediators from purinergic, nitrergic and peptidergic neurons.

Pathophysiology of the coronary circulation

The main pathological condition is *atherosclerosis*, in which atheromatous plaque forms within the arteries; this narrows them and decreases perfusion of the myocardium. Plaque formation is initiated by endothelial damage. A simplified explanation of this process has three steps:

1. Platelets, macrophages and low-density lipoprotein (LDL) adhere to the damaged endothelium.
2. Macrophages release free radicals; these cause lipid peroxidation of the LDL, which the macrophages then ingest.
3. Macrophages release inflammatory cytokines and growth factors, which cause proliferation of smooth muscle and fibroblasts.

Plaque-mediated decreased perfusion of the myocardium causes *angina pectoris*, which is pain caused by the action on nociceptors of chemicals released from the ischaemic heart muscle. The pain is usually in the chest, is constricting in type and radiates down the left arm. *Stable angina* occurs with a constant amount of exercise; ceasing exertion at the appropriate moment can prevent its onset. Angina that occurs with decreasing amounts of exertion, finally coming on at rest, is termed *unstable angina* and is an indication that a thrombus has formed on the plaque (refer to Fig. 15.9 in Chapter 15), which may have ruptured. It can presage infarction. *Variant angina* (rare) is caused by coronary artery spasm.

Complete block of a coronary artery is usually a sudden, often dramatic event and results in *myocardial infarction*, which can result in death or damage of the tissue supplied by the blocked blood vessel. It is a very common cause of death in the developed world.

ANGINA

The therapeutic aims in anti-anginal therapy are:
- to reduce cardiac work and, thus, metabolic demand,
- to increase perfusion of heart muscle,
- to prevent myocardial infarction.

The last aim may be achieved by several means (Fig. 14.4). *Lipid-lowering drugs*, particularly **statins** (see below) and *antiplatelet drugs*, especially **aspirin** (Chapter 15) and **platelet glycoprotein receptor (GPIIb/IIIa) antagonists** (see Chapter 15) can reduce the possibility of thrombosis but are only used via IV infusion to prevent restenosis after percutaneous coronary interventions. Aspirin is particularly important in the treatment of unstable angina (which requires hospitalization).

Drugs used in angina and atheromatous disease

- **Organic nitrates** have the first two actions specified under therapeutic aims.
- **Calcium antagonists** (calcium channel blockers) have the first two actions specified under therapeutic aims (see above); only aspects relevant to angina therapy are dealt with below.
- **β-adrenoceptor antagonists** have only the first action (see Chapter 11 for details; only aspects relevant to angina therapy are dealt with below).
- **Nicorandil**, a K⁺ channel activator, has both actions.
- **3-hydroxy-3methylglutaryl**-coenzyme A (HMG-CoA) inhibitors (statins) have the third action (above), and other lipid lowering drugs by reducing plaque development.

Organic nitrates

Examples: glyceryl trinitrate (nitroglycerin), isosorbide mononitrate.

The actions and mechanisms of action of nitrates are explained in Figs 14.4 and 14.5 (see above).

Pharmacokinetic aspects

Glyceryl trinitrate can be taken by sublingual tablet or spray, in which case its effects start within minutes and last approximately 30 min. Given by transdermal patch, its action lasts approximately 24 h. It can also be given intravenously. It cannot be given orally as it would be inactivated by first-pass metabolism in the liver.

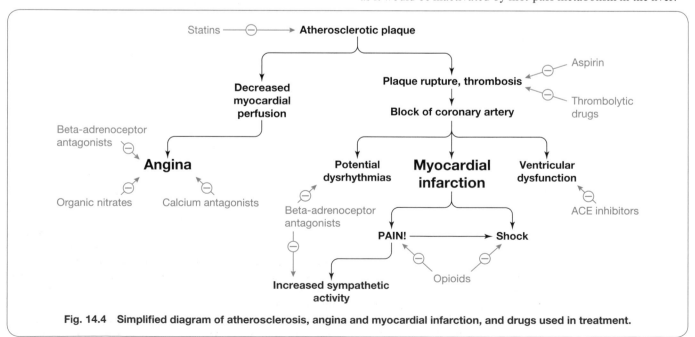

Fig. 14.4 Simplified diagram of atherosclerosis, angina and myocardial infarction, and drugs used in treatment.

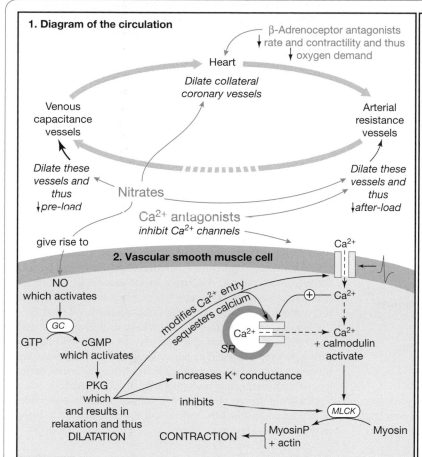

Fig. 14.5 **Pharmacological effects and mechanisms of action of the main antianginal drugs.** (Larger text size means more important actions.)

Isosorbide mononitrate is a longer-acting nitrate which is given orally. Its half-life is 4 h. A slow-release preparation is also available.

Clinical use of the organic nitrates

- **In the treatment of angina**: glyceryl trinitrate or isosorbide mononitrate is given sublingually to prevent or treat stable angina; glyceryl trinitrate is given intravenously to treat unstable angina.
- **In the treatment of chronic heart failure**: nitrates can be given to decrease venous return and thus reduce preload (see below).

Unwanted effects
Nitrates can cause headache because of the pronounced vasodilatation, and postural hypotension. Frequent use of isosorbide mononitrate can cause tolerance which is short lived, lasting only a day or so after administration of the nitrate is stopped.

Calcium antagonists (calcium channel blockers)
Examples: **nifedipine, amlodipine**, verapamil.

Actions and mechanisms of action
Calcium antagonists all act by blocking voltage-dependent L-type Ca^{2+} channels in vascular smooth muscle (see Fig. 14.5) and cardiac muscle. Some are more active on blood vessels; some are more active on the heart.

Actions on blood vessels
Nifedipine and amlodipine act mainly on arterial resistance vessels causing relaxation and vasodilatation (see Fig. 14.5 and above).

Actions on the heart
Verapamil acts mainly on the heart, slowing the rate by action on the SA and AV nodes. It inhibits the slow inward movement of Ca^{2+} during the plateau phase of the cardiac action potential (see Fig. 14.1). It has little useful effect on blood vessels. Verapamil is not used in angina because of the risk of heart failure or heart block from its inhibitory action on AV conduction.

Pharmacokinetic aspects
Calcium antagonists are given orally and are easily absorbed. Nifedipine has a short half-life (approximately 2 h); amlodipine is much longer acting (half-life of approximately 40 h). Verapamil undergoes fairly extensive first-pass metabolism and has a half-life of approximately 4 h.

Unwanted effects
The unwanted effects are extensions of the pharmacological actions. Nifedipine and amlodipine cause reflex tachycardia, headache and flushing due to the vasodilatation. Verapamil can cause constipation, possibly by inhibition of Ca^{2+} channels in intestinal smooth muscle.

Serious adverse effects do not generally occur.

Clinical use of calcium antagonists

- **In the treatment of angina:** amlodipine is used to prevent angina.
- **In the treatment of dysrhythmias:** verapamil, a class IV antidysrhythmic agent, is used to slow the heart in atrial fibrillation; it is also used to prevent supraventricular tachycardias (see above).
- **In the treatment of hypertension:** amlodipine can be used to lower the blood pressure.

β-Adrenoceptor antagonists

Examples: **atenolol**, metoprolol.

These reduce cardiac work and thus the heart's metabolic demand. Their action in angina is described in Figs 14.4 and 14.5. Other aspects of the pharmacology of β-blockers are covered in Chapter 11.

Cardiac uses of the β-adrenoceptor antagonists

- To prevent angina.
- Other uses are given in Chapter 11.

Nicorandil

Nicorandil, a potassium ion (K$^+$) channel activator with some nitrate-like actions, dilates both arteries and veins. It is given orally and can cause headache, giddiness and flushing.

Lipid-lowering drugs

Several drugs with different mechanisms of action can decrease plasma LDL cholesterol. They are used in conjunction with dietary management and correction of other cardiovascular risk factors.

Statins: HMG-CoA reductase inhibitors

The statins are among the most valuable of the cholesterol-reducing drugs introduced in the past decade and are proving to be very important in the treatment of cardiovascular disease. Examples of such drugs include **simvastatin** and **pravastatin**. Their main overall effect is to reduce plasma LDL cholesterol and total cholesterol. They also decrease plasma triglyceride and increase HDL cholesterol.

Mechanism of action Statins inhibit cholesterol synthesis in the liver by specific, reversible competitive inhibition of HMG-CoA reductase. Falling cholesterol concentrations increase expression of the LDL receptor gene and thus augment synthesis of LDL receptors, leading to increased clearance of LDL.

Pharmacokinetic aspects Statins are given orally and are well absorbed. They are extracted by the liver and undergo first-pass metabolism. Simvastatin is inactive until biotransformed in the liver.

Unwanted effects Unwanted effects of statins are mild and include GI disturbances, increased liver transaminases in the plasma, rash and insomnia. There is a low incidence of a more severe adverse effect – myositis (inflammation of the muscles) – and combining statins with fibrates increases this risk.

Fibrates

Examples of fibrates include **fenofibrate** and **gemfibrozil**. The main overall effect of fibrates is a marked reduction in plasma triglyceride, but the drugs also decrease LDL cholesterol and increase HDL cholesterol.

Mechanism of action Fibrates bind to and activate a nuclear transcription factor termed *peroxisome proliferator-activated receptor alpha (PPARα)*, which results in stimulation of the β-oxidation of fatty acids and an increase in lipoprotein lipase synthesis. This latter action leads to greater plasma clearance of triglycerides.

Pharmacokinetic aspects Fibrates are given orally and are well absorbed if given with food. They are metabolized to glucuronate conjugates, which are excreted by the kidneys.

Unwanted effects Fibrates may cause a myositis-like syndrome, and combining them with statins can potentiate this action. Fibrates can also increase the risk of gallstones.

Drugs that interfere with the absorption of cholesterol

Ezetimibe The drug ezetimibe *specifically* inhibits the transporter pathway by which cholesterol is absorbed from the intestine.

Mechanism of action Ezetimibe blocks a sterol carrier protein (NPC1L1) in the brush border of the intestinal enterocytes and effectively reduces the amount of dietary and biliary cholesterol delivered to the liver via chylomicrons. This reduces the liver's cholesterol store and increases hepatic LDL activity and clearance of LDL cholesterol from the circulation. Ezetimibe has no effect on the absorption of triglycerides, bile acids or the fat-soluble vitamins A, D and E.

Pharmacokinetic aspects Ezetimibe is given orally and is absorbed and metabolized in the liver to give a pharmacologically active metabolite. The parent drug and the metabolite reach maximum concentration within 2 hours, after which they undergo enterohepatic recycling and are gradually eliminated.

Unwanted effects Ezetimibe is well tolerated, though GI tract disturbances, headaches, hypersensitivity reactions (e.g. rashes), fatigue and myalgia may occur.

Bile acid binding resins

Examples of bile acid binding resins include **cholestyramine** and **colestipol**. Their overall effect is to decrease LDL cholesterol.

Mechanism of action Bile acid binding resins are positively charged drugs that bind the negatively charged bile acids in the gut to inhibit their absorption, which diminishes the pool of bile acids in the liver. This stimulates the synthesis of bile acids, thus decreasing the hepatic store of cholesterol, which the resins also lower by reducing its absorption from the gut. This, in turn, stimulates the synthesis of LDL receptors. As with statins, this increases LDL uptake, reducing the plasma concentration of LDL. There can be some temporary increase in plasma triglycerides.

Pharmacokinetic aspects and unwanted effects Bile acid binding resins are given orally and, because they are not absorbed, systemic adverse effects do not occur. Within the bowel, they interfere with the absorption of fat-soluble vitamins and some drugs. They are likely to produce bloating and dyspepsia. Their use has decreased since the introduction of ezetimibe.

MYOCARDIAL INFARCTION

Drugs used to treat myocardial infarction

This is a medical emergency requiring hospitalization. The therapeutic aims are:

- to alleviate the pain: **opioids** (Chapter 13)
- to improve oxygenation of the myocardium: **oxygen**
- to open the blocked artery by reducing thrombus size and limiting its extension:
  - **thrombolytic drugs** (see Chapter 15) are effective if given within 12 h of onset
  - **anticoagulants** (Chapter 15)
  - **antiplatelet drugs** especially aspirin (see Chapter 15)

- to improve survival: **angiotensin-converting enzyme** (ACE) **inhibitors** (see above) have been shown to have this effect if given soon after the infarct occurs
- to reduce the possibility of re-infarction: **aspirin** (Chapter 15) and **β-adrenoceptor antagonists** (see above).

Cardiac output and cardiac failure

One of the main pathophysiological conditions affecting the heart is *heart failure*. To understand the basis of this and how it is treated it is necessary to understand the mechanism of *contraction* of cardiac muscle and the factors that determine *cardiac output*. In heart failure, the cardiac output is inadequate for bodily needs.

Cardiac contraction

Cardiac contraction requires an increase in intracellular Ca^{2+}, which then activates the contractile mechanism. Fig. 14.6 shows the role of Ca^{2+} in contraction, the action of NA and the sites of action of some drugs.

Cardiac output

The main factors that determine cardiac output include plasma volume, venous pressure, SV and the actions of the sympathetic and parasympathetic nervous systems. The interaction of these factors is shown in Fig. 14.7.

The autonomic nervous system in the control of cardiac output

The sympathetic nervous system:
- Increased force of contraction through effect on Ca2+ channels.
- Increased rate.
- Increased oxygen consumption (decreased efficiency).

In cardiac failure, increased sympathetic activity increases the vicious cycle of events in that it increases rate and force

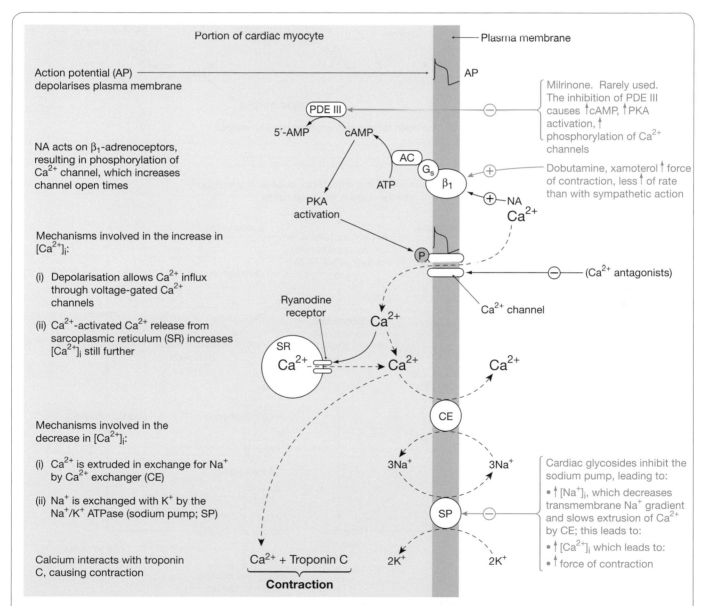

Fig. 14.6   Cardiac contraction, the role of calcium ion (Ca^{2+}) and noradrenaline (NA) and the action of drugs. The site of action of the calcium antagonists is shown, *but these are not used for the treatment of heart failure*. *AC*, Adenylate cyclase; *G*, G-protein; *PDE III*, phosphodiesterase III; *PKA*, protein kinase A; →, acts on; --->, moves to or is converted to.

and increases peripheral resistance, which increases after-load (Fig. 14.8).

The parasympathetic nervous system:

- Decreased rate and automaticity through the action of acetylcholine on M_2 receptors in nodal tissues increasing K^+ permeability.
- Decreased force of contraction mainly in atria through inhibition of adenylate cyclase and, therefore, decreased protein kinase A activation and decreased phosphorylation of Ca^{2+} channels.

Cardiac failure

Cardiac failure is essentially a reduction of cardiac output in spite of adequate venous filling, the reduced output becoming insufficient to perfuse the tissues. Cardiac failure can result

from several factors, such as myocardial disease, hypertension or valvular disease. The interaction of these factors is shown in Fig. 14.8. Note that the factors specified as increasing pre-load (along with increased sympathetic activity) are initially compensatory, maintaining cardiac output. However, eventually they, and the factors increasing after-load, result in exacerbation of the situation, and the clinical signs and symptoms of failure become evident.

Drugs used to treat heart failure
Diuretics

Diuretics are dealt with in Chapter 18; only actions relevant for the treatment of heart failure are given here.

Diuretics are first choice drugs for heart failure; a loop diuretic is usually used (e.g. **furosemide** (frusemide)) though a thiazide

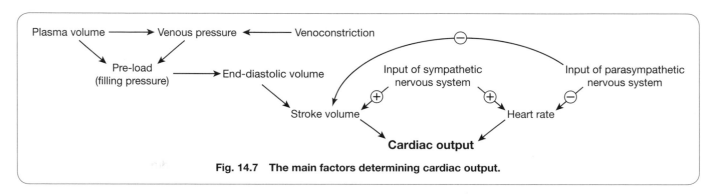

Fig. 14.7 The main factors determining cardiac output.

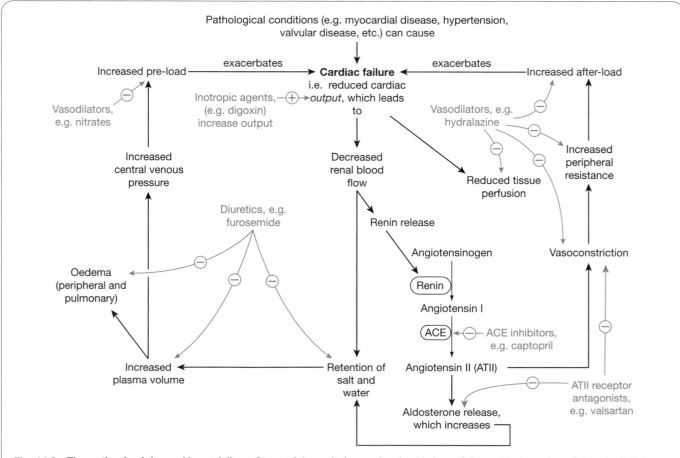

Fig. 14.8 The pathophysiology of heart failure. Some of the main factors involved in heart failure with the action of the principal drugs used in treatment. *ACE*, Angiotensin-converting enzyme; *AT* II, angiotensin II.

(e.g. **bendroflumethiazide** (bendrofluazide)) may be used instead. The action is shown in Fig. 14.8; diuretics decrease pre-load by increasing salt and water excretion.

Angiotensin-converting enzyme (ACE) inhibitors
Examples are **captopril** and **enalapril**. These are dealt with above; only actions relevant to the treatment of heart failure are given here.

ACE inhibitors are used with a diuretic if the diuretic alone is not effective. They inhibit formation of AT II and thus reduce not only peripheral resistance (and, therefore, after-load), but also the release of aldosterone. This results in reduction of salt and water retention and, therefore, decreased plasma volume leading to decreased pre-load.

Angiotensin II receptor antagonists
AT II acts on AT II (subtype AT_1) receptors. Antagonists at this receptor, such as **valsartan**, reduce not only peripheral resistance (and, therefore, after-load) but also the release of aldosterone – with the results described above (see Fig. 14.8).

β-Adrenoceptor antagonists
Sympathetic nervous system action increases cardiac contraction; in the early stages of failure this is compensatory. Accordingly, it has been thought that blocking this would worsen the failure. Paradoxically, however, sympathetic *overactivity* can be an exacerbating factor in established cardiac failure and in this circumstance the use of β-adrenoceptor antagonists would seem to be a logical step. Some light has been shone on this problem because it has been reported recently that β-blockers (e.g. **metoprolol**) used carefully, along with other agents, can prolong survival.

Digitalis glycosides
The digitalis glycosides are third-line drugs; the main example is **digoxin**.

Pharmacological actions and mechanisms of action
- An increase in the force of contraction without increasing oxygen consumption; this is their main action in heart failure.
- A decrease in rate mainly by an action on the vagus, which reduces AV conduction; there is an increase in the refractory period in the AV node and the bundle of His (the rate decrease allows for better filling and this, with the increased force of contraction, increases cardiac output).

- An increased possibility of disturbances of rhythm:
  - Digoxin inhibits the sodium pump (which normally tends to cause hyperpolarization by the $3Na^+/2K^+$ exchange mechanism), causing depolarization.
  - Digoxin increases $[Ca^{2+}]i$, thus increasing after-depolarization; if this reaches threshold, an action potential is generated leading to ectopic beats.

Pharmacokinetic aspects
Digoxin is given orally, usually with a loading dose (except in mild failure) and is excreted largely unchanged by the kidney. It has a half-life of 36 h.

Unwanted effects
- Dysrhythmias; ventricular fibrillation with high doses.
- Nausea and vomiting.
- Confusion.
- Disturbances in colour vision.

Vasodilators
Vasodilators also have a role in the treatment of heart failure:
- **Nitrates** (see above for details): actions relevant to the treatment of heart failure are shown in Fig. 14.8.
- **Hydralazine**: only used if it is not possible to use ACE inhibitors (see Fig. 14.8 for site of action; mechanism of action unknown).

Drugs used in acute severe cardiac failure
The term cardiac failure is usually used to refer to chronic congestive cardiac failure. This develops slowly, fluid retention occurring first as indicated by an increase in weight, before actual oedema, breathlessness and decreased exercise tolerance are evident. The cardiac output is, however, sufficient for the patient to pursue most daily activities for several years.

However, the heart can fail more suddenly (e.g. with myocardial infarction), producing all the features of heart failure while the patient is at rest. This is acute severe cardiac failure. **Dobutamine**, a β$_1$-agonist (see Fig. 11. 14), can be effective in this clinical setting because its effect on cardiac contractility is believed to be greater than its effect on cardiac rate. Dobutamine's effect on the heart also has a place in the treatment of hypovolaemic shock.

Acute severe heart failure is also treated by intravenous infusion with dobutamine; the drug is a β$_1$-adrenoceptor agonist and increases sympathetic input (Fig. 14.8).

Due to the fact that blood is a liquid, it can sometimes be overlooked as an organ. Blood has multiple tasks: delivering oxygen and nutrients to tissue, taking waste products for disposal, embodying the immune response to pathogens and preventing haemorrhage after injury (which has the added benefit of creating a rapid barrier to the external environment when trauma has occurred). Blood accomplishes these tasks through the physiological processes of haematopoiesis (the production of blood cells) and haemostasis (the maintenance of vascular integrity). The first part of this chapter will discuss how blood cell production occurs and how this can be modified pharmacologically, whilst the second part of the chapter will discuss haemostasis, and the importance of pharmacology to prevent thrombosis or to modulate bleeding disorders.

THE HAEMATOPOIETIC SYSTEM

The term *haematopoiesis* covers red blood cell generation (erythropoiesis), platelet production (thrombopoiesis) and white blood cell generation (leukopoiesis). Normal haematopoiesis requires certain exogenous substances (haematinic agents e.g. iron, folic acid, vitamin B_{12}) and various endogenous haematopoietic growth substances (e.g. colony-stimulating factors, erythropoietin, thrombopoietin). Thus dependent on these signals and other environmental cues, pluripotent stem cells residing in the bone marrow continually generate progeny that give rise to mature red blood cells, leukocytes and platelets (although recent data suggests that platelet production may also occur from megakaryocytes that have travelled to the pulmonary vascular bed) that egress from the bone marrow and circulate.

Erythropoiesis
The main function of the red blood cells (erythrocytes) is to carry oxygen.

Pathophysiology
The main disorders of erythropoiesis are the *anaemias*, which are classified according to the changes in the erythrocytes:
- Hypochromic, microcytic anaemia (small red cells with low haemoglobin) due to deficiency of iron, the main cause being chronic blood loss.
- Macrocytic anaemia (large red cells, few in number) due to deficiency of folic acid and/or vitamin B_{12}.
- Normochromic normocytic anaemia (fewer normal-sized red cells with normal haemoglobin) usually due to acute excessive destruction of red blood cells – haemolytic anaemia.

Haematinic agents
Iron
Iron is essential for haemoglobin production. A summary of its distribution in the body, transfer in the plasma, storage, movement between compartments and removal from the body is shown in Fig. 15.1. Iron is readily available for transfer to the plasma from ferritin stores in the liver.

The main preparation of iron is **ferrous sulphate**, given orally. A preparation for deep intramuscular use is **iron sorbitol**.

Unwanted effects
The main unwanted effect of iron salts is dose-related gastrointestinal (GI) tract disturbance: nausea, epigastric pain, abdominal cramps, diarrhoea. Acute iron toxicity with necrotizing gastritis and cardiovascular collapse can occur if large amounts of iron salts are ingested; chronic iron toxicity can follow repeated blood transfusions. Both are treated with an iron chelator: **desferrioxamine**.

Clinical uses of iron salts

- For iron-deficiency anaemia caused by:
  - chronic blood loss, e.g. from excessive menstrual loss, haemorrhoids, etc.;
  - increased need for iron during pregnancy; or
  - reduced iron intake or absorption.

Folic acid and vitamin B_{12}
Both folic acid and vitamin B_{12} are essential for DNA synthesis and cell proliferation.

Pathophysiology
Deficiencies of folic acid and/or vitamin B_{12} lead to megaloblastic anaemia in which there are large, fragile, distorted red cells and abnormal precursors in the blood. Vitamin B_{12} deficiency also causes neurological disease.

The principal cause of vitamin B_{12} deficiency is decreased absorption of the vitamin either because of a lack of intrinsic factor (normally secreted by the stomach but missing in pernicious anaemia) or because of conditions that interfere with its absorption in the ileum. As there are large stores in the liver, the results of the deficiency can take a long time to manifest.

Folic acid deficiency results from dietary insufficiency, often associated with increased demand.

Folic acid
Folic acid (pteridine + *para*-aminobenzoic acid + glutamic acid) is essential for DNA synthesis and cell proliferation.

Actions
Folates, in the tetrahydrofolate (FH_4) polyglutamate form, are cofactors in the synthesis of purines and pyrimidines, being particularly important in thymidylate synthesis (Fig. 15.2).

Pharmacokinetic aspects
Folic acid is absorbed by active transport into intestinal cells where it is reduced by dihydrofolate reductase to FH_4 and then methylated to methyl-FH_4 which passes into the plasma. Eventually extra glutamates are added to give the active polyglutamate form.

Unwanted effects
These do not occur. However if folic acid alone is given in vitamin B_{12} deficiency, the blood picture may improve, but other lesions (e.g. neurological) will not improve.

Vitamin B_{12}
Actions
Vitamin B_{12} is important in reactions that enable folate to function in thymidylate synthesis (Fig. 15.2). The reactions convert

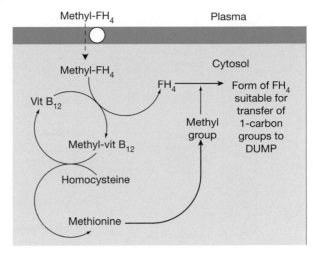

Fig. 15.3 The role of vitamin B$_{12}$ in reactions necessary for the eventual synthesis of thymidylate. Methyl-FH$_4$ enters cells from the plasma by carrier. The methyl group is transferred to homocysteine to form methionine via vitamin B$_{12}$, which is bound to a methyltransferase (not shown). Methionine donates the methyl group to FH$_4$. *DUMP,* 2'Deoxyuridylate.

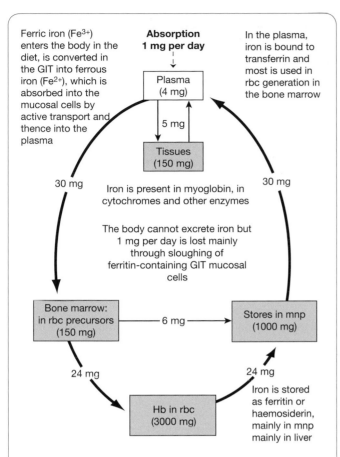

Fig. 15.1 The homeostasis of body iron. The distribution and daily movement between tissues is shown; the darker the colour, the higher the concentration of iron. *GIT,* gastrointestinal tract; *Hb,* haemoglobin; *MNP,* mononuclear phagocytes; *RBC,* red blood cells.

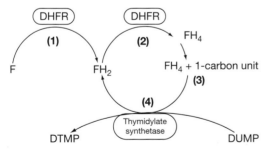

Fig. 15.2 Simplified diagram of the role of a folate in thymidylate synthesis. (1) Folate is reduced to dihydrofolate (FH$_2$) by dihydrofolate reductase (DHFR). (2) Dihydrofolate (FH$_2$) is reduced to tetrahydrofolate (FH$_4$) by DHFR. (3) The FH$_4$ functions as a carrier of a one-carbon unit, providing the methyl group necessary for (4) the conversion of 2'deoxyuridylate (DUMP) to 2'deoxythymidylate (DTMP) by thymidylate synthetase. During the transfer of the one-carbon unit, FH$_4$ is oxidized to FH$_2$, which must be reduced by DHFR to FH$_4$ (step 2) before it can act again. The thymidylate synthetase action is rate limiting in DNA synthesis. Note that in all the actions of folates it is the polyglutamate form that is most active.

5-methyl-FH$_4$ (a functionally inactive form of folate carried in the plasma) to the form of folate (FH$_4$) that can carry the one-carbon unit necessary for the formation of 2'deoxythymidylate (DTMP) from 2'deoxyuridylate (DUMP) (Fig. 15.2). The mechanism of action is shown in Fig. 15.3.

Administration
Vitamin B$_{12}$ is given intramuscularly and is stored in the liver.

Unwanted effects
There are none.

Clinical uses of folic acid and vitamin B$_{12}$

- Folic acid is used mainly:
  - to treat anaemias caused by folic-acid deficiency, or
  - in prophylaxis if there is potential for developing deficiency, as in pregnancy.
- Vitamin B$_{12}$ is used for pernicious anaemia.

Haematopoietic growth factors
Various haematopoietic growth factors are responsible for the division of pluripotent stem cells in the bone marrow and the multiplication and maturation of their progeny. Erythropoietin, produced in the kidney, controls red cell production; myeloid growth factors, produced by many cell types, control the production of monocytes and polymorphonuclear leukocytes; interleukins control lymphocyte production and thrombopoietin controls platelet production (Fig. 15.4).

Erythropoietin
Recombinant erythropoietin (**epoetin**) is available for therapeutic use. It can be given intravenously, subcutaneously or intraperitoneally.

Unwanted effects
Include flu-like symptoms, a dose-related increase in blood pressure and encephalopathy.

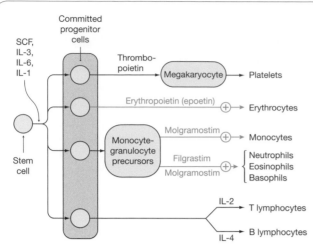

Fig. 15.4 Growth factors controlling haemopoiesis. *IL*, Interleukin; *SCF*, stem cell factor.

Clinical use of haematopoietic growth factors

- Epoetin is used mainly for the treatment of anaemia associated with chronic renal failure.
- Filgrastim is used in some cases of neutropenia.
- Molgramostim is used to shorten neutropenia after procedures such as cancer chemotherapy or autologous bone marrow transplantation.
- Filgrastim can be used to mobilize haematopoietic stem cells in the circulation that are then harvested via leukapheresis for stem cell transplantation of leukaemia patients.

Myeloid growth factors

Recombinant forms of the two main myeloid growth factors are available for therapeutic use. Granulocyte colony-stimulating factor (G-CSF) is available as **filgrastim** and granulocyte-macrophage colony-stimulating factor (GM-CSF) is available as **molgramostim**.

Filgrastim stimulates only polymorphonuclear development; molgramostim stimulates the development of all myeloid cells. Both can be given either intravenous (IV) or subcutaneous (SC). Both require specialist administration.

CXCR4 antagonism

Stem cells and leukocytes are retained in the bone marrow via a chemokine-chemokine receptor axis (SDF-1α – CXCR4 retention mechanism). Disruption of this axis with a CXCR4 antagonist (**plerixafor**) can be used in patients with leukaemia to boost the mobilization of stem cells required for harvesting. In particular, plerixafor can be used in combination with G-CSF to act in synergy and greatly mobilize the number of stem cells required for successful bone marrow transplantation procedures where donors or patients may be refractory to G-CSF therapy.

HAEMOSTASIS AND THROMBOSIS

Haemostasis is the arrest of blood loss from damaged blood vessels and is essential to life. During haemostasis a haemostatic plug is formed, the main processes being:

- adhesion and activation of platelets, and
- activation of clotting factors leading to blood coagulation (fibrin formation) (Figs. 15.5 and 15.7).

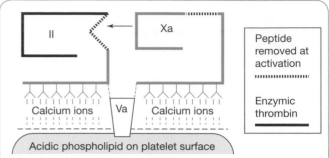

Fig. 15.5 The activation of prothrombin (factor II) by factor Xa. Factor Va complexed with a negatively charged phospholipid surface (both partly supplied by aggregated platelets) forms a binding site for factor Xa and prothrombin. Platelets thus serve as a localizing focus. Calcium ions form a bridge between the γ-carboxylated glutamate residues and the phospholipid surface. When factor X is activated it activates prothrombin, liberating enzymic thrombin.

Thrombosis is a pathological condition – the formation of a haemostatic plug associated with arterial disease or with stasis of blood in the veins or the atria of the heart. A **thrombus** in the coronary arterial circulation may lead to a myocardial infarction. An **embolus** is a portion of a thrombus that breaks away into the circulation. If it derives from a venous thrombus, it may lodge in the lungs to form a pulmonary embolism; if it comes from a thrombus in the left heart, it may lodge in the brain (stroke) or other organs.

Therapy to promote haemostasis with procoagulant drugs is rarely employed but might be necessary in patients with rare clotting factor disorders or deficiencies. However, drug therapy of thromboembolic disease (with anticoagulant drugs, antiplatelet agents, fibrinolytic drugs) is extensively used because these diseases are the major cause of death in developed countries.

Procoagulant drugs
Vitamin K

Examples: natural fat-soluble **vitamin K** (phytomenadione), synthetic water-soluble **menadiol**.

Mechanism of action

Vitamin K, when reduced, acts as a cofactor in the post-translational γ-carboxylation of a cluster of glutamic acid (Glu) residues in factors II, VII, IX and X (Fig. 15.6).

Administration and pharmacokinetic aspects

Vitamin K preparations can be given orally, intramuscularly (IM) or IV. Phytomenadione requires bile salts for oral absorption; menadiol does not. Vitamin K is metabolized in the liver and excreted in bile and urine.

Drugs decreasing thrombosis

The selection of antiplatelet and anticoagulant drugs to be used is determined by the type of thrombus (arterial versus venous) the patient is at risk from. Arterial thrombi are induced by plaque rupture around sites of atherosclerosis and these have a large platelet component (a so-called white thrombus). Patients prone to venous thrombosis (induced by Virchow's Triad: blood stasis, hypercoagulability or endothelial disturbance) have a red thrombus. The decision to use antiplatelet and/or anticoagulant therapies is taken with caution and there is a need to determine the probability of an adverse or life threatening cardiovascular event occurring versus bleeding risk (which can also lead to death).

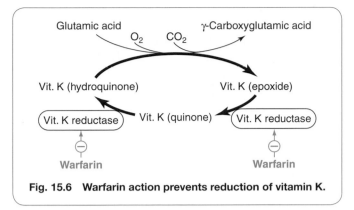

Fig. 15.6 Warfarin action prevents reduction of vitamin K.

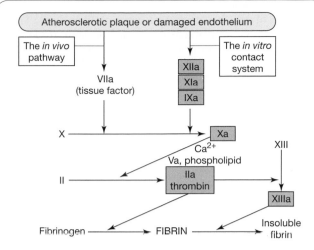

Fig. 15.7 Sites of action of heparin and low-molecular-weight heparins (LMWHs). Heparin (plus antithrombin III) acts on the enzymic forms of the factors (blue boxes). LMWHs act only on Xa.

Therefore these drugs tend to be given in patients for secondary prevention and prescribed only to individuals with a very high risk of a primary cardiovascular event.

Clinical uses of anticoagulants, antiplatelet agents and fibrinolytic drugs

- Anticoagulants (warfarin, direct acting oral anticoagulants (DOACs)) are primarily used in the prevention of stroke and systemic embolism, as options for the treatment of pulmonary embolism (PE) and deep vein thrombosis (DVT) and as prophylaxis of venous thromboembolism after surgery. Sometimes anticoagulants are administered with Rivaroxaban as an option for prophylaxis of atherothrombotic events (with aspirin alone or with aspirin and clopidogrel).
- Heparin and low-molecular-weight heparin (LMWH) are for short-term use.
- Oral antiplatelet drugs are used in secondary prevention of atherothrombotic events in people after myocardial infarction (MI), acute coronary syndrome (ACS), angina, peripheral arterial disease (PAD), stent implantation or transient ischaemic attack (TIA). Intravenous antiplatelet drugs are used in the prevention of atherothrombotic events in people undergoing percutaneous coronary intervention (PCI).

Injectable anticoagulants
Examples: heparin, low-molecular-weight heparins (LMWHs).

Mechanism of action
Heparin accelerates the action of antithrombin III, which inactivates factors XIIa, IXa, Xa and IIa (Fig. 15.7).

Administration and pharmacokinetic aspects
Heparin is a sulphated mucopolysaccharide. It is given IV (where it acts immediately) or SC (where it acts after 1 h). It has a two-phase elimination: first rapid then slow. The effect of heparins is monitored by the activated partial thromboplastin time (APTT). Examples of LMWHs are **dalteparin** (a heparin fragment) and **fondaparinux** (a synthetic pentasaccharide). LMWHs tend to be used more frequently than heparin; they can be given SC and have a longer half-life. Furthermore, blood monitoring is not routinely required. They are eliminated by the kidney.

Unwanted effects
The main hazard with the use of anticoagulants is bleeding; the effects of heparins can be treated with IV **protamine sulphate**, a strongly basic protein that neutralizes heparin. Osteoporosis may occur with long-term heparin therapy and hypo-aldosteronism has also been reported. Paradoxically, thrombosis associated

with heparin-induced thrombocytopenia (an immune response in certain individuals) can occur; this is rare and can be treated with an antithrombotic drug, danaparoid, which is also used to prevent postsurgical deep vein thrombosis.

Oral anticoagulants: warfarin
Mechanism of action
Warfarin inhibits the reduction of vitamin K and thus inhibits the necessary γ-carboxylation of the Glu residues in factors II, VII, IX and X (Fig. 15.6).

Administration and pharmacokinetic aspects
Warfarin is given orally and has a small distribution volume. Onset of effect takes several days because the circulating γ-carboxylated factors have first to be degraded. The effects of warfarin must be carefully monitored by the prothrombin time. Warfarin is metabolized in the liver.

Unwanted effects
Bleeding (into bowel or brain) is the main problem. It is treated by giving natural vitamin K (orally, IV or IM), fresh plasma or coagulation factor concentrates.

Drug interactions
These are important as some drugs potentiate the effects of warfarin, increasing the risk of bleeding (e.g. cimetidine, imipramine, ciprofloxacin, carbenicillin, aspirin, cephalosporins, etc.). In contrast some drugs lessen the anticoagulant action, increasing the risk of clotting (e.g. rifampicin, carbamazepine, etc.).

Oral anticoagulants: direct acting oral anticoagulants (DOACs)
Rivaroxaban, **apixaban** and **edoxaban** are examples of directly acting factor X inhibitors. In contrast to heparin, these drugs act directly on factor X, rather than the activation of antithrombin III. **Dabigatran** is a direct thrombin inhibitor (DTI). DTIs act by inhibiting the active site of thrombin (that is, the site that binds to factors V and X), rather than the fibrin binding site (exosite 1) or the exosite 2 that recognizes platelet protease activated receptor (PAR). DTIs inhibit both clot-bound and free thrombin. Of the DOACs, only dabigatran has an antidote (idarucizumab), although this drug class has favourable safety profiles compared to warfarin and heparin and do not require frequent blood monitoring.

Antiplatelet agents

The action of antiplatelet agents is summarized in Fig. 15.8.

Aspirin irreversibly inactivates cyclooxygenase (COX) and alters the balance between thromboxane A_2 (TXA_2), which promotes platelet adhesion and aggregation, and prostaglandin I_2 (PGI_2) (prostacyclin), which inhibits it. Vascular endothelium can synthesize more COX enzyme so that in time the effects of aspirin can be overcome by allowing new PGI_2 to be synthesized. Platelets, however, have no nucleus and thus cannot synthesize new COX, meaning that the pro-aggregatory TXA_2 is inhibited for the lifespan of the platelet. Thus platelet TXA_2 is restored only when existing platelets are replaced. Intermittent small doses given orally decrease platelet TXA_2 without significantly reducing endothelial PGI_2.

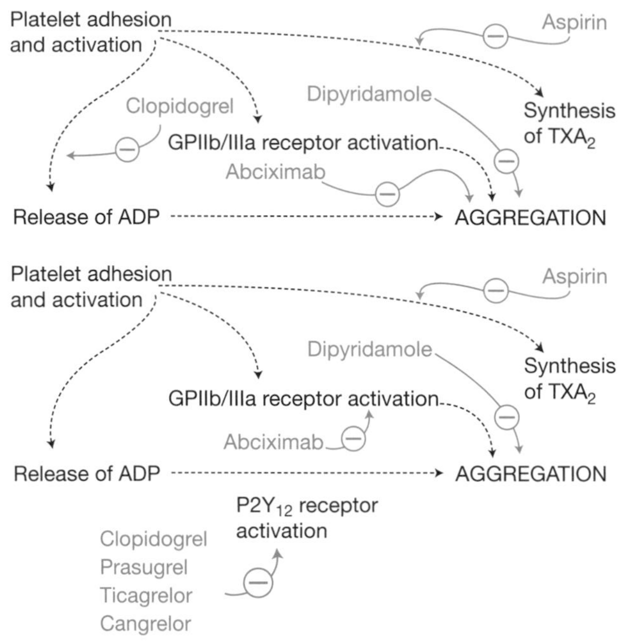

Platelet aggregation inhibitors

Clopidogrel, **prasugrel** and **ticagrelor** are platelet $P2Y_{12}$ receptor antagonists and inhibit aggregation to most platelet agonists (adenosine diphosphate (ADP) activation of $P2Y_{12}$ is required as a final common pathway towards platelet aggregation). Ticagrelor has a favourable safety and pharmacokinetic profile compared to clopidogrel and prasugrel. **Dipyridamole** is another antiplatelet drug that inhibits platelet phosphodiesterases non-selectively and **cilostazol** is a selective phosphodiesterase $(PDE)_3$ inhibitor. $P2Y_{12}$ antagonists and PDE inhibitors are given orally, long term and often in combination with aspirin to provide a greater inhibition of platelet activation (so-called dual antiplatelet therapy).

GPIIb/IIIa receptor antagonists include **abciximab** (antibody Fab fragment against the receptor) and **tirofiban** (a cyclic peptide fragment of a ligand for the receptor) block the linking of platelets by fibrinogen. These are given by IV infusion and are for specialist use only because the risk of bleeding is high.

Fibrinolytic drugs

Examples and antidotes are given in Fig. 15.9. Most have a short half-life (**reteplase** is long-acting) and are given IV, mainly by infusion. Their effectiveness is very time-dependent after myocardial infarction (MI) (up to 12 h) and stroke (up to 3 h). The main unwanted effect is bleeding. Surgery is often now used as a more effective measure to removing blood clots.

Fig. 15.8 Antiplatelet agents. *ADP*, Adenosine diphosphate; *TXA₂*, thromboxane A₂.

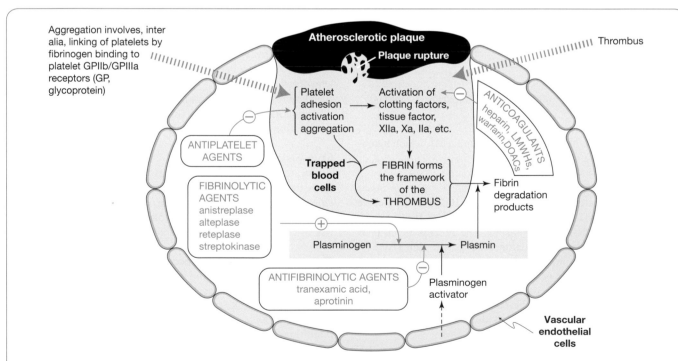

Fig. 15.9   Diagram of a thrombus showing the interaction of the platelet activation system, the coagulation cascade and the fibrinolytic (thrombolytic) system along with the action of drugs on these systems. *DOACs,* Direct acting oral anticoagulants; *GP,* glycoprotein; *LMWHs,* low-molecular-weight heparins.

Clinical uses of anticoagulants, antiplatelet agents and fibrinolytic drugs

- Anticoagulants are used in the prevention of stroke and systemic embolism, as options for the treatment of pulmonary embolism (PE) and deep vein thrombosis (DVT) and as prophylaxis of venous thromboembolism after surgery. Sometimes anticoagulants are Rivaroxaban, an option for prophylaxis of atherothrombotic events (with aspirin alone or with aspirin and clopidogrel).
- Heparin and low-molecular-weight heparins (LMWH) are for short-term use.
- Oral antiplatelet drugs are used in secondary prevention of atherothrombotic events in people with after myocardial infarction (MI), acute coronary syndrome (ACS), angina, peripheral arterial disease (PAD), stent implantation or transient ischaemic attack (TIA).
- Intravenous antiplatelet drugs are used in the prevention of atherothrombotic events in people undergoing percutaneous coronary intervention (PCI).
- Fibrinolytic agents are used in acute myocardial infarction (AMI) and stroke as an option to dissolve blood clots.

The term *acute inflammatory reaction* refers to the local events which occur in response to a disease-causing organism (pathogen). It consists of the *innate* immune response (non-memory) and may have an immunologically specific reaction superimposed on top (adaptive immune responses, where the host has memory of the pathogen through previous exposure and accelerates the acute inflammatory reaction, see below). These reactions are critical for host defence. However, if they are inappropriately deployed, as occurs in many diseases, they are deleterious. It is, therefore, important to understand the mediators which control these responses since many drugs currently used or in development are directed at influencing the generation and/or action of these mediators.

The *innate acute inflammatory reaction* involves both vascular events (vasodilatation, increased permeability of the postcapillary venules, exudation of fluid) and cellular events. The *cells* involved are (1) white blood cells (neutrophils, monocytes, lymphocytes, natural killer lymphocytes), which accumulate in the area of inflammation and are activated, some to ingest microorganisms or kill infected cells and some to release mediators, and (2) tissue cells (vascular endothelial cells, mast cells, macrophages). The mediators derived from cells include eicosanoids, cytokines, histamine, neuropeptides and many others; those derived from plasma include complement components and components of the kinin cascade such as bradykinin.

The *adaptive immune response* consists of two phases: an **induction phase** and an **effector phase**, the latter consisting of an *antibody-mediated* component and a *cell-mediated* component. Various cytokines control these phases. The key cells are the *lymphocytes* of which there are two main types, B cells and T cells.

(A third type, natural killer lymphocytes, participates in innate immune responses.) There are several subtypes of T cells (Fig. 16.1). Precursor T cells (ThP) give rise to Th0 cells (not shown in figure), which can be stimulated to develop into helper T cells (Th). The cytokine interleukin-2 (IL-2) drives the differentiation of ThP and Th1 cells (Fig. 16.1). On first exposure to antigen, memory B cells and T cells are produced; these speed up the response when that antigen is encountered again:

- **Th1** cells activate and participate in the pathway to **cell-mediated immunity.**
- **Th2** cells activate the pathway to **humoral (antibody-mediated) immunity** by stimulating the proliferation of B cells that mature to plasma cells (P) which generate antibodies. (But note that not all B cell responses are dependent on interaction with Th2 cells.)

Immune responses, meant for defence, can themselves cause damage if inappropriately triggered. Many diseases are caused by, or have a component of, inappropriately induced immune/inflammatory reactions. Some are associated with Th1 responses (e.g. rheumatoid arthritis, multiple sclerosis, aplastic anaemia, insulin-dependent diabetes), and the Th1 pathway is also involved in allograft rejection. Inappropriate Th2 responses are implicated in various allergic (hypersensitivity) conditions. The term *autoimmune disease* is applied to conditions in which the immune response is directed against the body's own tissues. Conversely, some cancers are now being treated with drugs (**immunostimulants**) that boost the adaptive immune response to lead to better cancer cell killing.

The eventual outcome of inflammation can be resolution and healing (possibly with scarring) or – if the pathogen or eliciting agent persists – the development of a *chronic inflammatory reaction*.

MEDIATORS OF INFLAMMATION AND THE DRUGS AFFECTING THEM

Eicosanoids and platelet-activating factor
Eicosanoids (prostanoids, leukotrienes) and platelet-activating factor are generated from phospholipids and are implicated in many physiological and pathological processes. Many drugs target steps in their production (Fig. 16.2). An important enzyme is cyclooxygenase (COX), which occurs in two main forms: COX-1 (a constitutive enzyme expressed in most cells and involved in tissue homeostasis) and COX-2 (which is induced in activated inflammatory cells). A COX-3 enzyme has also been described.

Bradykinin
Bradykinin is a nonapeptide clipped out of a plasma α-globulin. Its actions in inflammation are:
- vasodilatation (mediated by released nitric oxide (NO) and prostaglandin I_2 (PGI_2),
- increased vascular permeability, and
- stimulation of pain nerve endings (this is potentiated by prostaglandin (PGs)).

Histamine
Histamine is released from mast cells by a complement component C3a or, in type I hypersensitivity, by an antigen–antibody reaction on the cell surface.

Nitric oxide
Most inflammatory cells express the inducible form of NO synthase when activated by cytokines. NO dilates blood vessels, increases vascular permeability and stimulates PG release.

Cytokines
Cytokines are a large family of peptide mediators that are released or generated in inflammatory and immune reactions and which control the actions of inflammatory and immune cells by autocrine or paracrine mechanisms. They include interleukins (IL) (some of relevance to drugs include IL-2, tumour necrosis factor α (TNF-α) and IL-5), chemokines (mediators that attract and activate motile inflammatory cells such as polymorphs and macrophages), colony-stimulating factors (e.g. G-CSF), growth factors (VEGF, TGFβ) and many others.

ANTI-INFLAMMATORY DRUGS

The principal anti-inflammatory agents are:
- the glucocorticoids, and
- the nonsteroidal anti-inflammatory drugs (NSAIDs).
Others that are disease specific are:
- antirheumatoid drugs, and
- drugs used in the treatment of gout.

NONSTEROIDAL ANTI-INFLAMMATORY DRUGS

The degree to which NSAIDs inhibit the two COX enzymes varies as follows:

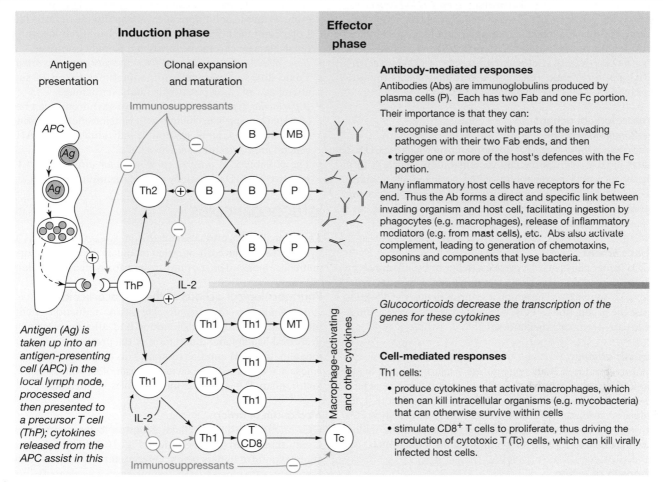

Fig. 16.1 Simplified outline of the immune response and the sites of action of immunosuppressant drugs. The antibody and cell-mediated responses shown above are protective in nature. When these are inappropriately deployed, they lead to disease; see Pathophysiology section. CD8 is a protein marker (defined by monoclonal antibody) of the precursor of cytotoxic T cells. *IL-2*, Interleukin-2; *MB*, memory B cells; *MT*, memory T cells.

Induction phase

Effector phase

Antigen presentation

Clonal expansion and maturation

Immunosuppressants

Antigen (Ag) is taken up into an antigen-presenting cell (APC) in the local lymph node, processed and then presented to a precursor T cell (ThP); cytokines released from the APC assist in this

IL-2

Immunosuppressants

Antibody-mediated responses

Antibodies (Abs) are immunoglobulins produced by plasma cells (P). Each has two Fab and one Fc portion.

Their importance is that they can:

- recognise and interact with parts of the invading pathogen with their two Fab ends, and then
- trigger one or more of the host's defences with the Fc portion.

Many inflammatory host cells have receptors for the Fc end. Thus the Ab forms a direct and specific link between invading organism and host cell, facilitating ingestion by phagocytes (e.g. macrophages), release of inflammatory mediators (e.g. from mast cells), etc. Abs also activate complement, leading to generation of chemotaxins, opsonins and components that lyse bacteria.

Glucocorticoids decrease the transcription of the genes for these cytokines

Cell-mediated responses

Th1 cells:

- produce cytokines that activate macrophages, which then can kill intracellular organisms (e.g. mycobacteria) that can otherwise survive within cells
- stimulate CD8⁺ T cells to proliferate, thus driving the production of cytotoxic T (Tc) cells, which can kill virally infected host cells.

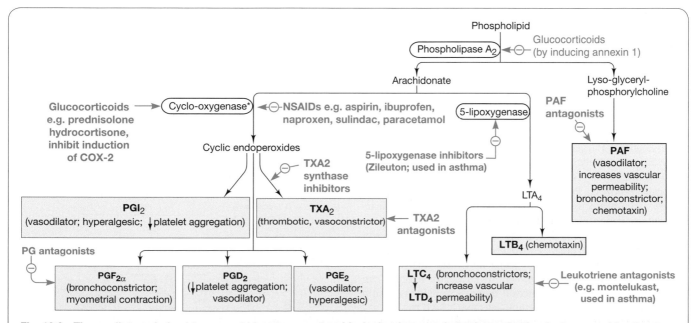

Fig. 16.2 The mediators derived from arachidonate – prostanoids, leukotrienes and platelet-activating factor – provide sites for anti-inflammatory drugs to act. *There are two forms of cyclooxygenase: COX-1, a constitutive enzyme expressed in most cells and involved in tissue homeostasis, and COX-2, which is induced in activated inflammatory cells. *LT*, Leukotriene; *PAF*, platelet-activating factor; *PG*, prostaglandin; *TX*, thromboxane; →, gives rise to. Important anti-inflammatory drugs are in larger type.

- *Highly COX-1-selective*: ketorolac; *very COX-1-selective*: flurbiprofen; *weakly COX-1-selective*: indometacin, ibuprofen, aspirin, naproxen, paracetamol. Paracetamol may also inhibit COX-3 in the central nervous system (CNS).
- *Very COX-2-selective*: etoricoxib; *weakly COX-2-selective*: piroxicam, diclofenac, celecoxib. (Note that agents that are weakly COX-2 selective also inhibit COX-1.)

Pharmacological actions

Anti-inflammatory actions

NSAIDs reduce those aspects of inflammation in which the COX-2 products have a role, specifically vasodilatation, which in turn facilitates increased permeability of the postcapillary venules. Some are strongly anti-inflammatory (e.g. naproxen, piroxicam, celecoxib), and some moderately so (e.g. ibuprofen). Some have little anti-inflammatory effect (e.g. paracetamol).

Analgesic actions

NSAIDs reduce pain caused by tissue damage or by inflammatory mediators that act on nerve endings (bradykinin, 5-hydroxytryptamine; see Chapter 13). The action is indirect in that the NSAIDs decrease the production of PGs, which sensitize the nerve endings to these pain-producing mediators.

Antipyretic actions

NSAIDs reduce fever. Body temperature is controlled by a hypothalamic 'thermostat' which ensures that heat production and heat loss are in balance around a set-point. Fever occurs when IL-1, an inflammatory mediator, generates, in the hypothalamus, E-type PGs that disturb the hypothalamic thermostat, elevating the set-point. NSAIDs act by interrupting the synthesis of the relevant PGs.

Mechanism of action

All NSAIDs act mainly by inhibiting COX enzymes (see above). With most agents, the effect is reversible; the exception is aspirin which causes irreversible inactivation of the enzymes.

Pharmacokinetic aspects

NSAIDs are usually given orally. Naproxen and indometacin can be given by rectal suppository, piroxicam by intramuscular (IM) injection or suppository, diclofenac by IM, intravenously or rectal suppository. Some have a short half-life of 1–4 h (aspirin, paracetamol ibuprofen); some have a rather longer half-life (e.g. naproxen 14 h, celecoxib 11 h); some have a very long half-life (piroxicam 45 h). Note that aspirin's action lasts longer because it acetylates the COX enzymes.

Unwanted effects

Adverse effects (largely due to COX-1 actions) are frequently reported, particularly if large doses are taken over a long period.

- *Gastrointestinal (GI) disturbances* are the most common. Locally produced PGs inhibit acid secretion in the stomach, have a cytoprotective effect by stimulating mucus and bicarbonate secretion and cause vasodilatation. NSAIDs decrease the synthesis of PGs and thus can cause mucosal damage and bleeding. The risk is greatest with piroxicam, less with naproxen and diclofenac, less still with ibuprofen and least with the COX-2 inhibitors. **Misoprostol**, a synthetic PG receptor agonist, can prevent NSAID-induced mucosal damage in patients with a peptic ulcer who need to take non-selective NSAIDs.
- *Skin reactions* are fairly common, particularly with sulindac.
- *Adverse renal effects* occur because NSAIDs decrease local renal PG levels. These PGs increase blood flow and promote natriuresis. NSAIDs can produce reversible renal insufficiency by

decreasing PG-induced compensatory vasodilatation, an effect more serious in conditions such as liver disease or heart failure. Long-continued NSAID consumption can result in significant renal damage: chronic nephritis and papillary necrosis.

- *Bone marrow depression and liver disorders* are less frequent. Toxic doses of paracetamol, sometimes taken in suicide attempts, can cause potentially fatal liver damage.
- *A particular type of encephalitis* (Reye's syndrome) can be precipitated by aspirin in children with viral infections. Aspirin may cause *bronchospasm* in susceptible individuals and NSAIDs in general are contraindicated in asthma.
- The possibility of *adverse cardiovascular effects* with COX-2 selective NSAIDs especially requires caution.

GLUCOCORTICOIDS

The adrenal cortex produces endogenous *glucocorticoids* (GC) (e.g. hydrocortisone and cortisone) that modulate the inflammatory and immune response. The starting substrate for synthesis is cholesterol.

Pharmacological actions of the glucocorticoids

Anti-inflammatory and immunosuppressive: reduction in chronic inflammation and in autoimmune and allergic reactions but decreased healing and diminution of the protective effects of the inflammatory and immune responses (as in infection). Mediators whose activity is reduced include eicosanoids, platelet-activating factor, many ILs, cell adhesion molecules, nitric oxide.

Mechanism of action

GCs interact with intracellular receptors belonging to a superfamily that control transcription (Fig. 16.3). The GC–receptor complexes form dimers before entering the nucleus (not shown). Some genes are repressed (i.e. transcription is prevented) some are induced (i.e. transcription is initiated).

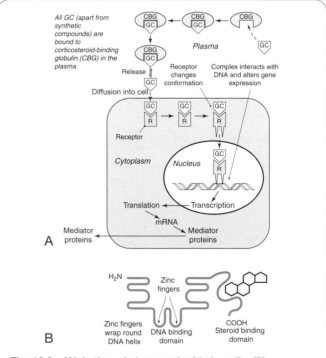

Fig. 16.3 (A) Action of glucocorticoids in cells. (B) The main domains of the glucocorticoid receptor. *GC*, glucocorticoids; *R*, receptors.

For anti-inflammatory and immunosuppressive actions:
- Inhibition of transcription of the genes for cyclooxygenase 2, cytokines (e.g. the ILs), the inducible form of nitric oxide synthase, etc.
- Block of vitamin D_3-mediated induction of the osteocalcin gene in osteoblasts and modification of transcription of the collagenase genes.
- Increased synthesis of lipocortin 1, which has a role in the negative feedback effects and may have anti-inflammatory actions.

Repression of genes involves inhibition of various transduction factors (AP-1, NF-κB).

Main glucocorticoid drugs

Prednisolone, hydrocortisone and **dexamethasone** can be given orally, parenterally or topically. **Beclometasone** and **Fluticasone** are given by inhalation for the treatment of asthma (see Chapter 19).

Unwanted effects

Unwanted effects of GCs are seen mainly with prolonged systemic use as anti-inflammatory or immunosuppressive agents (in which case all the metabolic actions are unwanted) but not usually with replacement therapy. The most important (with the most common in italics) are:
- suppression of response to infection,
- suppression of endogenous GC synthesis (the negative feedback effect); after prolonged use the drugs must be withdrawn gradually to prevent the precipitation of adrenal insufficiency,
- metabolic actions (see above),
- iatrogenic Cushing's syndrome (Fig. 16.4),
- growth suppression in children, and
- *osteoporosis* (a limitation to long-term therapy).

Pharmacokinetic aspects

GCs can be given orally, topically, by injection and by inhalation. They are metabolized principally in the liver and the metabolites excreted in the urine. The plasma half-lives are short (e.g. 90 min for hydrocortisone) but the main biological effects occur only after 2–8 h because protein synthesis of enzymes and mediators is required. Cortisone is inactive until converted to hydrocortisone.

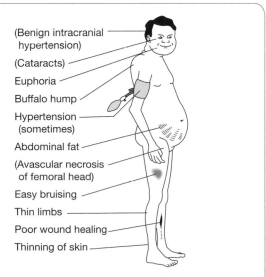

Fig. 16.4 Iatrogenic Cushing's syndrome (less frequent events in parentheses).

(Benign intracranial hypertension)
(Cataracts)
Euphoria
Buffalo hump
Hypertension (sometimes)
Abdominal fat
(Avascular necrosis of femoral head)
Easy bruising
Thin limbs
Poor wound healing
Thinning of skin

DRUGS USED FOR GOUT

Gout is a chronic disease caused by over-production of purines. Crystals of sodium urate precipitate in the joints evoking an inflammatory response.

Allopurinol reduces uric acid synthesis by competing with xanthines for xanthine oxidase. It is given orally, has a half-life of 2–3 h and is excreted in the urine. It is used only for long-term therapy; it can exacerbate the acute attack.

Colchicine inhibits migration of neutrophils into the joint by binding to tubulin. It is given orally and is excreted in the GI tract and the kidney. Its peak effect is in 1 h. It can both relieve and prevent an acute attack but can cause GI disturbances.

Probenecid acts on the proximal tubule of the nephron to increase uric acid excretion. It is given orally and its peak effect is in 3 h. It is used only to prevent attacks.

NSAIDs (diclofenac, naproxen and piroxicam, but not ibuprofen) are used for the pain of the acute attack.

Clinical uses of NSAIDs

- Analgesia, e.g. in musculoskeletal pain, dysmenorrhoea, postoperative pain, cancer metastases to bone:
  - short-term analgesia: **ibuprofen**, naproxen,
  - non-inflammatory pain (e.g. headache): **paracetamol**, and
  - chronic pain: diflunisal; **piroxicam.**
- Anti-inflammatory action in rheumatoid arthritis and other connective tissue disorders: ibuprofen or **naproxen** to start with, longer-acting agents (e.g. **piroxicam**) if necessary. Higher dosage and long-term use mean more likelihood of unwanted effects. Cyclooxygenase (COX)-2 inhibitors (e.g. **etoricoxib**) are used mainly in patients with high risk of gastrointestinal (GI) toxic effects.
- Fever reduction: **paracetamol.**
  (Note: aspirin is now used mainly as an antiplatelet agent in cardiovascular disease.)

Clinical uses of GLUCOSTEROIDS

- Anti-inflammatory/immunosuppressive therapy:
  - in asthma (by inhalation or, in severe cases, systemically),
  - in hypersensitivity states, e.g. severe allergic reactions to drugs or insect venom,
  - in miscellaneous diseases with autoimmune and inflammatory components, e.g. rheumatoid arthritis and other connective tissue diseases,
  - in various inflammatory conditions of skin, eye, ear or nose (given topically),
  - to prevent graft-versus-host disease following organ or bone marrow transplantation, and
  - in various neoplastic diseases, often in combination with cytotoxic drugs.
- Replacement therapy for patients with adrenal failure, e.g. Addison's disease (a mineralocorticoid (MC) will also be necessary).

DRUGS USED TO MODULATE IMMUNE RESPONSES

Antihistamines

Histamine is a mediator in both acute inflammation and the immediate hypersensitivity response. In the latter, a non-noxious antigen (e.g. grass pollen) evokes a special type of immunoglobulin (IgE), which is displayed on mast cells. On subsequent contact with

Table 16.1   Some Examples of H₁ Receptor Antagonists

	Promethazine	Cyclizine	Cetirizine
Anti-allergic action	+ + +	+ + +	+ + +
Sedation	+ +	+ +	--
Antimuscarinic effect	+ +	+ +	--
Anti-emetic effect	+ +	+ +	--
Duration of action	4–6 h	4–6 h	12–24 h

that antigen, the mast cell releases various mediators including histamine. Examples of immediate hypersensitivity reactions are hay fever and urticaria.

Pharmacological actions of histamine

There are two main types of histamine receptor, H_1 and H_2, and antihistamine drugs can target each receptor type.

H_1 *receptor activation* causes vasodilatation, increased permeability of postcapillary venules and contraction of some smooth muscle (e.g. bronchospasm; see Chapter 19). These actions are relevant in immediate hypersensitivity responses and can be modified by H_1-receptor antagonists. (For details of H_2-receptors, see Chapter 21.)

H₁ receptor antagonists

All H_1 receptor antagonists are competitive at H_1 receptors. Some detail of their actions is given in Table 16.1.

Unwanted effects

The sedative CNS actions may be unwanted in some situations but useful in others. The antimuscarinic effects (dry mouth, blurring of vision, constipation, urine retention) are always unwanted. GI disturbances are common.

Clinical uses of H₁ receptor antagonists

- Immediate hypersensitivity reactions such as hay fever, insect bites, urticaria, drug allergies: **cetirizine** (does not cross blood–brain barrier so avoids sedative actions).
- Sedation (e.g. **promethazine**, see Chapter 12).
- Motion sickness (see Chapter 21).

Immunosuppressants

The main action of immunosuppressants is to inhibit clonal expansion of lymphocytes and the production of inflammatory cytokines and chemokines required for the adaptive immune response.

Glucocorticoids are described above.

Anticytokine agents, such as **Anakinra,** have anti-IL-1 action. Two compounds target the action of TNF-α, an important mediator in rheumatoid arthritis (RA): **infliximab** (a monoclonal antibody against TNF-α) and **etanercept** (a TNF receptor joined to the Fc domain of an IgG molecule). **Mepolizumab** has anti-IL-5 action and is used in the treatment of certain eosinophilic asthma phenotypes.

Anti-IgE therapy. Omalizumab monoclonal antibody recognizes unbound IgE, used in the treatment of severe atopic asthma.

Ciclosporin and tacrolimus both act mainly by selective inhibition of IL-2 gene transcription. Both bind with and inhibit proteins that would normally activate calcineurin, a phosphatase necessary for activation of the relevant transcription factors. Ciclosporin is given orally or intravenously and has a half-life of 24 h; it accumulates in high concentration in the tissues. Tacrolimus has a half-life of 7 h. The main *unwanted effect* is nephrotoxicity, which is common and severe with ciclosporin, less so with tacrolimus.

Rapamycin inhibits IL-2 signal transduction.

Azathioprine is a cytotoxic drug which has antiproliferative action. It is also used in cancer chemotherapy (see Chapter 33).

Mycophenolate mofetil has a selective action on T and B cell proliferation by inhibiting an enzyme necessary for purine synthesis.

Rituximab and **Ofatumumab** are examples of anti-CD20 antibodies used to treat B-cell tumours.

Clinical use of immunosuppressants

- Inhibition of rejection of transplanted organs and tissues.
- Apoptosis to B cells.
- Suppression of graft-versus-host disease in bone marrow transplants.
- Treatment of various conditions that have an autoimmune component, e.g. rheumatoid arthritis (RA).
- Well-defined phenotypes of asthma: e.g. severe eosinophilic asthma.

Disease-modifying antirheumatoid drugs (DMARDS)

Disease-modifying antirheumatoid drugs (DMARDS) are used to alleviate the symptoms of RA but do not stop the progress of the disease. Immunosuppressants such as glucocorticoids and anticytokine agents are used (described above). Other DMARDs include those listed below.

Sulfasalazine is often a first-choice agent. Given orally, it is split into sulphapyridine and salicylate in the bowel. Common side effects are GI disturbances, malaise and headache. It can cause skin lesions and low white blood cell count.

Gold compounds include **auranofin** and sodium aurothiomalate. These cause the symptoms and signs of RA to decrease slowly over 3–4 months. Auranofin is given orally, sodium aurothiomalate by deep intramuscular injection. The compounds concentrate in the tissues, particularly in the joints. The half-life is initially 7 days but gradually increases.

Unwanted actions

These include skin rashes, blood dyscrasias, peripheral neuropathy and encephalopathy; they occur in 30% of patients treated with aurothiomalate but are less frequent with auranofin.

Penicillamine can chelate metals and also substitute for cysteine in cysteine disulphide. It is given orally and about 75% of patients with RA respond, though the effects are not seen for several months.

Chloroquine is an antimalarial drug (see Chapter 32) that can cause remission of RA. Given orally, it acts only after 30 days.

Immunostimulants

A newer class of drugs has recently entered the armoury of the clinician, and they are used to boost host defence. These immunostimulants have been developed to treat cancer but show future application in the treatment of difficult infections and sepsis. Immunostimulants currently used are classed as *checkpoint inhibitors* (drugs that suppress negative regulation of T cell activation):

- Programmed cell death protein 1 (PD-1) and PD ligand (PD-L) inhibitors (e.g. **Nivolumab, Pembrolizumab**) are monoclonal antibodies. The transmembrane PD-1 is activated by PD-L to induce apoptosis of antigen-specific T cells whilst reducing apoptosis of regulatory T cells (cells that suppress the adaptive immune response, thus reducing autoimmunity. However, upregulation of PD-1 in tumours can prevent tumour cell apoptosis by immune cell activation. Inhibitors of PD-1 and PD-L therefore suppress this negative regulation.

• CTLA-4 blockers (**Ipilimumab**) lead to enhanced antigen specific T-cell dependent immune reactions and killing of cancer cells, since CTLA-4 is a negative regulator of T cells.

Other immune-stimulants, for example toll like receptor (TLR) 7 TLRs recognize protein sequences of pathogen derived molecules) and ligands (Imiquimod, Resiquimod) activate immune cells and show promise in the treatment of cancers, viruses and bacterial infections.

The endocrine and metabolic systems of the body consist of glands with organs that secrete hormones into the circulation. Thus secreted hormones modulate tissue function elsewhere in the body, and these effects will be relatively slow compared to other communication processes (e.g. neurons). Glands include the hypothalamus, pituitary, thyroid, adrenals, gonads, pancreatic islets of Langerhans and parathyroids. Seven major physiological functions are regulated, and these are control of blood sugar levels, growth and development (growth hormone-insulin growth factor, IGF axis), metabolic rate (thyroid hormone), ion (calcium ion, Ca^{2+}) homeostasis, reproduction function (sex steroids), adaption to physiologic stress (glucocorticosteroids), and circulatory volume (Table 17.1). This chapter discusses the function and pharmacology of the thyroid, the adrenal cortex, the pancreas and blood sugar and the reproductive systems. Ca^{2+} homeostasis is discussed in Chapter 20 (Drugs and the musculoskeletal system), and circulatory volume in Chapter 18 (Drugs and the renal system) and Chapter 14 (Drugs and the cardiovascular system). Additional discussion on disorders of the genitourinary system is found in Chapter 22 (Drugs and the genitourinary system).

THE HYPOTHALAMIC-PITUITARY AXIS

The hypothalamus and pituitary glands integrate physiological signals and release hormones that then regulate the production of hormones affecting the function of other glands, for example adrenocorticotropin (ACTH) acting on the adrenal cortex, thyroid stimulating hormone (TSH) acting on the thyroid, growth hormone (GH) acting on the liver, and prolactin, follicle-stimulating hormone (FSH) and luteinizing hormone (LH) acting on the female reproductive system (Fig. 17.1).

THE ADRENAL CORTEX

The adrenal cortex produces steroids. Principal adrenal steroids are the *glucocorticoids* (GC) (e.g. hydrocortisone and cortisone) and the *mineralocorticoids* (MC) (e.g. aldosterone). Some *sex steroids* (mainly androgens) are also secreted. Synthetic steroids have been developed in which the GC and the MC actions have been separated. Examples are prednisolone (GC > MC), fludrocortisone (MC > GC).

Glucocorticoids

GCs are not stored pre-formed but are released when needed. The controlling factors are shown in Fig. 17.2. The starting substrate for synthesis is cholesterol.

Pharmacological actions of the glucocorticoids

- *Regulatory*: Negative feedback effects on anterior pituitary and hypothalamus (prolonged therapy can cause atrophy of adrenal cortex).
- *Metabolic*:
  - carbohydrates: decreased uptake and utilization of glucose, increased gluconeogenesis (thus tendency to hyperglycaemia);
  - protein: increased catabolism and decreased synthesis; and
  - fat: permissive effect on the lipolytic hormones.

(These actions are only made use of therapeutically in replacement therapy.)

Table 17.1 Functional Anatomy of the Endocrine and Metabolic Systems

Endocrine function	Regulatory factors	Endocrine organ/hormone	Target tissues
Availability of metabolic energy (fuel)	Serum glucose, amino acids, enteric hormones (somatostatin, cholecystokinin, gastrin, secretin), vagal reflex, sympathetic nervous system	Pancreatic islets of Langerhans/insulin, glucagon	All tissues, especially liver, skeletal muscle, adipose tissue, indirect effects on brain and red blood cells
Metabolic rate	Hypothalamic thyrotropin-releasing hormone (TRH), pituitary thyrotropin (TSH)	Thyroid gland/triiodothyronine (T_3)	All tissues
Circulatory volume	Renin, angiotensin II, hypothalamic osmoreceptor	Adrenals/aldosterone Pituitary/vasopressin	Kidney, blood vessels, central nervous system (CNS)
Somatic growth	Hypothalamic growth hormone-releasing hormone (GHRH), somatostatin, sleep, exercise, stress, hypoglycemia	Pituitary/growth hormone Liver/insulin-like growth factors (IGFs)	All tissues
Calcium homeostasis	Serum calcium ion (Ca^{2+}) and magnesium ion (Mg^{2+}) concentration	Parathyroid glands/ parathyroid hormone, calcitonin, vitamin D	Kidney, intestines, bone
Reproductive function	Hypothalamic gonadotropin-releasing hormone (GnRH), pituitary follicle-stimulating hormone (FSH) and luteinizing hormone (LH) inhibins	Gonads/sex steroids Adrenals/androgens	Reproductive organs, CNS, various tissues
Adaptation to stress	Hypothalamic corticotropin-releasing hormone (CRH), pituitary adrenocorticotropic hormone (ACTH), hypoglycemia, stress	Adrenals/glucocorticosteroids, epinephrine	Many tissues: CNS, liver, skeletal muscle, adipose tissue, lymphocytes, fibroblasts, cardiovascular system

Endocrine and metabolic systems regulate seven major bodily functions. For each target tissue effect, endocrine glands release hormones in response to regulating factors, which include physiologic (e.g. sleep and stress), biochemical (e.g. glucose and calcium ion (Ca^{2+})) and hormonal (e.g. hypothalamic and enteric hormones) stimuli.

From Page C, Curtis M, Walker M, Hoffman B. *Integrated Pharmacology*. 3rd ed. Philadelphia: Elsevier; 2006.

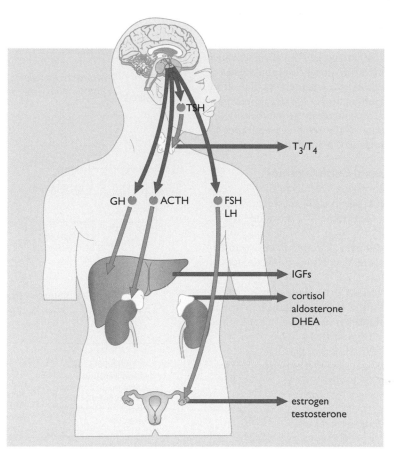

Fig. 17.1 The hypothalamic-pituitary axis. *ACTH*, Adrenocorticotrophin; *DHEA*, dehydroepiandrosterone; *FSH*, follicle stimulating hormone; *GH*, growth hormone; *IGFs*, insulin growth factors; *LH*, luteinizing hormone; *T3*, triiodothyronine; *T4*, thyroxine; *TSH*, thyroid stimulating hormone. (From Page C, Curtis M, Walker M, Hoffman B. *Integrated Pharmacology.* 3rd ed. Philadelphia: Elsevier; 2006.)

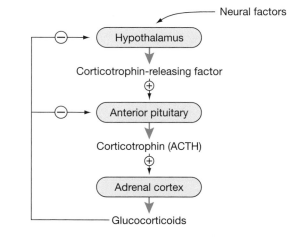

Fig. 17.2 Factors controlling the synthesis and release of glucocorticoids. Blue arrows, releases; black arrows, acts on.

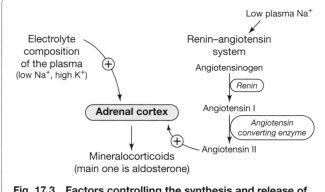

Fig. 17.3 Factors controlling the synthesis and release of mineralocorticoids.

For metabolic actions, most of the mediator proteins induced are enzymes, e.g. cyclic adenosine monophosphate (cAMP)-dependent kinase.

Mineralocorticoids

The synthesis and release of the MCs is shown in Fig. 17.3.

Pharmacological actions

The MCs are critically important for water and electrolyte balance. Aldosterone acts on the distal renal tubules to cause increased sodium ion (Na^+) reabsorption, with concomitant increased excretion of potassium ion (K^+) and hydrogen ion (H^+).

- Anti-inflammatory and immunosuppressive: A physiological role, and important pharmacological interest is the use of glucocorticoids in the treatment of inflammatory diseases (see Chapter 16).

Mechanism of action

The interaction of GCs with intracellular receptors belonging to a superfamily that control transcription is discussed elsewhere (see Chapter 16).

Mechanism of action

The mechanism of action is the same as that of the GCs (see Chapter 16) but aldosterone receptors occur virtually only in the kidney. (Spironolactone is a competitive antagonist of aldosterone at these receptors, see Chapter 18.) GCs enter renal cells but are inactivated by an enzyme (11-β-hydroxysteroid dehydrogenase) and thus have little or no action on these receptors (see Chapter 18). The effect of the mediator(s) produced by interaction of the steroid-receptor complex with the DNA is initially to increase the number of Na^+ channels in the apical membrane of the renal cell and later to increase the number of Na^+ pumps in the basolateral membrane.

Pathophysiology of the Adrenal Corticosteroids

* Excess production of endogenous GCs results in *Cushing's disease*. (Prolonged therapy with exogenous GCs can give a similar picture, *Cushing's syndrome*, see Chapter 16, unwanted effects of glucocorticoids.)
* Decreased GC production results in *Addison's disease* (muscular weakness, low blood pressure, depression, anorexia, loss of weight, hypoglycaemia).
* Excess production of MCs, termed *hyperaldosteronism*, causes marked Na^+ and water retention, with resultant increase in the volume of extracellular fluid, hypokalaemia, alkalosis and hypertension.

Clinical uses of adrenal steroids

Glucocorticoids
* Anti-inflammatory/immunosuppressive therapy:
  * in asthma (by inhalation or, in severe cases, systemically) in hypersensitivity states, e.g. severe allergic reactions to drugs or insect venom;
  * in miscellaneous diseases with autoimmune and inflammatory components, e.g. rheumatoid arthritis and other connective tissue diseases;
  * in various inflammatory conditions of skin, eye, ear or nose (given topically);
  * to prevent graft-versus-host disease following organ or bone marrow transplantation; and
  * in various neoplastic diseases, often in combination with cytotoxic drugs.
* Replacement therapy for patients with adrenal failure, e.g. Addison's disease (a mineralocorticoid (MC) will also be necessary).

Mineralocorticoids
* Replacement therapy in adrenal insufficiency (**fludrocortisone** orally with a glucocorticoid (GC)).
* **Spironolactone** is a competitive antagonist of aldosterone used as an antihypertensive drug (see Chapter 22). **Eplerenone** has fewer side effects as it has lower affinity for sex hormone receptors.

THE THYROID

The main thyroid hormones are thyroxine (T_4) and triiodothyronine (T_3). They are critically important for normal growth and development and for energy metabolism (see Fig. 17.4 for their regulation). The functional unit of the thyroid is the follicle. Each follicle consists of a single layer of epithelial cells around a cavity, the follicle lumen, which is filled with a thick colloid containing thyroglobulin (TG). The sequence of events in the thyroid is shown in Fig. 17.5. Unlike other endocrine secretions, the thyroid retains a store of precursors. More T_4 is released than T_3.

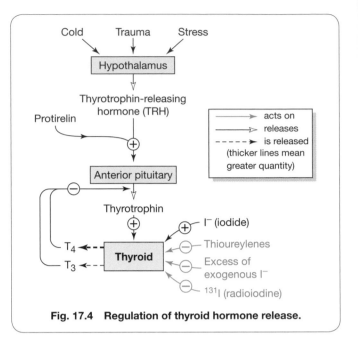

Fig. 17.4   Regulation of thyroid hormone release.

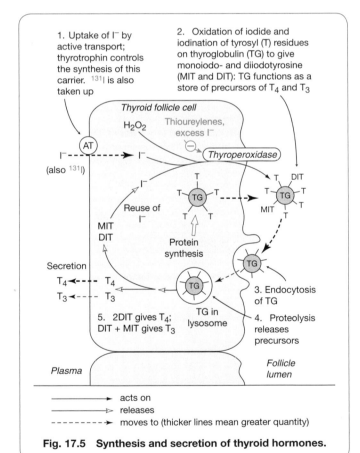

Fig. 17.5   Synthesis and secretion of thyroid hormones.

The action of the thyroid hormones

* On metabolism:
  * increased oxygen consumption and increased heat production leading to increase in basal metabolic rate (not in brain and gonads); and
  * increase in metabolism of carbohydrates, fats and proteins by modulation of the action of glucocorticoids, catecholamines, insulin and glucagon.

- On growth and development:
  - essential for normal growth by direct action on cells and potentiation of growth hormone, and
  - essential for maturation of the central nervous system (CNS) and for skeletal development.
- *Cellular action:* T_4 is converted to T_3, which binds to specific receptors on DNA. These receptors, when unbound, repress basal transcription. T_3 binding activates transcription, resulting in mRNA generation and protein synthesis.

Synthesis and secretion of the thyroid hormones and sites of drug action

The sequence of events leading to the production and release of T_4 and T_3 is shown in Fig. 17.5. There is a large pool of T_4 in the body; it has a low turnover rate and is found mainly in the circulation where it is bound to thyroxine-binding globulin. There is a small pool of T_3 in the body; it has a fast turnover rate and is found mainly intracellularly in the target organs.

Pathophysiology
Hyperthyroidism

Hyperthyroidism (**thyrotoxicosis**) results from overactivity of the thyroid. There is a high metabolic rate and an increase in temperature, sweating, nervousness, tremor, tachycardia, fatigability and increased appetite, but loss of weight occurs. The main types are the following:
- *Diffuse toxic goitre* (Graves' disease or exophthalmic goitre): Caused by an immunological action against the thyrotrophin receptor; patients have protrusion of the eyeballs (exophthalmos) and there is increased sensitivity to catecholamines.
- *Toxic nodular goitre:* Caused by a benign tumour; there is no exophthalmos.

Hypothyroidism

Hypothyroidism is a condition that results from decreased activity of the thyroid; it has several causes. The main types are the following:
- *Myxoedema,* which is immunological in origin, its manifestations include low basal metabolic rate (BMR), slow speech, deep hoarse voice, lethargy, bradycardia, sensitivity to cold, mental impairment and a thickening of the skin.
- *Cretinism* (hypothyroidism in childhood); manifestations are retardation of growth and mental deficiency.
- *Hashimoto's thyroiditis,* an autoimmune disease in which there is an immune reaction against TG, can lead to hypothyroidism.
- *Radioiodine therapy* induced hypothyroidism.

Simple, non-toxic goitre

Simple goitre is caused by dietary deficiency of iodine, which causes a rise in plasma thyrotrophic hormone and eventually an increase in the size of the gland. Normal amounts of thyroid hormone are produced, but eventually hypothyroidism may occur.

Drugs used in hyperthyroidism

The main drugs are the thioureylenes (e.g. **carbimazole**, propylthiouracil) and **radioiodine**. Iodide/iodine is also used.

The thioureylenes
Mechanism of action

Thioureylenes act on the thyroid to decrease hormone output (Fig. 17.5).

Actions and pharmacokinetic aspects

The drugs gradually decrease the thyroid hormone output and reduce the signs of thyrotoxicosis over 3–4 weeks.

All are given by mouth. Carbimazole is converted to methimazole (the active compound), which has a half-life of 16 h and causes 90% inhibition of the oxidation of iodine (organification of iodine) within 12 h. The clinical action is delayed until the store of hormones in the follicle lumen has been depleted, which may take several weeks. Propylthiouracil acts a little more quickly because it also inhibits the conversion of T_4 to T_3. The thioureylenes have no effect on the exophthalmos.

Unwanted effects
- Granulocytopenia (rare but serious)
- Rashes (more common)
- Headache, nausea, jaundice and joint pain (occasionally)

Radioiodine

Given orally, iodine-131 (^{131}I) is taken up by the thyroid and processed in the same way as I⁻, becoming incorporated into TG. It emits both β-particles and X-rays. The X-rays pass through the tissue, but the short range β-radiation causes significant destruction of nearby thyroid cells. Radioiodine has a radioactive half-life of 8 days. It is used in one single dose; its effect on the gland is delayed for 1–2 months and reaches maximum after 4 months.

Hypothyroidism occurs eventually and will need replacement therapy with levothyroxine (synthetic T_4).

Iodide/iodine

Iodide/iodine given orally in high doses temporarily reduces thyroid hormone secretion (mechanism not clear) and decreases the vascularity of the gland.

Other miscellaneous drugs

The **β-adrenoceptor antagonists** decrease signs and symptoms such as tachycardia, dysrhythmias, tremor and agitation.

Drugs used in hypothyroidism

The main drugs are **levothyroxine** (T_4) and **liothyronine** (T_3).

The actions and mechanism of action are the same as the natural hormones.

Unwanted effects

The thyroid hormones increase heart rate and output, cause dysrhythmias and the signs and symptoms of hyperthyroidism.

Clinical use of drugs acting on the thyroid

- Radioiodine:
  - treatment of relapse of hyperthyroidism after thioureylene therapy or surgery, and
  - as first-line treatment for hyperthyroidism (particularly in the United States); recurrence is rare.
- Thioureylenes:
  - hyperthyroidism (diffuse toxic goitre), at least 1 year of treatment being necessary; recurrence can occur but is susceptible to further treatment,
  - before surgery for toxic goitre, and
  - as part of the treatment of thyroid storm (very severe hyperthyroidism); carbimazole is preferred.
- Thyroid hormones:
  - levothyroxine (T_4) is the standard replacement therapy for hypothyroidism, and
  - liothyronine (T_3) is used to treat myxoedema coma.

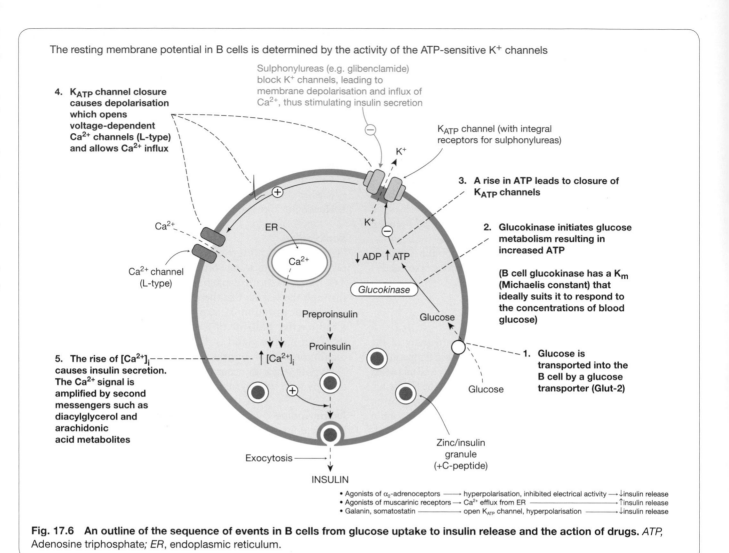

The resting membrane potential in B cells is determined by the activity of the ATP-sensitive K⁺ channels

Sulphonylureas (e.g. glibenclamide) block K⁺ channels, leading to membrane depolarisation and influx of Ca^{2+}, thus stimulating insulin secretion

4. K_{ATP} channel closure causes depolarisation which opens voltage-dependent Ca^{2+} channels (L-type) and allows Ca^{2+} influx

K_{ATP} channel (with integral receptors for sulphonylureas)

K⁺

3. A rise in ATP leads to closure of K_{ATP} channels

2. Glucokinase initiates glucose metabolism resulting in increased ATP

(B cell glucokinase has a K_m (Michaelis constant) that ideally suits it to respond to the concentrations of blood glucose)

Ca^{2+}

ER

K⁺

Ca^{2+}

Ca^{2+} channel (L-type)

Ca^{2+}

↓ ADP ↑ ATP

Glucokinase

Preproinsulin

Glucose

5. The rise of $[Ca^{2+}]_i$ causes insulin secretion. The Ca^{2+} signal is amplified by second messengers such as diacylglycerol and arachidonic acid metabolites

↑ $[Ca^{2+}]_i$

Proinsulin

1. Glucose is transported into the B cell by a glucose transporter (Glut-2)

Glucose

Exocytosis

Zinc/insulin granule (+C-peptide)

INSULIN

- Agonists of α₂-adrenoceptors ⟶ hyperpolarisation, inhibited electrical activity ⟶ ↓insulin release
- Agonists of muscarinic receptors ⟶ Ca^{2+} efflux from ER ⟶ ↑insulin release
- Galanin, somatostatin ⟶ open K_{ATP} channel, hyperpolarisation ⟶ ↓insulin release

Fig. 17.6   An outline of the sequence of events in B cells from glucose uptake to insulin release and the action of drugs. *ATP,* Adenosine triphosphate; *ER,* endoplasmic reticulum.

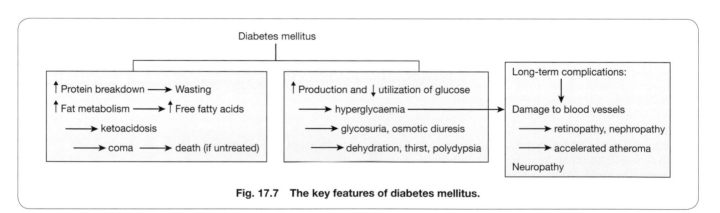

Diabetes mellitus

↑ Protein breakdown ⟶ Wasting

↑ Fat metabolism ⟶ ↑ Free fatty acids

⟶ ketoacidosis

⟶ coma ⟶ death (if untreated)

↑ Production and ↓ utilization of glucose

⟶ hyperglycaemia

⟶ glycosuria, osmotic diuresis

⟶ dehydration, thirst, polydypsia

Long-term complications:

Damage to blood vessels

⟶ retinopathy, nephropathy

⟶ accelerated atheroma

Neuropathy

Fig. 17.7   The key features of diabetes mellitus.

THE PANCREAS, BLOOD SUGAR AND DIABETES

Blood glucose concentrations are predominantly under the control of the pancreatic hormones *insulin* and *glucagon*. The pancreatic islets of Langerhans contain B cells, which secrete insulin and A, D and PP cells, which secrete glucagon, somatostatin and pancreatic polypeptide, respectively. Insulin exerts a major control over the metabolism of carbohydrates, fats and proteins and is the main regulator of blood glucose.

Insulin release is primarily regulated by glucose, although other fuels (fatty acids and amino acids) will also modify release. Change in B cell adenosine triphosphate (ATP) concentration as

a consequence of glucose metabolism is a key factor in insulin release (Fig. 17.6).

Glucagon causes a rise in blood glucose by initiating glycogenolysis and gluconeogenesis and inhibiting glycogen synthesis.

Pathophysiology of diabetes mellitus

Deficient secretion of insulin results in diabetes mellitus (Fig. 17.7), of which there are two types:

- *Type 1* (also known as *insulin-dependent diabetes mellitus (IDDM)* or juvenile-onset diabetes) in which the B cells have been completely destroyed by an autoimmune process and insulin replacement therapy is essential.

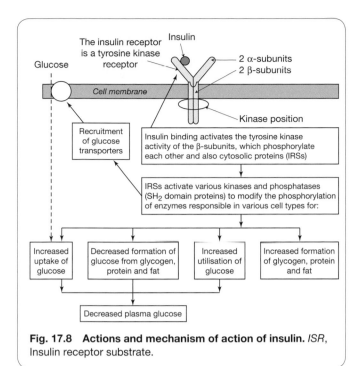

Fig. 17.8 **Actions and mechanism of action of insulin.** *ISR,* Insulin receptor substrate.

- *Type 2* (also known as *non-insulin-dependent diabetes mellitus* (NIDDM) or maturity-onset diabetes) in which individuals are insulin resistant and fail to secrete sufficient hormone.

DRUGS USED TO TREAT DIABETES

Insulin

The actions of insulin are shown in Fig. 17.8. Note that insulin also has a role in the synthesis of the enzymes implicated in glucose metabolism. Insulin receptor substrates (IRSs) activity may initiate the cascade: activation of the rat sarcoma (RAS – cell growth regulator) system → activation of mitogen-activated protein (MAP) kinases → DNA transcription → RNA production → enzyme synthesis.

Insulin preparations

- Short, rapid acting: **soluble insulin, insulin lispro** (an insulin analogue in which a lysine and a proline residue are interchanged), **insulin aspart.**
- Intermediate acting: **isophane insulin** (a suspension of a complex of insulin with protamine).
- Long acting: **insulin zinc suspension, insulin glargine.**

Human insulin, made in bacteria by recombinant DNA technology, has largely replaced insulin extracted from bovine or porcine tissues.

Insulin administration and pharmacokinetic aspects

Insulin is inactive by mouth owing to the proteolytic action of digestive enzymes and must be given by injection. Various regimens are used.

Day-to-day control of blood glucose in type 1 diabetes Patients can optimize control of their blood glucose by adjusting the timing of injections and proportions of soluble to long-acting insulin. A typical regimen would be twice daily subcutaneous injection of soluble insulin (peak effect 2–4 h, duration of action 6–8 h) combined with an intermediate or long-acting preparation. For tight control, soluble insulin or insulin lispro can be given shortly before meals.

Hyperglycaemic emergencies Soluble insulin is given intravenously (IV) (rapid but short action, inactivated in liver and kidney, half-life – 10 min).

Unwanted effects and their treatment

The most important untoward action is hypoglycaemia which occurs if the dose exceeds the requirement for the food intake and/ or amount of exercise. An excessively low blood glucose can lead to unconsciousness and possible brain damage. If the patient is conscious, a sweet drink, glucose tablet or snack may suffice. If the patient is unconscious, IV glucose or intramuscular **glucagon** will be necessary.

Oral hypoglycaemic agents

- Sulphonylureas: examples are tolbutamide, glibenclamide, glipizide
- Biguanides: the only example is metformin
- Thiazolidinediones
- Meglitinides
- Acarbose

Actions and mechanism of action of sulphonylureas, biguanides and acarbose

The sulphonylureas act adequately only in patients with some functioning B cells. They increase appetite and may promote weight gain. They work by binding to the sulphonylurea receptor (SUR) associated with the K_{ATP} channel to inhibit channel opening (Fig. 17.6). Metformin has no effect on insulin release (and therefore does not cause hypoglycaemia) but it increases glucose uptake into tissues and inhibits gluconeogenesis. It can cause weight loss. Acarbose inhibits intestinal α-glucosidase, so delaying carbohydrate absorption and reducing the rise in blood glucose which follows a meal.

Pharmacokinetic aspects

Sulphonylureas are well absorbed by mouth and are well tolerated. They bind extensively to plasma albumin and may be displaced by other drugs given concomitantly. Their action is enhanced by reduced renal function associated with age or disease. Tolbutamide has a half-life of 4 h and glibenclamide 10 h; both yield active metabolites. Metformin has a half-life of approximately 3 h. Acarbose is taken with meals.

Unwanted effects

The sulphonylureas can cause hypoglycaemic attacks; this is more likely in elderly people and with the longer-acting drugs such as glibenclamide. Agents that inhibit the drug-metabolizing enzymes increase the likelihood of hypoglycaemia. Gastrointestinal (GI) tract upsets and skin rashes are seen in a small percentage of patients. Metformin tends to cause anorexia and diarrhoea and thus weight loss. A rare effect is potentially fatal lactic acidosis. Acarbose causes flatulence.

Newer oral hypoglycaemic drugs

Repaglinide and nateglinide (meglitinides), like the SURs, block K_{ATP} channels on B cells (but with greater selectivity compared to vascular smooth muscle K_{ATP} channels) and stimulate insulin secretion. They have a rapid onset and are eliminated quickly, with a lower risk of hypoglycaemia.

Thiazolidinediones (**pioglitazone**) lower blood glucose very slowly (over months) and enhance the effect of administered

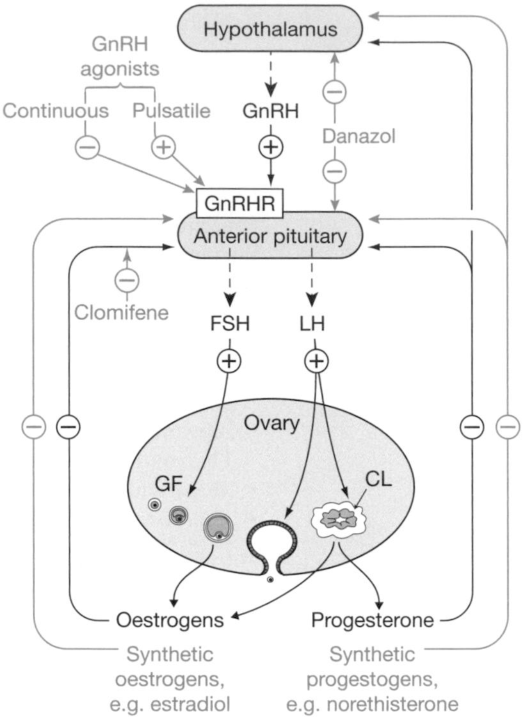

1. The menstrual cycle starts with the onset of menstruation, during which the top layer of the endometrium is shed. When bleeding ceases, the endometrium is regenerated during the rest of the cycle

2. Gonadotrophin-releasing hormone (GnRH) is released from the hypothalamus in pulsatile fashion to act on GnRH receptors (GnRHR) to stimulate release of glycoproteins: follicle-stimulating hormone (FSH) and luteinizing hormone (LH) from the anterior pituitary

3. In the initial phase of the cycle, FSH stimulates the development of the Graafian follicle (GF), which contains the ovum

4. FSH stimulates the granulosa cells surrounding the ovum to produce oestrogens (oestradiol, and some oestrone and oestriol), the secretion of which rises till mid-cycle. The oestrogens control the proliferative phase of endometrium renewal (from day 5 or 6 to mid-cycle) and act on the anterior pituitary to reduce gonadotrophin release

5. At mid-cycle, a surge of LH secretion stimulates ovulation

11. If the ovum does not implant, progesterone secretion ceases, triggering menstruation; in the absence of the negative feedback action the cycle begins again

10. Progesterone acts on the hypothalamus and anterior pituitary, reducing the secretion of GnRH and LH. It also raises body temperature by about 0.5 °C

9. Progesterone, acting on oestrogen-induced receptors, stimulates the secretory phase of endometrium regeneration, which prepares it for implantation of the ovum

8. The endogenous sex steroids act on nuclear receptors in target tissues, activating transcription of some genes and inhibiting transcription of others

6. Oestrogens promote progesterone receptor synthesis in peripheral target tissues, including the endometrium

7. The ruptured follicle, under the influence of LH, develops into the corpus luteum (CL), which secretes both oestrogen and progesterone

12. If the ovum implants, progesterone secretion continues and its negative feedback action on hypothalamus and anterior pituitary ensures that another menstrual cycle does not commence. The chorion and later the placenta secrete gonadotrophins (including human chorionic gondotrophin), progesterone and oestrogens; these hormones maintain the pregnancy

Fig. 17.9 Hormonal control of the menstrual cycle and the action of drugs.

insulin. Pioglitazone is an agonist to the peroxisome proliferator-activated gamma (PPARγ) nuclear receptor, which can be activated by endogenous agonists such as unsaturated fatty acids and derivatives (e.g. PGJ_2) and is involved in insulin signalling. However, a full mechanism of action on glucose haemostasis is not yet understood, since the receptors are found mainly on fat cells. Pioglitazone might therefore affect the glucose-fatty acid (Randle) cycle and reduce in free fatty acids. Onset is rapid but action is prolonged to 24 h for pioglitazone by an active metabolite.

Thiazolidinediones cause weight gain and fluid retention. Rosiglitazone and troglitazone are examples that were both withdrawn because of increased risk of heart attacks and liver damage respectively.

Hypoglycaemic agents that mimic Incretin

Exenatide and Liraglutide mimic the action of the gut hormone incretin glucagon-like peptide 1 (GLP-1), which stimulates insulin secretion to lower blood glucose. They reduce satiety and are associated with modest weight loss. They are recommended in obese patients who are refractory to dual therapy.

Gliptins (e.g. sitagliptin, vildagliptin) competitively inhibit dipeptidyl-peptidase-4 (DDP-4). This then lowers blood glucose by potentiating endogenous incretins (GLP-1) to stimulate insulin secretion. They do not affect weight.

Summary of drug use in diabetes

- Insulin:
  - For life-long treatment of type 1 diabetes.
  - In treatment of type 2 diabetes if oral drugs become less effective, e.g. during infections or major surgery.
  - Different formulations have different durations of action.
- Oral hypoglycaemic drugs:
  - For type 2 diabetes if needed as a supplement to dietary control.
  - **Sulphonylureas** are main agents; effective in 30% of patients.
  - Metformin is used in obese patients or if sulfonylureas are ineffective.
  - Acarbose is used in type 2 diabetes not controlled by other drugs.

THE REPRODUCTIVE SYSTEM

The control of the reproductive system in both the male and female involves sex steroids from the gonads, hypothalamic peptides and glycoprotein gonadotrophins from the anterior pituitary.

THE FEMALE REPRODUCTIVE SYSTEM

To understand drug action on the female reproductive system it is necessary to be familiar with the events of the menstrual cycle (Fig. 17.9).

Drugs acting on the female reproductive system
Oestrogens
The main example is **estradiol**; others are given below.

Pharmacological actions Estradiol's main action is to prevent pregnancy, i.e. to function as a contraceptive (discussed below). Other uses are conditional on age and state of sexual maturity. In prepubertal patients they stimulate the development of the secondary sex characteristics; in adult females with primary amenorrhoea, given with a progestogen, they induce an artificial menstrual cycle. Other effects include some degree of water retention, decreased bone resorption (see Chapter 20) and possibly some mild anabolic actions.

Mechanism of action Oestrogens bind to nuclear receptors in the cells of the target tissues (the reproductive organs and the anterior pituitary); the drug–receptor complexes then bind to steroid-response elements in the DNA and initiate transcription of some genes (e.g. for the synthesis of progesterone receptors) and repress transcription of others.

Pharmacokinetic aspects Oestrogens are well absorbed from the GI tract, the skin and mucous membranes. Natural oestrogens are quickly metabolized in the liver, the synthetic nonsteroidal oestrogen-like compounds less rapidly.

Unwanted effects These include nausea, salt and water retention and an increased risk of thromboembolism. Administered postmenopausally, oestrogens may cause endometrial thickening unless given with a progestogen. The unwanted effects of contraceptives are given below.

Raloxifene
This is a selective oestrogen receptor modulator that has anti-oestrogenic action on uterus and breast but oestrogenic action on bone, lipids and blood coagulation. It is used to treat postmenopausal osteoporosis.

Anti-oestrogens
These compete with natural oestrogens for target receptors (e.g. **tamoxifen**, a drug used in breast cancer therapy; see Chapter 33).

Progestogens
Progestational hormones have a mechanism of action similar to that of oestrogen (Fig. 17.9 and see Contraceptive drugs below). **Medroxyprogesterone**, a synthetic compound, can be given orally or by injection. Other progestogens are used in contraception (see below).

Antiprogestogens
Mifepristone may be used to terminate early pregnancy, acting by sensitizing the uterus to abortifacient prostaglandins (see below).

Therapeutic uses of female sex hormones
Female hormones are used for two main purposes: contraception and postmenopausal hormone replacement therapy (HRT). Other uses are less frequent and are mentioned above.

Contraceptive drugs
Contraception can be affected by both oral and injected agents.

The combined pill
The combined pill contains **ethinylestradiol** or **mestranol** with a *progestogen* (e.g. **norethisterone, desogestrel**).

Mechanism of action Oestrogen suppresses the development of the ovarian follicle by inhibiting FSH release.
- The progestogen prevents ovulation by inhibiting LH release; it also makes the cervical mucus less welcoming to the sperm.
- Together they render the endometrium less suitable for implantation of the ovum.

Unwanted effects These are infrequent but can include weight gain, flushing, mood changes, dizziness and sometimes acne or skin pigmentation and a transient rise in blood pressure. There is some risk of thromboembolism.

The progestogen-only pill
Agents used include **norethisterone** and **levonorgestrel** to inhibit secretion of LH. The pill is taken every day without a break. The contraceptive effect is mainly through making the cervical mucus unwelcoming to sperm, but the actions on the endometrium cited above may play a part. It is less reliable and irregular bleeding can occur.

Postcoital contraception
Emergency postcoital contraception can be effected with a large oral dose of **levonorgestrel**, with or without an oestrogen, taken within 72 hours of unprotected sex and repeated 12 hours later.

Postmenopausal hormone replacement therapy
A combination of an oestrogen and a progestogen is used for women with an intact uterus, an oestrogen alone in hysterectomized individuals. The doses used are much lower than those used for contraception. Examples of the oestrogens used are **conjugated oestrogens** or **estradiol** (given orally), oestriol (given intravaginally) and **estradiol** (implanted subcutaneously). Examples of the progestogens used are **norethisterone** and **medroxyprogesterone**. Tibolone has both oestrogenic and progestogenic action and is used on its own.

The main beneficial effects of HRT are:
- relief from menopausal symptoms (hot flushes, inappropriate sweating, paraesthesias, palpitations, atrophic vaginitis, etc.);
- a reduction in osteoporosis (controversial) (see Chapter 20; see also raloxifene); and
- a possible decrease in the risk of coronary artery disease (this has recently been questioned).

The unwanted effects of HRT are:
- a slightly increased risk of venous thromboembolism,
- a moderate increase in the risk of breast cancer, and
- an oestrogen-induced risk of endometrial cancer if a progestogen is not also used.

Gonadotrophins and gonadotrophin release
Endogenous gonadotrophin-releasing hormone (GnRH) stimulates secretion of both FSH and LH from the anterior pituitary (Fig. 17.9) and its action is inhibited by the sex steroids, mainly progesterone.

Long-acting *GnRH analogues* (e.g. **goserelin**) cause continuous stimulation and thus desensitization of the GnRH receptors; this results in suppression of gonadotrophin release and the suppression of the LH surge, promoting follicle maturation. They can be used in the treatment of infertility and for endometriosis and tumours of the breast or prostate.

GnRH antagonists (e.g. **ganirelix**) also decrease gonadotrophin release and are adjuncts in infertility treatments.

Clomifene, an antiestrogen, acts on the anterior pituitary to inhibit the negative feedback action of oestrogen, thus increasing gonadotrophin release; it is used to treat infertility and can result in multiple pregnancies. **Danazol** inhibits gonadal function by suppressing the mid-cycle surge of the gonadotrophins (Fig. 17.9); it is used for endometriosis.

Menotrophin, a preparation of the gonadotrophins FSH and LH, is used to treat infertility.

Drugs acting on the uterus

Uterine stimulants: examples are **oxytocin** (a synthetic preparation of the neurohypophyseal peptide), **ergometrine** (an ergot derivative), **dinoprostone** (prostaglandin E_2), **gemeprost** (a prostaglandin E_1 analogue), carboprost (an analogue of prostaglandin $F_{2\alpha}$). The prostaglandins contract the uterus but relax the cervix.

Uterine stimulants are used by obstetricians as follows:
- To augment or induce labour: dinoprostone (intravaginally); oxytocin (by infusion).
- For the management of the third stage of labour (ergometrine plus oxytocin).
- To treat postpartum haemorrhage: ergometrine plus oxytocin, carboprost if necessary.
- To terminate pregnancy: gemeprost (by vaginal pessary).

Uterine relaxants: the main drugs used are β-adrenoceptor agonists, e.g. **ritodrine**. These are given to delay preterm labour.

THE MALE REPRODUCTIVE SYSTEM

The hormonal control of the male reproductive system is outlined in Fig. 17.10. FSH acts on Sertoli cells to nurture gametogenesis. Interstitial cell-stimulating hormone (ICSH, the equivalent of LH) stimulates the interstitial cells to secrete *androgens* such as **testosterone**, which controls gametogenesis and the secondary sexual characteristics. Testosterone is converted by 5α-reductase to dihydrotestosterone, which is the main active male sex hormone. As with the female sex steroids, the androgens act on nuclear receptors to modify transcription. Testosterone preparations are used for replacement therapy in testicular failure.

Anti-androgens These (e.g. flutamide) are used in the chemotherapy of prostate cancer.

Drugs used in erectile dysfunction

Penile erection occurs when sexual stimulation causes relaxation of the arteriolar and non-vascular smooth muscle of the corpora cavernosa. This allows inflow of blood into the tissue which, in turn, compresses the venules and occludes venous outflow. The resulting pressure of the blood causes an erection. Nitrergic nerves have a key role in the process (Fig. 17.11).

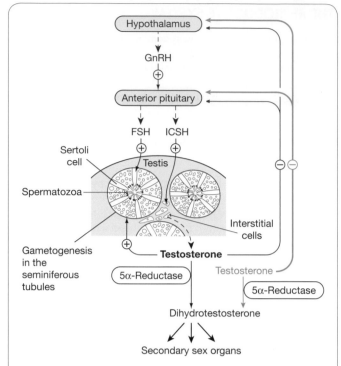

Fig. 17.10 Hormonal control of the male reproductive system and action of some drugs. *FSH,* Follicle-stimulating hormone; *ICSH,* interstitial cell-stimulating hormone.

Sildenafil

Sildenafil enhances penile erection in response to sexual stimulation but is also able to cause penile erection on its own. Its action in essence is the inhibition of phosphodiesterase type V, which normally reduces cyclic guanosine monophosphate (cGMP) concentration by converting it to 5'-GMP. The concentration of cGMP is increased, causing reduction of the contractile properties of smooth muscle and the promotion of its relaxation properties (Fig. 17.11). There is thus dilatation of the arterioles and relaxation of the trabecular smooth muscle, with the results described above.

Pharmacokinetic aspects Sildenafil is taken orally, giving a peak plasma concentration after 30–120 min unless absorption is delayed by food. It has the same mode of action as the organic nitrates (see Chapter 14) and so should not be used during therapy with these agents lest it exacerbates their effects.

Unwanted actions Unwanted actions are due to the action of the drug on other vascular beds and include a fall in blood pressure, headache and flushing.

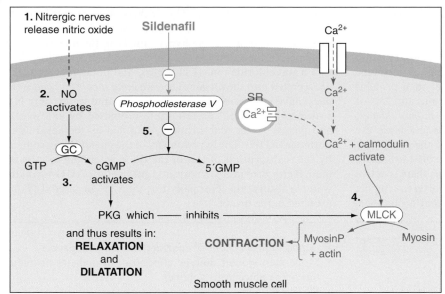

1. Nitrergic nerves release NO (see Chapter 14)

2. The released NO activates guanylate cyclase (GC) which increases cGMP

3. cGMP activates protein kinase G, which inhibits myosin light chain kinase (MLCK) which, with actin, would otherwise cause contraction (4). This action of PKG, along with actions that decrease intracellular calcium and increase K^+ conductance (not shown here, see Fig. 20.2) promotes relaxation of the smooth muscle

5. Normally cGMP is inactivated by phosphodiesterase V thus reducing cGMP concentration and promoting the contractile wing of the smooth muscle response

Sildenafil inhibits phosphodiesterase V, increasing cGMP and thus its relaxatory properties

Fig. 17.11   The mechanism of smooth muscle relaxation of the corpora cavernosa that is involved in penile erection, and the action of sildenafil in promoting this. In the figure the contractile elements that are inhibited by cyclic guanosine monophosphate (cGMP) are shown muted.

The main function of the kidney is the excretion of waste products; it is also important in the regulation of the salt and water content of the body and in acid–base balance. The main active transport mechanism in the renal tubule is the sodium pump (the Na^+/K^+ ATPase) in the basolateral membrane of the tubule cells. All the constituents of the plasma (other than protein) are filtered into the renal tubules at the glomerulus and 75% of the filtrate is reabsorbed isosmotically in the *proximal tubules*, bicarbonate in particular. Some organic acids and bases are secreted into the tubule. Water is absorbed in the *descending limb of the medullary loop* (Henle's loop). In the *thick ascending limb of the loop*, which is impermeable to water, there is active reabsorption of salt via a $Na^+/K^+/2Cl^-$ cotransporter (a symport in which transport of one ion is coupled to that of another) in the luminal membrane. This reabsorption of salt from the filtrate into the cells and from there into the interstitium is a major factor in producing hypertonicity in the interstitium in this area. In the *distal tubule*, more absorption of sodium ions (Na^+) and chloride ions (Cl^-) occurs, and potassium ions (K^+) are secreted into the filtrate. The *collecting tubule* and *collecting ducts* have low permeability to both salts and water; here Na^+ reabsorption and K^+ excretion are promoted by aldosterone and passive water reabsorption promoted by the antidiuretic hormone (ADH). The hypertonicity of the interstitium produced by the reabsorption of salt in the thick ascending loop is the main factor providing the osmotic gradient for ADH-mediated water reabsorption. Normally less than 1% of filtered Na^+ is excreted in the urine.

DRUGS ACTING ON THE KIDNEY

- Diuretics
- Drugs affecting urinary pH (see lower right of Fig. 18.1)
- Drugs that can alter the excretion of organic molecules: e.g. probenecid

Diuretics

Diuretics are drugs that increase Na^+ (and thus water) excretion by a direct action on the kidney. They do this mainly by reducing the absorption of salt from the filtrate, the increase in water loss being secondary to the increased salt loss.

Loop diuretics
Examples: **furosemide**, torasemide.

Pharmacological actions
- Very potent diuretics causing a profuse flow of urine
- K^+ and hydrogen ion (H^+) loss
- Decreased excretion of uric acid
- Increased excretion of calcium ions (Ca^{2+}) and magnesium ions (Mg^{2+})
- Moderate vasodilator effect

Mechanism of the diuretic action
See Fig. 18.1.

Pharmacokinetic aspects
Loop diuretics are given orally or intravenously (IV) and are secreted into the proximal tubule. The fraction not secreted is metabolized in the liver. Furosemide has a half-life of 90 min and a duration of action of 3–6 h. Torasemide has a longer half-life and duration of action.

Unwanted effects
The main unwanted effects of this drug class are:
- hypokalaemia owing to K^+ loss,
- metabolic alkalosis owing to H^+ loss,
- depletion of Ca^{2+} and Mg^{2+}, and
- depletion of the extracellular fluid volume resulting in hypotension.

High IV doses can cause deafness. Nausea and hypersensitivity reactions can occur.

Thiazides and related diuretics
Examples of thiazides: **Bendroflumethiazide** and **hydrochlorothiazide**; examples of the related agents are chlortalidone, xipamide and adipiodone (indapamide).

Pharmacological actions of thiazides and their congeners
- Moderately potent diuretic effect (but in diabetes insipidus, thiazides reduce urine volume)
- K^+ and H^+ loss
- Decreased excretion of uric acid
- Decreased excretion of Ca^{2+}
- Increased excretion of Mg^{2+}
- Moderate vasodilator effect

Mechanism of the diuretic action
See Fig. 18.1.

Pharmacokinetic aspects
Given orally, thiazides and related agents are secreted into the proximal tubule (Fig. 18.1). With most agents, the diuresis starts within 2 h and lasts 8–12 h. Chlortalidone has a longer duration of action.

Unwanted effects of thiazides and related agents
The main unwanted effects are a result of renal actions are:
- hypokalaemia due to K^+ loss,
- metabolic alkalosis due to H^+ loss, and
- increased plasma uric acid (gout thus a possibility).
Other unwanted effects include possible hyperglycaemia (a problem in diabetes mellitus), increased plasma cholesterol (with long-continued use), male impotence (reversible) and allergic reactions. A rare but serious adverse effect is hyponatraemia.

Potassium-sparing diuretics
Examples: amiloride, spironolactone and triamterene.

These have only limited diuretic action and all act in the distal tubule and collecting tubules, the sites for the control of K^+ homeostasis.

Spironolactone is given orally and is rapidly metabolized to an active metabolite, canrenone. The onset of action is slow. It is an antagonist of aldosterone, inhibiting the Na^+-retaining, K^+-excreting effect of aldosterone. Eplerenone is similar but shorter acting. As these drugs are steroid-like, unwanted actions on other steroid receptors outside of the renal system can occur, resulting in gynaecomastia, testicular problems and menstrual disorders.

Triamterene and amiloride are both given orally, triamterene having a more rapid onset and shorter duration of action than amiloride. These drugs inhibit Na^+ reabsorption and reduce K^+ excretion.

Unwanted effects
All three agents can cause hyperkalaemia and may cause acidosis.

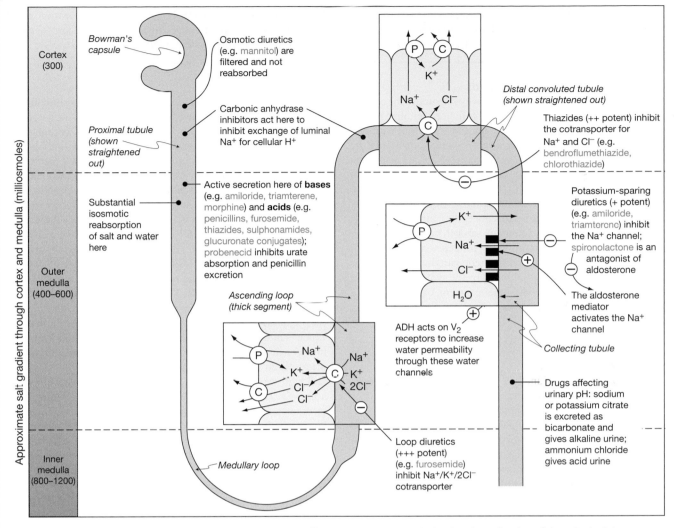

Fig. 18.1 Diagram of the nephron. The movement of ions in the main parts of the tubule, the sites of action of the principal drugs, some of the main agents secreted into the proximal tubule and the range of salt concentration from cortex to inner medulla are shown. *ADH*, Antidiuretic hormone; *C*, cotransporter; *P*, pump;.

Osmotic diuretics

Osmotic diuretics (e.g. **mannitol**) are drugs that pass into the tubules in the glomerulus and increase the osmotic pressure of the filtrate. They act mainly in the proximal tubule and the overall effect is to increase water excretion. They are usually given IV and the principal unwanted effects are a temporary expansion of the extracellular fluid compartment and hyponatraemia, resulting from osmotic extraction of intracellular water.

Clinical uses of diuretic agents

Simplified indication of clinical uses. The thickness of the lines indicates approximate importance.

Thiazides and related agents	Hypercalciuria
	Diabetes insipidus
	Hypertension
Loop diuretics	Oedema of chronic heart failure
	Acute pulmonary oedema
	Ascites
	Oliguria of renal failure
	Nephrotic syndrome
	Hypercalcaemia
Spironolactone	Hyperaldosteronism
Amiloride Triamterene	Maintenance of K+ balance with K+-losing diuretics
Mannitol	Cerebral oedema
	Increased intraocular pressure

The chief functions of respiration are to supply oxygen (O_2) and remove carbon dioxide (CO_2) from the body. The main disorders of the respiratory system are *asthma* and *chronic obstructive pulmonary disease* (COPD), but respiratory depression can be caused by overdosage of many drugs that have a depressive effect on the central nervous system (CNS).

Control of airway muscle and glands

Airway smooth muscle The upper airways are under the control of the parasympathetic nervous system with acetylcholine (ACh) acting on muscarinic M_3 receptors on airway smooth muscle leading to contraction. The lower airways can be constricted by excitatory non-adrenergic, non-cholinergic (NANC) transmitters (e.g. inflammatory peptides released from sensory neurons) and are relaxed by inhibitory NANC transmitters (e.g. nitric oxide). Airway smooth muscle contraction can also be inhibited by circulating adrenaline acting on β_2-adrenoceptors, although there is no sympathetic nerve supply to airway smooth muscle. However, sympathetic nerve fibres can indirectly influence airway smooth muscle tone by inhibiting parasympathetic ganglia.

Glands Mucus secretion is inhibited by the sympathetic system and is stimulated by the parasympathetic system, by inflammatory mediators and by chemical (e.g. air pollutants) and physical (e.g. cold air) stimuli.

ASTHMA

Asthma is a syndrome in which there are recurrent attacks of reversible airway obstruction – caused by bronchoconstriction and mucus secretion – occurring in response to stimuli that are not in themselves noxious due to underlying bronchial hyperresponsiveness. Asthma is recognized as a chronic inflammatory condition (Fig. 19.1) with an asthma attack being characterized by difficulty breathing out, wheezing and cough. Many asthmatics have associated allergic diseases, whilst others have so-called intrinsic asthma where allergy is not thought to play a major role. Certain subjects can also have asthma attacks precipitated by exposure to aspirin or tartrazine.

Drugs used in the treatment of asthma

Two main types of drug are used:
- Bronchodilators
- Anti-inflammatory agents

Bronchodilators

β_2-adrenoceptor agonists
Examples: **salbutamol** and terbutaline (both short acting, peak action in 30 min, duration 4–6 h) are used for symptomatic relief by relaxing airway smooth muscle. Longer acting β_2 agonists such as **salmeterol** (longer acting, duration 12 h) or indacaterol (duration 24 h) are used for maintenance treatment to prevent symptoms, usually administered in combination with an inhaled corticosteroid (see below).

Mechanism of action All act as physiological antagonists to counter the airway smooth muscle contraction induced by various spasmogenic mediators released during an asthma attack, e.g. histamine and cysteinyl-leukotrienes (Fig. 19.1). They have no effect on bronchial hyperresponsiveness or the inflammatory components of asthma.

Pharmacokinetic aspects Usually given by inhalation but can be given orally or by injection. Salbutamol can be given intravenously (IV) for the treatment of acute severe asthma.

Unwanted effects The main unwanted effect during asthma treatment is tremor. Other effects that can occur if the drugs are absorbed are given in Chapter 11, with hypokalemia and tachycardia being the most serious.

Xanthines
Examples: the methylxanthines **theophylline, doxophylline** and **aminophylline** (theophylline ethylene diamine).

Pharmacological actions Xanthines are now recognized as having both bronchodilator and anti-inflammatory actions.

Mechanism of action Xanthines have traditionally been considered to work as non-selective phosphodiesterase (PDE) inhibitors that result in an increase in cyclic nucleotides, cyclic adenosine monophosphate (cAMP) and cyclic guanosine monophosphate (cGMP). In airway smooth muscle it is the inhibition of PDE_3 that leads to relaxation, with inhibition of PDE_4 contributing to the anti-inflammatory effects of xanthines. Theophylline, but not doxophylline, is also known to act as an adenosine receptor antagonist, although this action is more likely the cause of the side effect profile of this drug.

Pharmacokinetic aspects Theophylline is given orally as a sustained-release preparation and acts for up to 24 h depending on the preparation. It is useful for nocturnal asthma. Aminophylline, which is more soluble, is given by a slow IV injection (at least 20 min) for the treatment of acute severe asthma. The xanthines are metabolized in the liver with a half-life of approximately 8 h, although this varies widely among individuals. Xanthines have a narrow therapeutic window with 5–10 ug/mL in plasma being recommended for maintenance treatment, although higher plasma levels are often required for acute bronchodilation. Above 20 ug/mL plasma levels serious side effects can occur (see below) and so measurement of plasma levels of theophylline is recommended. A number of drug-drug interactions occur with xanthines which can become clinically important in view of the narrow range of safe plasma concentrations. Some drugs increase the plasma xanthine concentration (e.g. oral contraceptives, erythromycin, ciprofloxacin, cimetidine, some calcium channel blockers), whilst some decrease it (e.g. rifampicin, carbamazepine).

Unwanted effects of the xanthines Xanthines have stimulant effects on the heart and the CNS and cause gastrointestinal (GI) tract disturbances. Xanthines are also mild diuretics and can cause sleep disturbance.

Muscarinic receptor antagonists
Muscarinic receptor antagonists are also used in the treatment of asthma. They antagonize the effects of ACh released from the parasympathetic nerves carried in vagus nerve X that innervate the lung and thus reduce airway smooth muscle contraction and mucous secretion. Short-acting muscarinic receptor antagonists are exemplified by **ipratropium bromide** are used for the acute treatment of asthma exacerbations, often in combination with salbutamol. Longer acting muscarinic receptor antagonists such as tiotropium bromide that have been widely used in the treatment of COPD are now being more frequently used in the treatment of asthma, often in combination with a long-acting β_2 agonist. This class of drug has no anti-inflammatory actions.

Cysteinyl leukotriene receptor antagonists and 5-lipoxygenase inhibitors
Montelukast blocks the $CysLT_1$ receptor and reduces the effects of leukotrienes released during an asthma attack. **Zileuton** is a 5-lipoxygenase inhibitor that inhibits the production of leukotrienes. These drugs are used in prevention of exercise

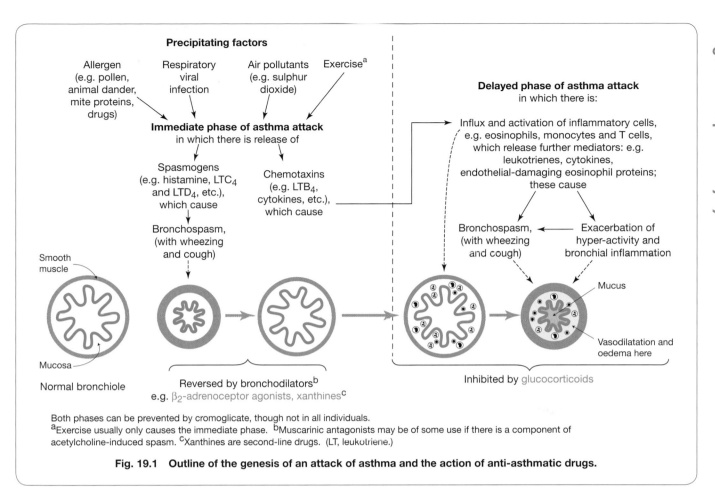

Fig. 19.1 Outline of the genesis of an attack of asthma and the action of anti-asthmatic drugs.

induced bronchospasm and are often used by paediatricians in patients who do not take their glucocorticoids (steroid phobia), although they have at best very modest anti-inflammatory actions. Montelukast is administered orally once daily and may provide additional improvement in lung function when used along with other drug classes. Unwanted effects include headache and GI tract disturbances.

Anti-inflammatory agents
Glucocorticoids
Examples used in the treatment of asthma include **beclomethasone diproprionate, budesonide,** fluticasone propionate and mometasone (all given by inhalation), **prednisolone** (given orally) and **hydrocortisone** (given IV for the treatment of acute severe asthma). These drugs are ineffective for relieving acute symptoms as they have no bronchodilator activity, but they are highly effective at reducing airway inflammation, particularly eosinophil infiltration. The mechanism of action is described in Chapter 16. Glucocorticoids also reduce the activation of inflammatory cells as well as the release of proinflammatory cytokines (Fig. 16.3) and other inflammatory mediators.

Unwanted effects Inhaled glucocorticoids may cause thrush (oropharyngeal candidiasis) and voice problems; spacing devices that reduce deposition of the drug in the pharynx and promote deposition in the smaller airways can ameliorate these effects. Systemic adverse effects (see Chapter 16) are rare with inhaled agents but can occur with regular large doses of oral agents.

Cromoglycate and nedocromil sodium
Mechanism of action Cromoglycate and nedocromil sodium are administered by inhalation of an aerosol or powder,

prophylactically to prevent allergic responses in the airways. It has been suggested that they work to reduce the release of inflammatory mediators from mast cells to reduce bronchoconstriction and airway inflammation, although they are not able to induce bronchodilation and so should not be used to treat acute attacks of asthma. These drugs are also able to inhibit the activation of sensory nerve fibres in the lung and can therefore reduce airway irritability and cough.

Unwanted effects These drugs have a very good safety profile but rarely cause irritation of the upper respiratory tract.

Antibody therapies Anti-immunoglobulin E (anti-IgE) and anti-interleukin-5 (anti-IL-5) antibodies may be administered by injection for patients with severe atopic asthma or certain eosinophilic asthma phenotypes and are described in Chapter 16.

Regimen for the treatment of asthma
Mild asthma is usually treated with inhaled β_2-agonists taken as required for symptomatic relief. With progressively more severe asthma, inhaled corticosteroids, long-acting β_2-agonists and xanthines are introduced on a prophylactic basis. Because of their more serious side effects, oral steroids are used only in severe asthma.

CHRONIC OBSTRUCTIVE PULMONARY DISEASE

COPD is a very common condition in which there is chronic inflammation of the airway that gives rise to chronic bronchitis and cough – at first intermittent, later chronic – with progressive breathlessness associated with the development of emphysema (damage to the alveoli) and eventually respiratory failure. Treatment is essentially palliative using muscarinic receptor antagonists such as the long-acting drug tiotropium bromide or the β_2-agonists discussed above. Increasingly these drugs are used in combination inhalers to provide dual bronchodilation or in so-called triple inhalers that also contain an inhaled corticosteroid. However, there is growing concern of the increased risk of pneumonia in patients with COPD treated regularly with inhaled steroids.

The orally active selective PDE_4 inhibitor roflumilast is used as add-on therapy to the standard of care described above to provide additional anti-inflammatory activity in patients with severe COPD.

Recent data have suggested that the orally active mucolytic agents N-acetyl-cysteine, erdosteine and carbocysteine have a role in reducing acute exacerbations in patients with mild to moderate COPD.

COUGH

Cough is usually caused by irritation (e.g. inflammation, neoplasia, COPD) in the bronchi and bronchioles. Antitussive drugs (drugs that relieve cough) include codeine (see Chapter 13),

dextromethorphan and levodropropizine, although the evidence for these drugs being effective is very poor.

Clinical use of drugs in airway disease

- β_2-receptor agonists: **Salbutamol** and the longer acting **salmeterol** are used:
  - to treat asthma, and
  - as palliative treatment in COPD.
- Methyl xanthines: Aminophylline is used with a glucocorticoid in asthma non-responsive to β_2-agonists. They can also be used in the treatment of acute severe asthma (status asthmaticus).
- Glucocorticoids: Beclomethasone diproprionate, budesonide, and prednisolone are anti-inflammatory drugs used to inhibit or prevent the inflammatory component that underlies asthma and COPD.
- Hydrocortisone given intravenously (IV) is used for acute severe asthma.

BONE METABOLISM

Bone is continuously remodelled throughout life, osteoclasts digesting it and osteoblasts laying down new bone (Fig. 20.1). Endogenous factors influencing the process include parathormone (PTH, parathyroid hormone), the vitamin D family, calcitonin and various cytokines. Exogenous factors include diet, exercise and drugs. Oestrogens, in particular, inhibit bone digestion. These factors are closely related to the control of calcium ion (Ca^{2+}) homeostasis.

Calcium homeostasis

In many cells, calcium influx into the cytoplasm is involved in signal transduction in many cell types and so plasma Ca^{2+} levels need to be controlled very precisely. Cytosolic $[Ca^{2+}]$ is about 100 nmol/L and plasma $[Ca^{2+}]$ is about 2.5 mmol/L. The factors controlling plasma $[Ca^{2+}]$ are outlined in Fig. 20.2.

Calcitonin

Calcitonin is produced by C cells in the thyroid follicles and its secretion is determined by plasma $[Ca^{2+}]$. Calcitonin decreases plasma $[Ca^{2+}]$ (Fig. 20.2).

Disorders of bone metabolism

- *Osteoporosis*: increased fragility resulting from distortion of the microarchitecture of bone. Main causes are postmenopausal oestrogen deficiency, excessive use of glucocorticoids or thyroxine.
- *Rickets*: defective bone mineralization caused by vitamin D deficiency.
- *Hypocalcaemia*: caused by hypoparathyroidism or vitamin D deficiency.
- *Hypercalcaemia*: caused by hyperparathyroidism and some cancers.
- *Hyperphosphataemia*: caused by renal failure.

Drugs used to treat disorders of bone metabolism
Bisphosphonates

Examples are disodium etidronate and alendronate.

These drugs prevent osteoclast-mediated bone resorption by inhibiting enzymes in the ruffled border (Fig. 20.1). In addition, bisphosphonates are incorporated into the bone matrix and ingested by the osteoclasts promoting osteoclast apoptosis.

Bisphosphonates are given orally (milk impairs absorption) and 50% of the absorbed drug concentrates at sites of bone mineralization for a long period of time.

Unwanted effects

Gastrointestinal (GI) tract disturbances (alendronate can cause oesophagitis) and bone pain.

The bone remodelling cycle:

Bone resorption

1. The precursor cell releases cytokines (e.g. interleukin-6 (IL-6)) that recruit osteoclasts (OCs). **Parathormone** (PTH) and vitamin D product **calcitriol** promote this; **bisphosphonates (BPs)** inhibit it

2. OCs digest bone, releasing embedded cytokines, particularly insulin-like growth factor (IGF). **Bisphosphonates** and **oestrogens** inhibit this action

Bone formation

3. IGF promotes the differentiation of osteoblasts (OBs) from precursor cells (not shown). Bone morphogenic proteins (BMPs) (osteogenic proteins) promote this; **glucocorticoids** in pharmacological concentrations inhibit it

4. IGF promotes the action of OBs in secreting osteoid (bone matrix), which consists mainly of collagen but also osteocalcin, phosphoproteins, etc. IGF molecules are embedded in the osteoid. **Glucocorticoids** in pharmacological concentrations inhibit this

5. Mineralization of the osteoid occurs (i.e. complex calcium phosphate crystals (hydroxyapatite) are deposited)

6. IL-6 released from OBs can recruit OCs (not shown) and the cycle can start again

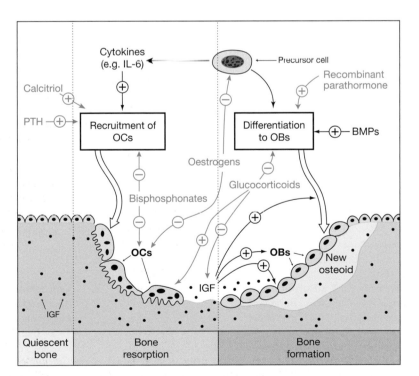

Fig. 20.1   The sequence of events in the bone remodelling cycle and the sites of action of drugs.

Clinical use of drugs affecting bone metabolism

Bisphosphonates
- Paget's disease of bone
- Malignant hypercalcaemia
- Postmenopausal osteoporosis (either alone or with oestrogens)
- Glucocorticoid-induced osteoporosis

Vitamin D
- Rickets
- Hypocalcaemia associated with hypoparathyroidism
- Osteodystrophy of renal failure

Calcitonin
- Paget's disease of bone
- Hypercalcaemia to lower blood calcium ion (Ca^{2+})
- Part of the treatment of glucocorticoid-induced osteoporosis

Calcium salts
- Hypocalcaemia (given orally)
- Hypocalcaemic tetany (given intravenously (IV))
- Postmenopausal osteoporosis (with oestrogen and calcitonin or a bisphosphonate)
- Hyperkalaemia-induced cardiac dysrhythmias

Cinacalcet
- Hyperparathyroidism

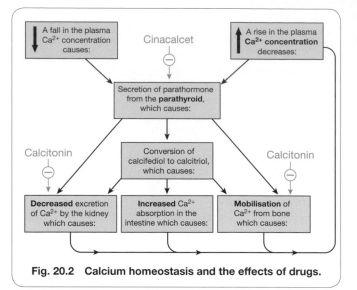

Fig. 20.2   Calcium homeostasis and the effects of drugs.

The vitamin D family

Vitamin D is a prehormone that is metabolized to give several biologically active substances (Fig. 20.3), the main ones being *calcifediol*, which is the principal metabolite in the plasma (not shown), and the more biologically potent *calcitriol*. These are considered true hormones.

The vitamin D in the body is derived from the following:
- Dietary ergosterol obtained from plants (gives rise to vitamin D_2).
- Cholesterol gives rise to 7-dehydrocholesterol, which, in the skin, is converted to cholecalciferol (vitamin D_3) (Fig. 20.3). The cholecalciferol enters the liver where it is converted to calcifediol (a secosteroid, a steroid in which one of the rings has undergone fission); this, in turn, is converted to calcitriol (also a secosteroid) in the kidney.

Factors controlling the synthesis of calcitriol
- Negative feedback control by plasma calcitriol.
- PTH secretion of this being controlled by the plasma $[Ca^{2+}]$ and the calcitriol level in the blood.
- The plasma phosphate concentration (not shown in Fig. 20.3).

Actions
The main action is the maintenance of plasma $[Ca^{2+}]$ which involves:
- increasing Ca^{2+} absorption in the intestine,
- mobilizing Ca^{2+} from bone, and
- decreasing renal Ca^{2+} excretion.

Preparations and unwanted effects
Ergocalciferol (vitamin D_2) is the main drug used. It is given orally and needs bile salts for absorption because it is fat soluble. **Calcitriol** and alfacalcidol are also available and can be administered orally or by injection.

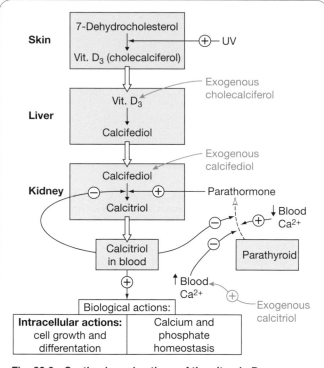

Fig. 20.3   Synthesis and actions of the vitamin D hormones.

Calcitonin
The preparations for clinical use are salcatonin (synthetic) and calcitonin (natural porcine). They are given subcutaneously (SC), IV or by nasal spray.

Calcium salts
Preparations used therapeutically include calcium gluconate, calcium lactate and hydroxyapatite. They are administered orally, and unwanted effects include gut disturbances.

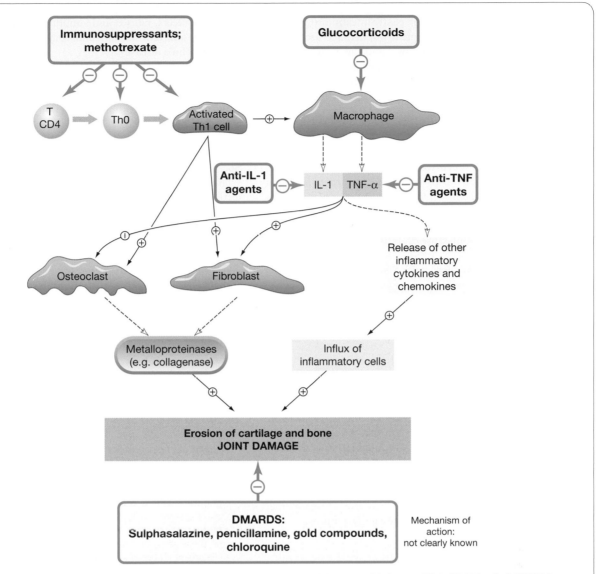

Fig. 20.4 The pathogenesis of rheumatoid joint damage and the action of antirheumatoid drugs. *CD4*, CD4 T cell; *DMARDS*, disease modifying antirheumatic drugs; *IL-1*, interleukin-1; *T*, T cell; *Th0*, T helper type 0 cell; *Th1*, T helper type 1 cell; *TNF*, tumour necrosis factor.

Cinacalcet

This is a calcimimetic compound that activates the calcium-sensing receptor in parathyroid cells decreasing secretion of parathormone (Fig. 20.2).

Drugs affecting skeletal muscle contraction

Nicotinic receptor and antagonists that inhibit the actions of acetylcholine (ACh) at the skeletal muscle junction and other drugs influencing cholinergic transmission at the skeletal neuromuscular junction are discussed in Chapter 11.

Drugs affecting joints

Drugs influencing diseases of joints such as rheumatoid arthritis are summarized in Fig. 20.4 and discussed fully in Chapter 16.

21 Drugs and the gastrointestinal tract

The main physiological aspects of gastrointestinal (GI) tract function that are of pharmacological importance are gastric acid secretion, the motility of the bowel and the excretion of its contents; the main pathophysiological conditions of the GI tract are peptic ulcers, nausea and vomiting, diarrhoea, constipation, gallstones and chronic inflammatory bowel disease (ulcerative colitis, Crohn's disease).

GASTRIC SECRETION AND PEPTIC ULCER

Pathogenesis of peptic ulcer
In peptic ulceration the balance between mucosal-damaging processes (excessive secretion of acid and pepsin) and mucosal-protective mechanisms (secretion of bicarbonate and mucus) is altered. The bacillus *Helicobacter pylori* is likely to be a major cause of the swing towards mucosal damage by increasing gastrin secretion. Nonsteroidal anti-inflammatory drugs (NSAIDs) are an additional important cause of gastric ulceration.

Drugs used to treat peptic ulcer, with their mechanisms of action
The main approaches are (1) to reduce acid secretion (this is the most important), (2) to treat *H. pylori* infection and (3) to protect the gastric mucosa.

Drugs used to reduce acid secretion (Fig. 21.1)
- Histamine H_2 antagonists (e.g. **cimetidine**, **ranitidine**) or proton pump inhibitors (e.g. **omeprazole**) are the most effective agents.
- Selective muscarinic M_1 antagonists (e.g. **pirenzepine**) also reduce acid secretion, but less effectively than H_2 antagonists. (There are no clinically useful gastrin antagonists.)
- Antacids (e.g. **magnesium trisilicate, aluminium hydroxide**) simply neutralize the acid in the stomach.
- **Misoprostol**, a prostaglandin $(PGE)_2$ analogue, not only reduces gastric acid secretion, but may also increase bicarbonate and mucus secretion by epithelial cells. Its main use is to counteract the damaging effects of NSAIDs on the gastric mucosa.

Drugs used to treat H. pylori infection
H. pylori infection is treated with a combination of a proton pump inhibitor or H_2 antagonist with two antibiotics (**amoxicillin** is commonly used with either **metronidazole** or **clarithromycin**). **Bismuth** chelate, which has an antibacterial action plus a mucosa-protective effect, can also be used.

Drugs used to protect the gastric mucosa
Sucralfate (a complex of aluminium hydroxide and sulphated sucrose) can form complex gels with mucus to enhance its protective effect on the mucosa. Bismuth chelate is also protective.

Pharmacokinetic aspects and unwanted actions
H_2 antagonists are readily absorbed after oral administration. Both cimetidine and ranitidine can inhibit renal tubular secretion of basic drugs. Cimetidine, importantly, can inhibit cytochrome P450 and so potentiate the actions of many drugs including oral anticoagulants, phenytoin and aminophylline. Omeprazole has a half-life of only 1 h but its concentration in the parietal cell canaliculus allows its action to persist for 2–3 days. Most of a sucralfate dose remains in the gut, where it can reduce the absorption of other drugs (e.g. digoxin, tetracycline and theophylline).

Clinical use of anti-emetic drugs

- 5-hydroxytryptamine ($5-HT_3$) receptor antagonists (e.g. **ondansetron**): Emesis caused by cancer chemotherapy agents (drugs of choice), postoperative and radiation-induced vomiting.
- Dopamine D_2 receptor antagonists (e.g. **domperidone, phenothiazines**): Emesis caused by uraemia, radiation, gastrointestinal (GI) tract disorders, viral gastroenteritis.
- Muscarinic receptor antagonists (e.g. **scopolamine**): motion sickness (drug of choice).
- Histamine H_1 receptor antagonists: **cyclizine** (motion sickness), **cinnarizine** (Ménière's disease).
- Cannabinoids (e.g. nabilone): Emesis caused by cytotoxic drugs.

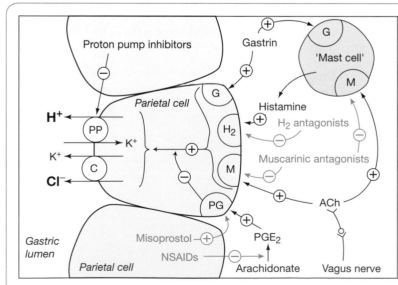

Control of acid secretion

HCl is secreted by the parietal cells within the gastric glands and passes into the stomach lumen producing a pH of ~1. Secretion is stimulated by histamine H_2 receptors, acting via an increase in cAMP within the cell, and by acetylcholine (ACh) and gastrin acting on muscarinic and gastrin receptors, respectively. ACh and gastrin may act directly on the parietal cell (increasing cell $[Ca^{2+}]$) (one-cell hypothesis) or can act indirectly via release of histamine from mast cell-like cells (two-cell hypothesis). Rises in cAMP and $[Ca^{2+}]$ in the parietal cell activate a proton pump (PP), which exchanges H^+ in the cell with K^+ in the lumen of the gastric gland. The cotransporter (C) moves Cl^- into the lumen with K^+. Activation of prostaglandin receptors (possibly EP_3) by PGE_2 inhibits HCl secretion.

Fig. 21.1 Control of acid secretion and drug actions. *ACh,* Acetylcholine; *NSAIDs,* nonsteroidal anti-inflammatory drugs; *PGE₂,* prostaglandin E₂.

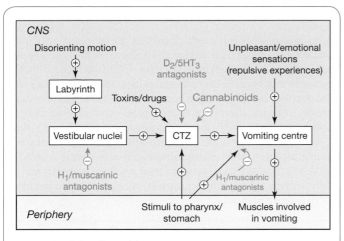

Fig. 21.2 Stimuli resulting in emesis and the action of anti-emetic drugs. *CNS*, Central nervous system; *CTZ*, chemoreceptor trigger zone; *HT*, hydroxytryptamine.

EMESIS AND ANTI-EMETIC DRUGS

Pathophysiology

Vomiting is a complex act involving the coordinated activity of the involuntary muscles of the GI tract and the somatic respiratory and abdominal muscles. It is controlled by two centres in the medulla:
- the vomiting centre, and
- the chemoreceptor trigger zone (CTZ).

Many stimuli can give rise to emesis (Fig. 21.2):
- Input from higher centres, e.g. repulsive sights or smells, pain, emotional factors
- Impulses from the labyrinths and/or vestibular nuclei (e.g. in motion sickness, Ménière's disease)
- Endogenous blood-borne factors (e.g. in uraemia)
- Drugs (e.g. cancer chemotherapy agents, particularly platinum salts); the toxic effects of many drugs result in nausea and emesis
- Stimuli acting in the pharynx or stomach

The main receptors involved in the control of vomiting include histamine H_1, muscarinic, dopamine D_2 and 5-hydroxytryptamine (5-HT_3). Opioid, neurokinin-1 and endocannabinoid receptors may also have a role.

Anti-emetic drugs

The selection of agents depends on the cause of vomiting and in particular on the relative importance of the vestibular nuclei, CTZ and vomiting centre:
- Older H_1 antagonists (e.g. cyclizine, promethazine, cinnarizine):
  - effective against vestibular apparatus stimuli and local gut stimuli, and
  - ineffective against direct CTZ stimuli.
- Muscarinic receptor antagonists (e.g. **scopolamine**, **hyoscine**):
  - effective against vestibular apparatus stimuli and local gut stimuli, and
  - ineffective against CTZ stimuli.
- D_2 antagonists (e.g. **prochlorperazine, domperidone**, metoclopramide):
  - effective against CTZ stimuli, and
  - ineffective against local gut stimuli.
- 5-HT_3 antagonists (e.g. **ondansetron**, granisetron):
  - effective against CTZ stimuli, and

- effective against local gut stimuli.
- Cannabinoids (e.g. **nabilone**) inhibit the effect of CTZ stimulants.
- Neurokinin antagonists (e.g. **aprepitant**) used with dexamethasone or 5-HT_3 antagonists to control nausea and emesis associated with chemotherapy.

> **Summary of drugs used to treat peptic ulcer**
>
> - Histamine H_2 antagonists: **cimetidine**, ranitidine.
> - Proton pump inhibitors: **omeprazole**.
> - Antacids: **magnesium trisilicate, aluminium hydroxide**.
> - Antibacterial agents effective against *H. pylori*: **clarithromycin, metronidazole, amoxicillin, bismuth chelate**.
> - Mucosal protectants: **sucralfate**, bismuth chelate.

Pharmacokinetic aspects and unwanted effects of anti-emetics

H_1 receptor antagonists such as scopolamine can be taken orally to prevent nausea, but once vomiting ensues there is obviously a difficulty in using this route. Transdermal preparations of hyoscine have been developed that circumvent this problem, particularly for the treatment of motion sickness. H_1 receptor antagonists such as scopolamine cause drowsiness and scopolamine has many other side effects owing to its muscarinic receptor antagonistic activity inhibiting the parasympathetic nervous system (e.g. dry mouth, blurring of vision). The D_2 antagonists can be given orally, rectally or parenterally. Important side effects are the extrapyramidal effects on movement and increased prolactin release, resulting in galactorrhoea. GI disturbances can occur. Domperidone has fewer extrapyramidal effects because of its reduced penetration of the blood–brain barrier.

OTHER GASTROINTESTINAL CONDITIONS

Diarrhoea

Diarrhoea caused by infectious agents (*Escherichia coli, Campylobacter*) will only require the use of antibiotics if severe. However, replacement of fluid and electrolytes is essential. Opiates and, less usefully, muscarinic receptor antagonists are used to reduce GI motility. Of the opiates, **loperamide** and **diphenoxylate** are used in preference to **codeine** because they have less action on the central nervous system (CNS). Opiates also have an antisecretory action.

Constipation

Bulk laxatives (e.g. dietary cellulose (bran) or methylcellulose) are not digested and increase the mass of material in the gut lumen so stimulating peristalsis. Osmotic purgatives (e.g. **magnesium sulphate**, lactulose) are not absorbed and retain water, by osmotic action, in the gut – the increased fluid volume stimulating peristalsis. Stimulant purgatives act by increasing mucosal secretion or by stimulating enteric nerves. Senna is a natural product containing anthracene derivatives that are metabolized by bacteria in the colon to produce the active stimulants.

Gallstones

Non-calcified cholesterol gallstones can be dissolved by oral administration of the bile acid ursodeoxycholic acid, which reduces the synthesis and secretion of cholesterol.

BENIGN PROSTATIC HYPERPLASIA

In men the most common cause of urinary retention is benign prostatic hyperplasia (BPH), due to the blocking of flow of urine out of the bladder. There are three classes of drugs used to treat BPH:
- Alpha1 receptor antagonists (alpha blockers)
- Parasympathomimetics
- Anti-androgens

Alpha blockers

Doxazosin and prazosin are alpha blockers that act by relaxing the smooth muscle at the opening of the urethra, increasing the flow of urine into the bladder. These drugs are generally well tolerated but can cause postural hypotension.

Parasympathomimetics

Bethanechol is a muscarinic receptor agonist that causes detrusor muscle contraction and the effect of this drug is most marked when there is bladder outlet obstruction, but it has no role in the relief of acute urinary retention. Muscarinic receptor agonists can produce a number of side effects including sweating, bradycardia and intestinal colic.

Anti-androgens

Finasteride is a specific inhibitor of 5 alpha reductase, an enzyme that converts testosterone to the more potent androgen, dihydrotestosterone, which leads to a reduction in prostate size and thus improves the flow of urine.

URINARY INCONTINENCE

Urinary incontinence is the involuntary leakage of urine and there are three main types:
- True incontinence (fistulous track)
- Stress incontinence (due to an incompetent sphincter)
- Urge incontinence (due to instability of the detrusor muscle)

Urge incontinence is the only cause that can be treated with drugs and the main drug class used for this purpose are muscarinic receptor antagonists. **Oxybutynin** is the most widely used drug, although newer examples are solifenacin and tolterodine. These drugs relax the detrusor muscle of the bladder and are usually administered orally. The side effects are those typical of muscarinic receptor antagonists such as dry mouth, constipation and blurred vision.

Duloxetine is a serotonin/noradrenaline uptake inhibitor which can be used to treat stress incontinence. Desmopressin is an ADH analogue used as a nasal spray to treat nocturnal enuresis and the selective beta agonist mirabegron has also been used as a treatment of overactive bladder.

ERECTILE DYSFUNCTION

Erectile dysfunction (impotence) can be caused as a side effect of certain drugs such as anti-hypertensives and as a complication of cardiovascular diseases such as diabetes and atherosclerosis. Following the discovery of nitric oxide as a neurotransmitter, it was established that the non-adrenergic, non-cholinergic (NANC) (nitrergic) neurotransmission is able to promote vasodilation in the corpus cavernosum leading to an erection. Nitric oxide elicits vasodilation by increasing cyclic guanosine monophosphate (cGMP) levels in vascular smooth muscle cells. cGMP is metabolized by phosphodiesterase 5 and inhibiting this enzyme leads to elevated levels of cGMP which in patients with reduced nitrergic transmission (e.g. patients with diabetes) leads to an erection that may otherwise not have been possible. The most widely used phosphodiesterase $(PDE)_5$ inhibitor is **sildenafil**, although vardenafil is a longer acting example of this drug class that has revolutionized the treatment of erectile dysfunction. Due to their mechanism of action, PDE_5 inhibitors must never be used with nitrovasodilators. Furthermore, sildenafil can also inhibit PDE_6 which is present in the retina and this can lead to colour disturbances in some patients' vision.

Papaverine, a non-selective PDE inhibitor, and the prostaglandin E1 (PGE_1) analogue alprostadil can be injected directly into the corpus cavernosum to cause vasodilation and an erection.

The most common skin diseases are dermatitis (eczema), acne, psoriasis, skin cancer (usually managed surgically), viral warts and urticarias (which can be allergic or non-allergic in nature).

DERMATITIS (ECZEMA)

Eczema is an inflammatory disease of the skin, defined by the presence of epidermal intercellular oedema or spongiosis, and can be the result of:
- exogenous irritants and contact allergens,
- infections, or
- adverse responses to certain drugs.

Drugs used to treat dermatitis and their targets are shown in Fig. 23.1.

ACNE

Acne affects the pilosebaceous unit and occurs in anatomical sites where these are most numerous, such as on the face, back and chest. Acne is characterized by the presence of keratin plugs in the sebaceous duct openings, known as *comedones*. Acne may also involve the presence of inflammatory papules, pustules, nodules, cysts and scars. Acne is stimulated by androgens, which is why it usually occurs in puberty, and why the antiandrogen cyproterone is often used in females with acne (see Chapter 17 for an understanding of drugs and endocrine function). The drugs used to treat acne and their targets are shown in Fig. 23.2.

PSORIASIS

Psoriasis is a genetic skin disorder that can be precipitated by stress, infection, damage from ultraviolet light or trauma. In psoriasis, the turnover rate of skin is much greater than normal, and this disease is characterized by the following:
- Thickened skin plaques
- Superficial scales
- Dilated capillaries in the dermis (these might act to initiate psoriasis or as nourishment for hyperproliferating skin)
- An infiltrate of inflammatory cells, especially lymphocytes and neutrophils, in the epidermis and dermis, respectively

Drugs used to treat psoriasis and their targets are shown in Fig. 23.3.

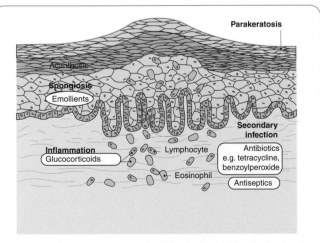

Fig. 23.1 Characteristics of eczema and point of action of its drug treatment. (Modified from Page C, Curtis M, Walker M, Hoffman B. *Integrated Pharmacology*. 3rd ed. Philadelphia: Elsevier; 2006.)

TREATMENT OF SKIN DISORDERS

Preparations of topical drugs for use on skin

Drugs applied to the skin are delivered by a variety of vehicles such as ointments, creams, pastes, powders, aerosols, gels, lotions and tinctures. The choice of the vehicle is dependent on a number of factors:
- The solubility of the active drug
- The ability of the drug to penetrate the skin
- The stability of the drug-vehicle complex
- The ability of the vehicle to delay evaporation, this being greatest for ointments and least for tinctures

Emollients

Emollients are used to soothe and hydrate the skin. A simple preparation is an aqueous cream, which is often as effective as more complex drugs. Most creams are thin emollients, whereas a mixture of equal parts soft white paraffin and liquid paraffin is a thick emollient. Camphor, menthol and phenol preparations have antipruritic effects, whereas zinc-based and titanium-based emollients have mild astringent (contracting) effects.

Mechanism of action – Emollients hydrate the skin and reduce transepidermal water loss.

Route of administration – Topical. Many emollients can be added to bath water.

Indications – Emollients are used for the long-term treatment of dry scaling disorders and should be used liberally in the management of eczema and psoriasis.

Contraindications – None.

Adverse effects – Some ingredients, such as lanolin or antibacterials, may induce an allergic reaction.

Corticosteroids

Examples of corticosteroids include clobetasol propionate, betamethasone, clobetasol butyrate and hydrocortisone (Table 23.1).

Mechanism of action – Corticosteroids suppress many aspects of the inflammatory reaction by both genomic effects (e.g. to reduce the synthesis of proinflammatory cytokines) and non-genomic (acute vasoconstriction to reduce "redness") (see Chapter 16 and Fig. 16.3).

Route of administration – Topical because of many adverse effects when administered systemically (see below); oral, intradermal or intravenous in severe disease.

Indications – Corticosteroids are used for the relief of symptoms associated with inflammatory conditions of the skin other than those caused by infection.

Contraindications – Rosacea, untreated skin infections.

Adverse effects – Most likely to occur with prolonged or high dose therapy. Local: spread or worsening of infection, thinning of the skin, impaired wound healing, irreversible striae atrophicae. Systemic: immunosuppression, peptic ulceration, osteoporosis, hypertension, cataracts.

Please note that withdrawal of corticosteroids after high doses or prolonged use should be gradual, even when used topically.

Dithranol

Dithranol is the most potent topical drug for the treatment of psoriasis.

Mechanisms of action – Dithranol modifies keratinization and has an immunosuppressive effect.

113

Route of administration – Topical.

Contraindications – Dithranol should not be given to people with hypersensitivity or acute and pustular psoriasis.

Adverse effects – Local skin irritation, staining of skin and hair.

Vitamin D analogues

Calcipotriol and tacalcitol are vitamin D analogue derivatives. Vitamin D analogues are keratolytics.

Mechanism of action – Inhibition of epidermal proliferation and induction of terminal keratinocyte differentiation.

Vitamin D analogues are also anti-inflammatory and inhibit T-cell proliferation and cytokine release, decrease the capacity of monocytes to stimulate T-cell proliferation and stimulate cytokine release from T cells. They can also inhibit neutrophil accumulation into psoriatic skin.

Route of administration – Topical.

Indications – Psoriasis.

Contraindications – Vitamin D analogues should not be given to people with disorders of calcium metabolism. They should not be used on the face because irritation may occur.

Adverse effects – Side effects of vitamin D analogues include local irritation and dermatitis. High doses may affect calcium homeostasis.

Tar preparations

Coal tar is made up of about 10,000 components, is keratolytic and is more potent than salicylic acid. It also has anti-inflammatory and antipruritic properties.

Mechanism of action – Coal tar modifies keratinization, but the mechanism is unclear (Fig. 23.3).

Route of administration – Topical.

Indications – Psoriasis and occasionally eczema.

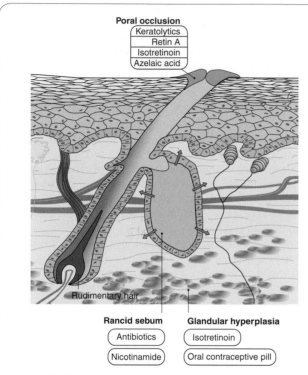

Fig. 23.2   Characteristics of acne and point of action of its drug treatment. (Modified from Page C, Curtis M, Walker M, Hoffman B. *Integrated Pharmacology*. 3rd ed. Philadelphia: Elsevier; 2006.)

Table 23.1   Potency of Some Topical Steroids (UK Classification and Nomenclature)

Group	Approved name	Proprietary name
I (very potent)	Clobetasol propionate	Dermovate
II (potent)	Betametasone valerate 0.1%	Betnovate
	Beclometasone dipropionate	Propaderm
	Hydrocortisone 17-butyrate	Locoid
III (moderately potent)	Clobetasone butyrate	Eumovate
IV (mild)	Hydrocortisone 1%	Various
	Hydrocortisone 2%	Various

Modified from Graham-Brown R and Bourke J. *Mosby's Color Atlas and Text of Dermatology*. St. Louis: Mosby; 1998.

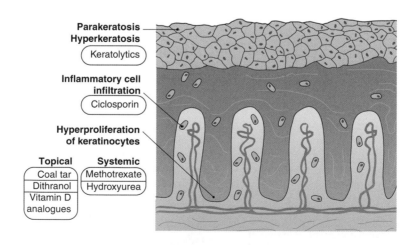

Fig. 23.3   Characteristics of psoriasis and point of action of its drug treatment. (Modified from Page C, Curtis M, Walker M, Hoffman B. *Integrated Pharmacology*. 3rd ed. Philadelphia: Elsevier; 2006.)

Contraindications – Coal tar should not be given to people with acute or pustular psoriasis or in the presence of an infection. It should not be used on the face or on broken or inflamed skin.

Adverse effects – Skin irritation and acne-like eruptions, photosensitivity, staining of the skin and hair.

Salicylates

Salicylic acid is keratolytic at a concentration of 3% to 6%.

Mechanism of action – Salicylic acid causes desquamation of the skin via the solubilization of cell-surface proteins that maintain the integrity of the stratum corneum.

Route of administration – Topical.

Indications – Hyperkeratosis, eczema, psoriasis (combined with coal tar or dithranol preparations) and acne, wart and callus eradication.

Contraindications – Sensitivity to the drug or broken or inflamed skin. High concentrations, such as those needed to treat warts, should not be given to people with diabetes mellitus or peripheral vascular disease because ulceration may be induced.

Adverse effects – Side effects of salicylic acid include anaphylactic shock in those sensitive to the drug, skin irritation and excessive drying. Salicylic acid can also have systemic effects if used long-term.

Other drugs used in skin disease

Several specific biologics that selectively target interleukins (IL) (e.g. ustekinumab that targets IL-12 for psoriasis) or tumour necrosis factor (TNF) (adalimumab or etanercept) are used in the treatment of psoriasis. In addition, apremilast, an orally active phosphodiesterase 4 inhibitor, has recently been approved for the treatment of severe psoriasis and psoriatic arthritis.

Treatment of Allergic Skin Disorders

Allergic reactions occur when the immune system mounts an inappropriate response to an innocuous foreign substance. Most common allergic disorders are caused by immunoglobulin E (IgE) – so-called mediated type I immediate hypersensitivity reactions that occur in a previously sensitized person re-exposed to the sensitizing antigen. Type I immediate hypersensitivity reactions are also known as atopic disorders. Patients with atopic diseases have an inherited predisposition to develop IgE antibodies to allergens that are normally innocuous in healthy subjects. These specific IgE antibodies become bound to high-affinity IgE receptors (FceRI) on the surface of tissue mast cells and blood basophils. The cross-linking of this cell-surface-bound IgE by antigen (allergens), on subsequent exposure, induces degranulation and release of mediators such as histamine, leukotrienes and prostaglandins. The released vasoactive and inflammatory mediators produce many local and systemic effects, including vasodilatation, increased vascular permeability, smooth muscle contraction, oedema, glandular hypersecretion and inflammatory cell infiltration.

Drug therapy of allergic disorders

The most effective therapy in hypersensitivity reaction is avoidance of the offending antigen or environment. When this is not possible, drug therapy can be used.

Histamine and H₁-receptor antagonists (antihistamines)

Histamine is a basic amine that is stored in mast cells and in circulating basophils; it is also found in the stomach and central nervous system (CNS). The effects of histamine are

Table 23.2 Effects at Histamine Receptors

Histamine receptor	Effect
H_1	Responsible for most of the actions of histamine in a type I hypersensitivity reaction: <ul><li>Capillary and venous dilatation (producing 'flare' or systemic hypotension)</li><li>Increased vascular permeability (producing 'wheal' or oedema)</li><li>Contraction of smooth muscle (producing bronchial and gastrointestinal contraction)</li></ul>
H_2	Regulation of gastric acid secretion: <ul><li>H_2-receptors respond to histamine secreted from the enterochromaffin-like cells that are adjacent to the parietal cell.</li></ul>
H_3	Involved in neurotransmission: <ul><li>The exact physiological role is not clear but there may be presynaptic inhibition of neurotransmitter release in the central and autonomic nervous system affecting itch and pain perception.</li></ul>

From Page C. *Crash Course: Pharmacology*. 5th ed. Philadelphia: Elsevier; 2019.

mediated by three different receptor types found on target cells (Table 23.2). As the major chemical mediator released during an allergic reaction, histamine produces a number of effects, mainly via action on H_1-receptors. Therefore H_1 antagonists (antihistamines) are of potential benefit in the treatment of allergic disorders.

H₁-receptor antagonists: antihistamines

There are two main types of H_1-receptor antagonists:
- 'Older' drugs that cross the blood brain barrier and therefore cause sedation, for example, chlorphenamine and promethazine.
- 'Newer' nonsedative types, for example, cetirizine and loratadine.

Mechanism of action – Antagonism of histamine H_1-receptors.

Indications – H_1 receptor antagonists are used for the treatment and prevention of allergic skin reactions such as urticarial rashes, pruritus and insect bites, and in the emergency treatment of anaphylactic shock. The older sedating H_1-receptor antagonists can also be used to reduce itching and scratching in young children with severe eczema.

Route of administration – Oral or topical. Intravenous chlorphenamine can be used in anaphylaxis.

Adverse effects – Older H_1 receptor antagonists produce quite pronounced sedation or fatigue, as well as anticholinergic effects such as dry mouth. The newer agents that do not cross the blood–brain barrier do this less.

Immunosuppressants

Deliberate pharmacological suppression of the immune system is used in the following three main clinical areas:
- To suppress inappropriate autoimmune responses (e.g. systemic lupus erythematosus or rheumatoid arthritis), where the host immune system is attacking host tissue.
- To suppress host immune rejection responses to donor organ grafts or transplants.
- To suppress donor immune responses against host antigens (prevention of graft-versus-host disease (GVHD) after bone marrow transplant).

The main pharmacological agents used for immunosuppression are as following:

- Calcineurin inhibitors
- Antiproliferatives
- Glucocorticoids (see Chapter 16).

Solid organ transplant patients require immunosuppression to prevent organ rejection. They are usually maintained on a corticosteroid combined with a calcineurin inhibitor (cyclosporine) or with an antiproliferative drug (azathioprine or mycophenolate mofetil), or with both.

Calcineurin inhibitors

The main drug in this class is cyclosporine.

Mechanism of action – Cyclosporine is a cyclic peptide, derived from fungi, that has powerful immunosuppressive activity. It has a selective inhibitory effect on T cells by inhibiting the T-cell receptor (TCR)-mediated signal transduction pathway. It is believed to exert its actions after entering the T cell and preventing the transcription of specific genes (Fig. 23.4). After entry into the T cell, cyclosporine specifically binds to its cytoplasmic binding protein,

cyclophilin. This cyclosporine-cyclophilin complex then binds to a serine-threonine phosphatase called calcineurin, inhibiting its phosphatase activity. Calcineurin is normally activated when intracellular calcium ion levels rise following TCR binding to the appropriate major histocompatibility complex: antigen complex. When calcineurin is active, it dephosphorylates the cytoplasmic component of the nuclear factor of activated T cells (NF-ATc) into a form that migrates to the nucleus and induces transcription of genes such as IL-2 that are involved in T-cell activation. Inhibition of calcineurin by the cyclosporine-cyclophilin complex therefore prevents the nuclear translocation of NF-ATc and the transcription of certain genes essential for the activation of T cells. Hence the production of IL-2 by T-helper cells, the maturation of cytotoxic T cells and the production of some other cytokines, such as interferon-Υ, are all inhibited. The overall action of cyclosporine is to suppress reversibly both cell-mediated and antibody-specific adaptive immune responses.

Indications – Cyclosporine is used for the prevention of graft and transplant rejection, and prevention of GVHD.

Route of administration – Oral, intravenous.

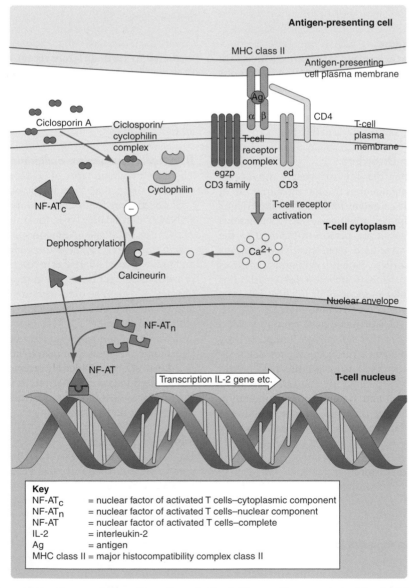

Fig. 23.4 Cyclosporine and T-cell suppression. (From Page C. *Crash Course: Pharmacology*. 5th ed. Philadelphia: Elsevier; 2019.)

Adverse effects – Unlike most immunosuppressive agents, cyclosporine does not cause myelosuppression. However, it is markedly nephrotoxic to the proximal tubule of the kidney, and renal damage almost always occurs. This may be reversible or permanent. Hypertension occurs in 50% of people. Less serious side effects include mild hepatotoxicity, anorexia, lethargy, gastrointestinal upsets, hirsutism and gum hypertrophy.

Therapeutic notes – Cyclosporine is often used as part of a post-transplantation triple therapy regimen with oral corticosteroids and azathioprine.

Antiproliferatives
Azathioprine
Mechanism of action – Azathioprine is a prodrug that is converted into the active component 6-mercaptopurine in the liver. Mercaptopurine is a fraudulent purine nucleotide that impairs DNA synthesis and has a cytotoxic action on dividing cells.

Indications – Azathioprine is used for the prevention of graft and transplant rejection and autoimmune conditions when corticosteroid therapy alone is inadequate.

Route of administration – Oral, intravenous.

Adverse effects – Side effects of azathioprine include bone marrow suppression, which can lead to leucopoenia, thrombocytopenia and sometimes anaemia. This is often the dose-limiting side effect. Increased susceptibility to infections (often opportunistic pathogens), and to certain cancers (lymphomas) can occur. Common side effects include gastrointestinal disturbances, nausea, vomiting and diarrhoea. Alopecia may be partial or complete but is usually reversible. Drug interaction with allopurinol necessitates lowering the dose of azathioprine.

Therapeutic notes – Azathioprine is used as part of a posttransplantation triple therapy regime with oral corticosteroids.

Mycophenolate mofetil
Mechanism of action – Mycophenolate mofetil is rapidly hydrolysed to mycophenolic acid, which is the active metabolite. Mycophenolic acid is a potent, uncompetitive and reversible inhibitor of inosine monophosphate dehydrogenase, and therefore inhibits the pathway critical for T-lymphocyte and B-lymphocyte proliferation. It is selective because other cells are not solely reliant on this enzyme and so are able to maintain their rapid proliferation.

Indications – Prophylaxis of acute renal, cardiac or hepatic transplant rejection (in combination with cyclosporine and corticosteroids).

Contraindications – Pregnancy and those with hypersensitivity to the drug.

Route of administration – Oral, intravenous.

Adverse effects – Side effects of mycophenolate mofetil include bone marrow suppression, which can lead to leucopoenia, thrombocytopenia and sometimes anaemia. Increased susceptibility to infections (often opportunistic pathogens) and to certain cancers (lymphomas) can occur. Common side effects include gastrointestinal disturbances, nausea, vomiting and diarrhoea. Alopecia may be partial or complete but is usually reversible.

The eye is a 25-mm sphere made up of two fluid-filled compartments (the aqueous humour and the vitreous humour) separated by a translucent lens, all encased within four layers of supporting tissue. These layers are:
- The cornea and sclera
- The uveal tract, comprising the iris, ciliary body and choroid
- The pigment epithelium
- The retina (neural tissue containing photoreceptors)

Light entering the eye is focused by the lens onto the retina, and the signal reaches the brain via the optic nerve.

GLAUCOMA

Glaucoma describes a group of disorders characterized by a loss in the visual field associated with cupping of the optic disc and optic nerve damage. Glaucoma is the second most common cause of blindness in the world and the most common cause of irreversible blindness. Glaucoma is generally associated with raised intraocular pressure (IOP) but can also occur when the IOP is within normal limits. There are two types of glaucoma: open-angle and closed-angle, the most common type being open-angle. It is caused by pathology of the trabecular meshwork that reduces the drainage of the aqueous humour into the canal of Schlemm. Treatment involves either reducing the amount of aqueous humour produced (Fig. 24.1) or increasing its drainage. Acute closed-angle glaucoma symptoms include painful, red eye and blurred vision. Acute closed-angle glaucoma is a medical emergency and requires admission to save sight. It is difficult for the patient to notice a gradual loss of visual fields associated with chronic open-angle glaucoma and so regular check-ups are vital for at risk groups, such as elderly people.

The most effective way of preventing damage to the eye is by lowering the IOP. Most drugs used to treat eye disease can be given topically in the form of drops and ointments. To enable these drugs to penetrate the cornea, they must be lipophilic or uncharged. Drugs used to treat open-angle glaucoma include beta-adrenoceptor antagonists timolol and betaxolol. Prostaglandin analogues are used as treatments for inhibiting aqueous production.

Beta-adrenoceptor antagonists

Beta-adrenoceptor antagonists block β_2-receptors on the ciliary body and on ciliary blood vessels, resulting in vasoconstriction and reduced aqueous production (Fig. 24.1).

Route of administration – These drugs are administered topically.

Contraindications – Beta-adrenoceptor antagonists should not be given to patients with asthma, bradycardia or heart block.

Adverse effects – Systemic side effects include bronchospasm in asthmatic patients, and potentially bradycardia owing to their nonselective action on beta-receptors. Other side effects include transitory dry eyes and allergic blepharoconjunctivitis.

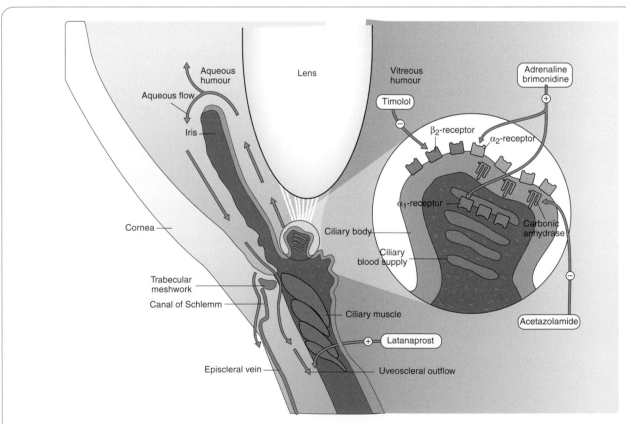

Fig. 24.1 Production and drainage of the aqueous humour. (Modified from Page C, Curtis M, Walker M, Hoffman B. *Integrated Pharmacology*. 3rd ed. Philadelphia: Elsevier; 2006.)

Prostaglandin analogues

Examples include latanoprost and travoprost.

Mechanism of action – Promote outflow of aqueous from the anterior chamber via an alternative drainage route, called the uveoscleral pathway.

Indications – Open-angle glaucoma, ocular hypertension.

Contraindication – Pregnancy.

Adverse effects – Brown pigmentation of the iris may occur.

Sympathomimetics (adrenoceptor agonists)

Adrenaline, dipivefrine and brimonidine are commonly used sympathomimetics.

Mechanism of action – Agonism at α-adrenoceptors is thought to be the principal means by which these agents reduce aqueous production from the ciliary body. Adrenaline may also increase drainage of aqueous humour.

Route of administration – Topical.

Indications – Open-angle glaucoma. Sympathomimetics are also used in the management of cardiac (see Chapter 14) and anaphylactic emergencies, and in the treatment of asthma and COPD (see Chapter 19).

Contraindications – Closed-angle glaucoma, hypertension, heart disease.

Adverse effects – Pain and redness in the eye.

Therapeutic notes – Adrenaline is not very lipophilic, and therefore it does not penetrate the cornea effectively. This can be overcome by administering dipivefrine hydrochloride, a prodrug that crosses the cornea and that is metabolized to adrenaline once inside the eye.

Carbonic anhydrase inhibitors

Acetazolamide and dorzolamide are carbonic anhydrase inhibitors (CAIs).

Mechanism of action – CAIs inhibit the enzyme carbonic anhydrase, which catalyses the conversion of carbon dioxide and water to carbonic acid, which dissociates into bicarbonate and hydrogen ions (H^+). Bicarbonate is required by the cells of the ciliary body, and underproduction of bicarbonate limits aqueous secretion (Fig 24.1). CAIs given systemically also have a weak diuretic effect (see Chapter 18).

Route of administration – Oral, topical, intravenous.

Indications – Open-angle glaucoma.

Contraindications – Hypokalaemia, hyponatraemia, renal impairment. These effects can be reduced if the drug is given in a slow-release form.

Adverse effects – Irritation of the eye, nausea, vomiting, diarrhoea, diuresis.

Drugs used to increase the drainage of aqueous humour

Miotics–muscarinic agonists

Pilocarpine is a muscarinic agonist.

Mechanism of action – Pilocarpine causes contraction of the constrictor pupillae muscles of the iris, thus constricting the pupil, allowing aqueous humour to drain from the anterior chamber into the trabecular meshwork (Fig 24.1).

Table 24.1 Mydriatic and Cycloplegic Effects of the Commonly Used Muscarinic Antagonists

Drug	Duration (h)	Mydriatic effect	Cycloplegic effect
Tropicamide	1-3	++	+
Cyclopentolate	12-24	+++	+++
Atropine	168-240	+++	+++

From Page C. *Crash Course: Pharmacology*. 5th ed. Philadelphia: Elsevier; 2019.

Route of administration – Topical.

Indications – Open-angle glaucoma.

Contraindications – Acute iritis, anterior uveitis.

Adverse effects – Eye irritation, headache and brow ache, blurred vision, hypersalivation. May exacerbate asthma.

Treatment of closed-angle glaucoma

Drugs to treat closed-angle glaucoma are used in emergencies as a temporary measure to lower IOP. Pilocarpine and a CAI are often first-line treatments, with mannitol and glycerol being administered systemically to reduce IOP for resistant or more serious cases. Yttrium-aluminium-garnet (YAG) laser surgery provides a permanent cure for closed-angle glaucoma. A hole is made in the iris (iridectomy) to allow increased flow of aqueous humour.

Examining the eye

Mydriatic drugs dilate the pupil, that is, cause mydriasis, whereas cycloplegic drugs cause paralysis of the ciliary muscle, that is, cycloplegia. Mydriatic and cycloplegic drugs are used in ophthalmoscopy to allow a better view of the interior of the eye. Mydriasis and cyclopegia reduce the drainage of the aqueous humour, and they should therefore be avoided in patients with closed-angle glaucoma.

Muscarinic antagonists

The most effective mydriatics are the muscarinic receptor antagonists. These block the parasympathetic control of the iris sphincter muscle. The type of muscarinic receptor antagonist chosen will depend on the length of the procedure and on whether or not cycloplegia is required. The most commonly used muscarinic receptor antagonists, their duration of action, and their mydriatic and cycloplegic effects are summarized in Table 24.1.

α-Adrenoceptor agonists

α-Adrenoceptor agonists can cause mydriasis by stimulating the sympathetic control of the iris dilator muscle. The sympathetic system does not control the ciliary muscle, however, and therefore these drugs do not produce cycloplegia. The α-agonist most commonly used to produce mydriasis is phenylephrine.

Muscarinic agonists and α-antagonists

A muscarinic agonist such as pilocarpine, or an α-receptor antagonist such as moxisylyte may be used to reverse mydriasis at the end of an ophthalmic examination, although this is not usually necessary.

PHYSIOLOGY OF THE EAR

The ear is a sensory organ that detects sound, head position and movement. The outer ear collects sound waves and directs them to the tympanic membrane that, along with the middle ear ossicular chain, amplifies sound vibration and transforms it into fluid shifts within the inner ear. The organ of Corti in the cochlea contains sensory receptor hair cells, which are set into motion by vibration of the cochlear duct basement membrane. Hair cell motion displaces the hair cell stereocilia projecting from the cell apex. This results in cellular depolarization produced by an inward cation current (calcium ion ($Ca2^+$), sodium ion (Na^+)) entering the apical end of the hair cell. The hair cell then releases a chemical transmitter from its basal end, leading to stimulation of the afferent bipolar neurons of the auditory nerve that connects to the central nervous system (CNS). Stereocilial deflection in the opposite direction results in hair cell hyperpolarization, which inhibits basal neurotransmitter release and suppresses auditory neurons, activity. Stereocilial oscillation therefore produces a train of excitatory and inhibitory impulses within the auditory nerve with the same frequency characteristics as the original sound. Balance depends on inputs from the vestibular, visual and proprioceptive sensory systems to the balance centres of the brain. The peripheral vestibular systems to the balance consist of the following:

- The otolithic organs, the utricle and saccule, which sense linear acceleration
- The semicircular canals, which sense angular acceleration or rotation

The sensory input from these organs is critical for maintaining equilibrium and stabilizing gaze with head movement. Depending on head position or movement, vestibular hair cells are either depolarized or hyperpolarized. Depolarization increases the basal release of neurotransmitter and the resting firing rate of the associated vestibular afferent neuron. Hyperpolarization has the opposite effect. Head movement and position are therefore resolved into stimulatory increases or inhibitory decreases of the resting firing rate of the vestibular nerve and its central connection.

DISEASES OF THE EAR

The main symptoms of ear disorders are hearing loss, tinnitus, vertigo, pain, pressure and itchiness.

Hearing loss

Hearing loss may be conductive (resulting from disorders of external or middle ear sound conduction) or sensorineural (resulting from abnormalities of the inner ear sensory cells and their connections with the CNS). Drugs which induce hearing loss as an adverse effect usually affect the sensorineural pathway.

Infections

Ear infections are extremely common and involve the outer ear (otitis externa), middle ear (otitis media) or inner ear (labyrinthitis).

Otitis externa

Otitis externa results from a bacterial or fungal infection of the soft tissue of the external ear canal. Common bacterial causes include *Pseudomonas aeruginosa*, *Proteus mirabilis*, staphylococci, streptococci and various Gram-negative bacteria. *Candida* and *Aspergillus* species are the most common fungal causes. Most pathogens are inhibited by an acidic medium, and a solution of equal parts of vinegar and isopropyl alcohol can be used to treat otitis externa. All infected debris and pus must be removed from the ear (otic toilet) before starting any medication. Moisture should be avoided. First-line treatment of otitis externa includes the use of topical preparations combining an appropriate antibiotic (e.g. neomycin and polymyxin) and a glucocorticoid (e.g. hydrocortisone). Topically applied polysorbate, gentian violet or nystatin may be used to treat fungal infections. Orally administered dicloxacillin, cephalexin, trimethoprim-sulfamethoxazole or ciprofloxacin are used to treat progressive cellulitis of the external ear canal, while intravenous cefazolin, dicloxacillin or ciprofloxacin may be needed for more severe cases. For the treatment of invasive skull base osteitis, combination therapy is required, preferably aztreonam with clindamycin or a combination of ciprofloxacin with one of the following antibiotics: ticarcillin, piperacillin, ceftazidime, imipenem, gentamicin, tobramycin or amikacin.

Otitis media

Acute purulent otitis media is caused by a bacterial infection of the middle ear. The usual pathogens are *Streptococcus pneumoniae*, *Haemophilus influenza*, and *Moraxella catarrhalis*. First-line therapy should include amoxicillin or erythromycin plus a sulphonamide or trimethoprim-sulfamethoxazole. Second-line therapy is directed at ß lactamase-producing organisms and is usually amoxicillin-clavulanate, cefaclor, cefuroxime, cefixime or clarithromycin.

Use of nasal spray containing a corticosteroid to promote drainage by opening the eustachian tubes can also be useful.

Chronic otitis media is defined by the presence of a perforated tympanic membrane in the presence of a middle ear infection caused by the presence of *P. aeruginosa*, *Proteus* spp. staphylococci, Gram-negative organisms, and/or anaerobes (*Klebsiella* spp., *Escherichia coli*, *Bacteroides fragilis*). Treatment includes use of ear drops containing neomycin and polymyxin and an oral antibiotic such as trimethoprim-sulfamethoxazole or cephalexin, though amoxicillin-clavulanate or ciprofloxacin with metronidazole is sometimes used. If pseudomonas is the cause of persistent otorrhea, combining two different ear drops, one containing ciprofloxacin and the other an aminoglycoside (gentamicin, tobramycin), may be effective. However, aminoglycosides can cause ototoxicity when applied to the middle ear, but this is rare in the presence of active infection.

Suppurative labyrinthitis

Bacterial infection of the spaces of the inner ear causes profound cochlear and vestibular destruction and loss of both hearing and vestibular function in the affected ear. Intralabyrinthine infection results from the spread of otitis media via the round or oval windows, a labyrinthine fistula or a lateral extension of meningitis through the cochlear aqueduct and cribriform plate at the lateral end of the internal auditory canal.

If infection is due to otitis media, treatment includes surgical drainage and intravenous antibiotics (ceftriaxone for acute otitis media, nafcillin with ceftazidime plus metronidazole for chronic otitis media). If infection is due to meningitis, the appropriate intravenous antibiotic should be given.

Hearing loss

Certain ototoxic drugs are common, e.g. aminoglycosides and certain macrolides.

Otosclerosis

Otosclerosis is characterized by idiopathic circumscribed endochondral otic capsule bone destruction and replacement with vascular bone and then dense lamellar bone in the anterior oval window niche, which results in stapes footplate fixation and a conductive hearing loss. Sensorineural hearing loss can result from a focus of otosclerosis adjacent to the endolymphatic space. Epidemiologic studies indicate a lower incidence of otosclerosis in regions with high fluoride concentrations in drinking water. However, the only widely recognized indication for using fluoride is progressive sensorineural hearing loss with a high risk of otosclerosis on taking the patient's history or upon examination. Calcium, 2–3 g daily, should be administered along with the fluoride.

Sudden sensorineural hearing loss

Sudden sensorineural hearing loss (SSHL) is usually unilateral, progresses within hours to days and is associated with tinnitus and, less frequently, vertigo. It can be caused by a viral infection, vascular disorder or inner ear membrane rupture. SSHL is a medical emergency and is usually treated by glucocorticoids tapered over 10 days to 2 weeks.

Autoimmune hearing loss

Autoimmune sensorineural hearing loss typically affects young adults, is slowly progressive over months and is not accompanied by other systemic disease or hereditary defects, but it is due to an autoimmune reaction to a specific inner ear antigen. There is no vertigo, but more severe disease causes ataxia in dim light. For more severe and bilateral cases, prednisone for 2–4 weeks is the treatment of choice. A second immunosuppressive agent may be needed if there is a good response and hearing recovers, but the patient becomes chronically dependent on glucocorticoids. Cyclophosphamide, methotrexate, or penicillamine are the drugs of choice.

Tinnitus

Tinnitus is the perception of sound in the absence of an external source. It may be objective and result from sounds generated within the body which are audible to an observer, or subjective and characterized by an auditory sensation in the absence of a physical sound.

Causes include musculoskeletal and vascular sounds producing objective tinnitus, and disorders of the peripheral and central auditory systems, which usually produce subjective tinnitus. The cause may be known (e.g. noise-induced, presbycusis). The first symptom of drug-induced ototoxicity is often tinnitus. Nonsteroidal anti-inflammatory drugs (NSAIDs), antibiotics and some antineoplastic agents can cause tinnitus. Most patients also have an irreversible high-frequency sensorineural hearing loss. Once an underlying disease has been excluded, the goal is to relieve the annoyance that tinnitus causes. If it is mild, patients may simply need to know its cause and that it is benign. Masking (the use of a noise generator to cover the subjective sound) is the prime treatment for more severe cases, although drugs may be needed to treat intractable tinnitus including local anaesthetics (procaine, lidocaine), benzodiazepines (diazepam, alprazolam, clonazepam) or γ-aminobutyric acid (GABA) agonists such as baclofen or tricyclic antidepressants (amitriptyline).

The treatment of tinnitus with local anaesthetics probably involves inhibition of the cochlear nerve and its brainstem connections. Lidocaine must be given intravenously and can produce a highly significant reduction in tinnitus. Benzodiazepines improve the patient's emotional response to tinnitus, but in some patients this may be a direct effect as the tinnitus may be due to insufficient inhibitory activity in the ascending auditory system. Benzodiazepines may act by enhancing the activity of the inhibitory neurotransmitter, GABA.

Vertigo, vestibular neuronitis and vestibular trauma

Vertigo is the hallucinatory perception of movement and can result from disorders of the peripheral or central vestibular systems. Peripherally induced vertigo is usually the more severe and associated with other aural symptoms such as hearing loss or tinnitus. Vertigo is produced by benign positional vertigo, which is either spontaneous or secondary to head trauma, occurs with motion of the head and usually lasts less than 30 seconds. There is a sensation of rotary motion, either of the world moving or one moving in the world. Malpositioning of otoliths is presumed to trigger an attack. It is treated by systematic head maneuvers and positioning to try to re-position the otoliths of the inner ear. Vertigo can also be caused by constant, often permanent, hypofunction of the affected labyrinth, for example acute vestibular neuronitis, suppurative labyrinthitis, and vestibular trauma. Transient fluctuations in vestibular neuron activity such as Ménière's disease and recurrent vestibulopathy can also lead to vertigo.

Vestibular neuronitis results in an acute decrease in vestibular function, which may be mild and reversible or profound and permanent. Symptoms include severe vertigo which can be accompanied by nausea and is probably caused by an unknown virus. Vestibular trauma can have a similar range of severity, depending upon whether there has been a brain concussion, total destruction of the vestibular structures or division of the vestibular nerve. Central adaptation must begin during the first month after onset. Patients must remain active, as forced inactivity may predispose to incomplete adaptation and permanent ataxia. Drugs such as dimenhydrinate are used to treat severe nausea, and the vestibular suppressants used for acute Ménière's disease (see below) can be used sparingly. No medication specifically promotes central adaptation.

Ménière's disease and recurrent vestibulopathy

Meniere's disease is a peripheral vestibular disorder associated with intermittent overaccumulation of endolymphatic fluid (endolymphatic hydrops). It causes episodes of severe rotary vertigo that continue for hours, hearing loss, tinnitus and a pressure sensation in the ear. Initially these symptoms occur in attacks, but eventually the condition burns out, leaving the patient with a stable severe sensorineural hearing loss and a permanent, usually well-compensated, decrease in peripheral vestibular function. Ménière's disease is managed with drugs, diets to restrict Na^+ intake and prevent hydrops and physical therapy to adapt to the loss of vestibular function. Drugs used to treat Ménière's disease include diuretics (e.g. hydrochlorothiazide, furosemide) to limit endolymphatic fluid accumulation, vestibular suppressants (sedatives, H_1 receptor antagonists, muscarinic receptor antagonists and narcotics) and vasodilating drugs or aminoglycosides to ablate peripheral vestibular function.

Hydrochlorothiazide prevents recurrent vertigo in many patients, but patients must be monitored for potassium (K^+) depletion by repeated measurements of serum K^+ and maintain a high potassium diet. Meclizine is useful to treat moderate acute attacks and it is likely that this occurs via its capacity to antagonize muscarinic receptors rather than H_1 histamine receptors. This is an example of a drug known to be in one class (H_1 receptor antagonism) which actually has its therapeutic benefit through another mechanism common to a different class of compounds (muscarinic receptor antagonists). If an attack becomes severe, a benzodiazepine such as diazepam or lorazepam not only provides sedation, but also acts directly on the medial and lateral vestibular nuclei to suppress otolithic and semicircular canal activity. Muscarinic receptor antagonists such as scopolamine have limited use because their adverse effects are more profound than those of meclizine. Some parenteral narcotics (e.g. fentanyl, droperidol) are potent vestibular suppressants and are occasionally needed for the treatment of an acute, incapacitating attack. Chemical ablation of vestibular function may be indicated for recurrent incapacitating vertigo that cannot be controlled by drugs; the patient with physician guidance must decide if it would be easier to cope with a permanent, medically induced loss of vestibular function. Streptomycin can be given parenterally for active disease in both ears and is carefully titrated to a point of symptom control, but all peripheral vestibular function must not be ablated as this can cause incapacitating oscillopsia and ataxia. For unilateral Ménière's disease, gentamicin can be injected directly into the middle ear, from where it is actively transported across the round window into the labyrinthine fluids. Here it probably acts on dark cells (thought to be important in the production of endolymph) and has a toxic effect on the vestibular hair cells. Most patients adapt well after unilateral destruction of vestibular function and have no further disabling spells of vertigo. Recurrent vestibulopathy, also known as vestibular Ménière's disease, presents with similar recurrent vertigo but with no auditory symptoms. The vertigo is typically more benign than that of Ménière's disease and is usually controlled with similar drugs.

Facial nerve palsy

Bell's palsy is acute unilateral facial weakness or paralysis without an identifiable cause, though herpes simplex virus type I has been implicated in this condition. Herpes zoster oticus (HZO) is acute facial paralysis with pain and varicelliform lesions, which often involves the conchal bowl, the concave central portion of the external ear. It is probably due to varicella-zoster virus infection of the geniculate ganglion and there is often eighth cranial nerve involvement, producing a profound sensorineural hearing loss and vestibular loss. Oedema traps the facial nerve as it passes through the narrow fallopian canal, resulting in ischemia and neural dysfunction. The use of glucocorticoids to treat acute facial paralysis is controversial and they are not indicated for incomplete facial paralysis, as this usually recovers fully without the need for treatment. When glucocorticoids are used for the treatment of complete facial paralysis due to Bell's palsy or HZO, they should be given within the first 10 days at a moderate dose, which is then tapered. Acyclovir (acycloguanosine), a nucleoside analogue that inhibits viral DNA replication, reduces functional deficits in immunocompromised patients with HZO but has no proven benefit in the treatment of Bell's palsy. Ideally treatment should be started as soon as possible after symptoms develop, up to about 72 hours after onset.

Motion sickness

Travel or motion sickness can be treated with older H_1 receptor antagonists such as hyoscine.

Ototoxic Drugs

Four clinically important classes of drugs can cause inner ear toxicity affecting both hearing and balance. Tinnitus is an additional symptom that often accompanies drug-induced ototoxicity.

Analgesics and antipyretics

The tinnitus characteristic of salicylate-induced ototoxicity is often accompanied by hearing loss, but the mechanism of salicylate ototoxicity is not fully understood. However, salicylates accumulate within extracellular fluid compartments and reduce prostaglandin synthesis within the stria vascularis by inhibiting cyclooxygenase which causes vasoconstriction within the stria vascularis, ischemia and inhibition of the cochlear nerve action potential. Salicylate ototoxicity occurs at serum concentrations over 0.35 mg/mL and is reversible within 48–72 hours of salicylate withdrawal.

Antibiotics

Aminoglycoside antibiotics have adverse effects on the kidney and inner ear: streptomycin and gentamicin are more vestibulotoxic; kanamycin, tobramycin and amikacin have more effect on cochlear hair cells. Gentamicin-induced ototoxicity occurs in approximately 5% of patients treated with this drug. Netilmicin has a reported prevalence of hearing loss in 1 per 250 patients and vestibular toxicity in 1 per 150 patients. Aminoglycosides first bind to the outer surface of the hair cell membrane and disturb Ca^{2+} membrane channels. They then bind to phosphatidylinositol bisphosphate on the inner surface of the cell membrane. Interference with intracellular Ca^{2+} and polyamine-regulated processes causes additional membrane damage, which eventually leads to cell death by apoptosis. Reversible ototoxicity can occur; however, severe, irreversible and untreatable hearing deficits are common. As patients requiring aminoglycosides often have debilitating medical conditions, early complaints of dizziness and tinnitus may be overlooked, especially in a bed-bound patient. Permanent disabling vestibulotoxicity often is only recognized when the mobile patient complains of movement intolerance, oscillopsia (difficulty in stabilizing gaze during head movement) and/or ataxia.

Glycopeptide antibiotics such as vancomycin are increasingly used clinically on account of increasing incidence of resistance to certain bacteria. Their mechanism of ototoxicity is not clear, but the pattern with outer hair cell loss preceding inner hair cell loss is similar to that seen with aminoglycosides, likely due to apoptosis. High-frequency sensorineural hearing loss, blowing tinnitus and vertigo can also follow large intravenous doses of erythromycin, a macrolide antibiotic. Although the mechanism of this ototoxicity is unknown, it is reversible on drug withdrawal.

Anticancer drugs

Cisplatin's ototoxic effect is probably due to local production of oxidants such as nitric oxide (NO) and induction of apoptosis with resulting labyrinthine hair cell degeneration. Cisplatin is primarily cochleotoxic, causing degeneration of the outer hair cells, spiral ganglion cells and cochlear neurons, with relative sparing of the vestibular system. The morphologic changes within the inner ear are similar to those of aminoglycoside ototoxicity. The outer hair cells of the basal turn of the cochlea are the most susceptible. Carboplatin also produces dose-dependent hearing loss, thought to result from generation of oxidative free radicals and subsequent apoptosis of cochlear cells.

Diuretics

Loop diuretics (furosemide and ethacrynic acid) inhibit chloride ion (Cl⁻) reabsorption at the distal loop of Henle and promote extra cellular fluid excretion. Within the inner ear they inhibit cell membrane K^+ transport within the stria vascularis and are principally cochleotoxic. Like aminoglycosides, loop diuretics have adverse effects on both the kidney and inner ear, and the toxic effects of these two medications can be synergistic. There is an increased risk of toxicity if the drug is given too rapidly by bolus injection, or if the patient is elderly or has renal failure. Tinnitus, hearing loss and vertigo may occur within minutes and can be reversible if the medication is withdrawn immediately.

LOCAL ANAESTHETICS

Local anaesthetics are drugs used primarily to inhibit pain by preventing impulse conduction along sensory nerves. They achieve this by blocking voltage-sensitive sodium ion (Na$^+$) channels in the cell membrane. Local anaesthetics are also used as antidysrhythmics (see Chapter 14) and in epilepsy (see Chapter 12).

The basic electrophysiology of neurons

Sodium channels (Figs. 26.1 and 26.2) can exist in three states: *resting* (i.e. closed), *activated* (i.e. open) and *inactivated* (i.e. blocked; explained below).

The resting cell

The action of the Na$^+$ pump in cell membranes normally maintains a high level of potassium ion (K$^+$) and a low level of Na$^+$ within the cell (see Chapter 4). In the resting cell, the membrane is more permeable to K$^+$ than to Na$^+$. The efflux of K$^+$ makes the cell interior negative with respect to the outside, giving a membrane potential between -60 and -90 mV. In the resting cell, the Na$^+$ channels are *closed*.

Activation – the action potential

When a nerve cell is stimulated locally (e.g. by noxious stimuli acting on a pain fibre or by neurotransmitter action on a receptor linked to a cation channel) the Na$^+$ channel opens, leading to a local increase in the membrane permeability to Na$^+$. The resultant increased influx of positive Na$^+$ causes membrane depolarization and an action potential is generated. This is a regenerative process, as the action potential itself causes more Na$^+$ channels to open, allowing its propagation along the nerve.

Inactivation

Within 5 ms the Na$^+$ channels are inactivated (i.e. they close and are transiently refractory to being opened again) allowing the cell to repolarize. (The delayed opening of K$^+$ channels in response to the membrane depolarization also contributes to repolarization.) The rapidity of the sequence of events means that repetitive firing can proceed at high frequency.

Local anaesthetics

Important examples are **lidocaine** (lignocaine), **tetracaine** (amethocaine), bupivacaine, procaine and prilocaine. Cocaine was the first local anaesthetic to be used but has few clinical applications now.

Mechanism of action

Local anaesthetics are nearly all weak bases (pK$_a$ 8–9) and have similar chemical structures (Fig. 26.3). They act by blocking Na$^+$ channels and stopping the propagation of action potentials in nerve. (Figs. 26.1 and 26.4). Local anaesthetics gain access to their binding site either from the cell interior or by lateral diffusion in the cell membrane. In both cases, it is essential for the drug to adopt its lipid-soluble, uncharged form to gain access (Fig. 26.4). This of course depends on pH and can explain the reduced activity of local anaesthetics in inflamed tissue, where the lower pH increases ionization. Many local anaesthetics show *use-dependence*, that is they are more effective in blocking channels once these have been activated. This may be because the drug's binding site is within the channel and accessible only when the channel opens, or it may result from greater affinity for the inactivated state of the channel.

Local anaesthetics usually block small diameter fibres at lower concentrations than large fibres. Accordingly, pain sensation is blocked before other sensory inputs, but it is not usually possible to achieve local anaesthesia without loss of other sensory modalities or local paralysis.

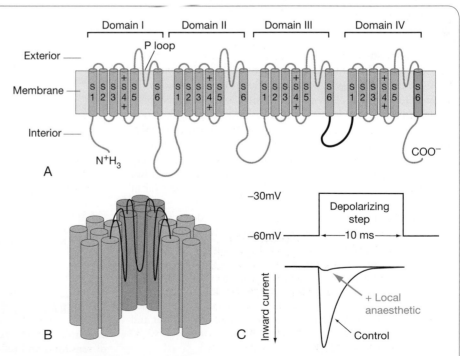

Sodium channels consist of one α subunit, which forms the aqueous channel, and one or two modulatory β subunits. The α subunit contains 4 linked domains each comprising 6 transmembrane helices (segments S1-S6); shown in A.

The S4 segments contain several positively charged amino acids and it is proposed that the outward movement of the S4 segments in response to membrane depolarisation causes a structural change which opens the channel.

Loops between S5 and S6 in each domain (labelled 'P loop' and shown as black lines in B) penetrate the membrane and line the outer part of the channel.

Inactivation of the channels is caused by the loop connecting domains III and IV — shown in black in A — folding up into the channel and blocking it like a trap door.

The local anaesthetic binding site is on S6 in domain 4 (which is shown in blue).

Fig. 26.1 Schematic diagram of sodium channel. (A) The four linked domains. (B) Suggested arrangement of the domains to form the channel (the front domain is omitted to show the pore). (C) Activation and inactivation of Na$^+$ current during a depolarizing voltage step.

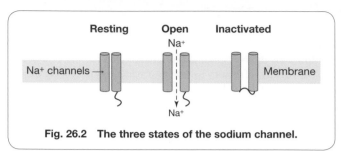

Fig. 26.2 The three states of the sodium channel.

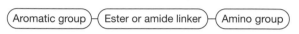

Fig. 26.3 Simplified outline of the structure of local anaesthetics.

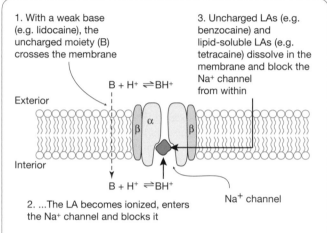

1. With a weak base (e.g. lidocaine), the uncharged moiety (B) crosses the membrane

3. Uncharged LAs (e.g. benzocaine) and lipid-soluble LAs (e.g. tetracaine) dissolve in the membrane and block the Na⁺ channel from within

$B + H^+ \rightleftharpoons BH^+$

Exterior

Interior

$B + H^+ \rightleftharpoons BH^+$

Na⁺ channel

2. ...The LA becomes ionized, enters the Na⁺ channel and blocks it

Fig. 26.4 Access of local anaesthetics (LAs) to channel-blocking site as uncharged species via the membrane or as charged species from the cell interior.

Pharmacokinetics

The plasma half-life of most local anaesthetics is 1–2 h, but their action persists for longer due to retention at the site of administration. The duration of action can be increased by the concomitant administration of a vasoconstrictor in the same formulation (epinephrine (adrenaline) or felypressin). The esters (tetracaine, benzocaine, procaine, cocaine) are hydrolysed rapidly by plasma esterases once they reach the bloodstream, whereas most amides (prilocaine, bupivacaine) are relatively resistant to plasma esterases and are subject to N-dealkylation and hydrolysis in the liver at a slower rate.

The variable lipid solubility of local anaesthetics determines the rate at which they penetrate tissues to cause nerve block and thus their suitability for action on mucous membranes.

Table 26.1 summarizes the properties of three local anaesthetics. Cocaine and lidocaine penetrate membranes readily; procaine does so poorly. Benzocaine differs from other local anaesthetics in lacking the basic amine side-chain; this results in increased lipophilicity and allows rapid entry into tissues, a fast onset and long duration of action.

Unwanted effects

The unwanted effects of local anaesthetics are due to their entry into the systemic circulation. Central nervous system (CNS) effects,

Table 26.1 Summary of the Pharmacokinetic Aspects of Some Local Anaesthetics (LAs)

LA	Onset of action	Duration of action	Metabolism
Lidocaine	Rapid	Moderate	Amide-linked LAs are degraded in the liver
Bupivacaine	Slow	Long	
Tetracaine	Slow	Long	Ester-linked LA, hydrolysed by plasma esterases

prominent with procaine, less with lidocaine and prilocaine, are paradoxically stimulatory and include restlessness and tremor, though larger doses are depressant. Respiratory depression may be a cause of death in overdose with these drugs. Local anaesthetics also cause myocardial depression and vasodilatation, which may result in a serious lowering of blood pressure. (Cocaine has additional effects related to its ability to inhibit monoamine uptake into nerve-endings (not shared by other local anaesthetics) – sympathomimetic effects arising in this way can include a dangerous rise in blood pressure leading to a hypertensive crisis). Hypersensitivity reactions, manifest as allergic dermatitis, may occur. **Levobupivacaine**, the *R*-isomer of bupivacaine (the racemate), has fewer CNS and cardiovascular effects than bupivacaine itself.

Clinical use and administration of local anaesthetics

- Surface anaesthesia: Lidocaine and tetracaine are used for local anaesthesia of skin, cornea and mucosal surfaces.
- Infiltration anaesthesia: Most local anaesthetics are suitable for this indication, administered by injection for minor surgery. Epinephrine (adrenaline) or felypressin may be co-administered to cause local vasoconstriction to prolong the retention of the local anaesthetic at the site of injury and also to reduce the amount gaining excess to the systemic circulation, thus reducing the likelihood of unwanted side effects.
- Intravenous regional anaesthesia: A pressure cuff maintains local concentration and prevents entry into the general circulation. Lidocaine and prilocaine are suitable for this use.
- Nerve-block anaesthesia: Most local anaesthetics are suitable for this purpose. Injection close to the nerve trunk produces regional anaesthesia for surgery or dentistry. Vasoconstrictors may be co-administered to enhance duration of action.
- Spinal anaesthesia: Lidocaine or tetracaine can be injected into the subarachnoid space to act on spinal roots and spinal cord. This is used for lower body surgery when general anaesthesia is undesirable.
- Epidural anaesthesia: Lidocaine or bupivacaine are injected into the epidural space. This is used for spinal anaesthesia and also in childbirth.

GENERAL ANAESTHETICS

General anaesthesia, by producing unconsciousness and loss of sensation and reflexes, facilitates surgery with much reduced distress to the patient. There are two broad categories of general anaesthetics: the inhalation anaesthetics (gases or volatile liquids) and intravenous agents.

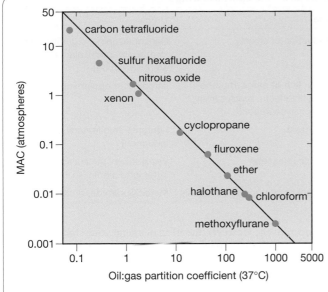

Fig. 26.5 Correlation of anaesthetic potency with oil:gas partition coefficient. Anaesthetic potency in humans is expressed as minimum alveolar partial pressure (MAC) required to produce surgical anaesthesia.

Table 26.2 Stages of Anaesthesia

Stage	Characteristics
I	*Analgesia*. Still conscious
II	*Excitement*. Loss of consciousness but responsive to painful stimuli; may move, have incoherent speech, vomiting and irregular breathing
III	*Surgical anaesthesia*. Reflexes disappear. Respiration initially more regular but depression develops with increasing depth of anaesthesia; muscle relaxation
IV	*Medullary depression*. Respiratory arrest and cardio-vascular collapse. Death

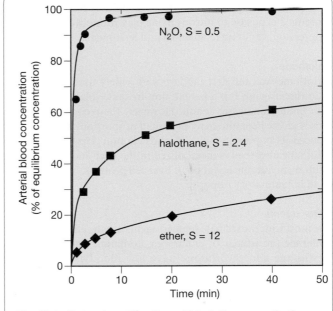

Fig. 26.6 Rate of equilibration of inhalation anaesthetics. S, Blood:gas partition coefficient.

Mechanisms of action
Inhalation anaesthetics
Unlike most drugs, the action of the inhalation agents does not seem to involve a well-defined receptor; the agents typically act at high concentration (for example, nitrous oxide acts at concentrations of 10 mmol or more, whereas atropine produces more than 50% block of muscarinic receptors at less than 10 nmol (a millionth of the concentration)). Neither is there a clear structure–activity relationship; most of the agents are small, unreactive molecules and even nitrogen produces anaesthesia in sufficiently high concentration. Their potency is well correlated with lipo-solubility (Fig. 26.5) so that cell membranes or, more likely, hydrophobic domains of proteins are possible sites of action.

Electrophysiological studies show that excitatory transmission (glutamatergic and nicotinic) may be inhibited, whereas inhibitory transmission at γ-aminobutyric acid (GABA$_A$) receptors is potentiated. In keeping with a particular interaction with ionotropic receptors, the stereoisomers of some inhalation anaesthetics (e.g. isoflurane) exhibit some differences in potency.

Intravenous anaesthetics
Barbiturates (e.g. thiopental), propofol and etomidate all potentiate the action of GABA on GABA$_A$ receptors, producing a CNS depression. Ketamine reduces neuronal excitability by blocking *N*-methyl-D-aspartate (NMDA) receptors (see Chapter 11).

Analgesic action
The analgesic action of these agents may involve the suppression of pain inputs at the spinal level, whereas the loss of consciousness probably involves an action on the reticular activating system and thalamocortical tract. The useful short-term amnesia caused by many anaesthetic agents may result from an effect on the hippocampus.

Stages of anaesthesia
The depression of CNS function commonly proceeds through well-defined stages as the concentration in the CNS rises

(Table 26.2). Modern practice allows a rapid transition to surgical anaesthesia so that the unwanted actions in stage II are often avoided.

Inhalation agents
Apart from nitrous oxide, all the currently used gaseous anaesthetics are halogenated ethers or hydrocarbons (all contain fluorine). All halogenated anaesthetics are prone to cause *malignant hyperthermia*.

Pharmacokinetic aspects
All of these agents are rapidly absorbed across the alveolar membranes of the lungs. The rate at which the body equilibrates with the inspired gas, however, varies considerably, as shown in Fig. 26.6. The rate of equilibration is determined mainly by the *blood:gas partition coefficient*. Agents with a low coefficient (e.g. nitrous oxide) equilibrate quickly and have a rapid effect, whereas agents with a high coefficient (e.g. ether) act more slowly.

Most of these agents are inert and undergo little metabolism; their elimination is mostly through exhalation via the lungs. The rate of elimination mirrors the rate of uptake, being quickest for nitrous oxide. In a long surgical operation, there is a slow but potentially large uptake of lipid-soluble agents (e.g. halothane) into adipose tissue. Slow release into the circulation when the anaesthetic is discontinued results in a sustained low level of CNS depression.

Ether

Ether is the archetypal inhalation anaesthetic; however, apart from being flammable, it is irritant to the airways and has mostly been replaced by superior agents.

Nitrous oxide

Nitrous oxide has a low potency, and inhalation at maximum possible concentrations will not produce surgical anaesthesia. It is, however, widely used in conjunction with other agents, allowing them to be administered at a lower concentration with a reduction in side effects. It has powerful analgesic actions and is used by itself (50% in oxygen) for pain relief in childbirth and accidents. Prolonged exposure to nitrous oxide may produce bone marrow suppression, resulting in anaemia and leukopenia.

Halothane

Halothane was the first modern and widely used halogenated anaesthetic agent. It is a potent, non-irritant, volatile anaesthetic with limited analgesic action. However, the recognition that it causes severe hepatotoxicity in a small proportion of patients has reduced its popularity and demands caution. Up to 20% of the halothane absorbed is metabolized in the liver and toxicity may result from fluoroacetylation of liver cell proteins, which can lead to an inflammatory response.

Other agents

The most widely used halogenated agents are the ethers **enflurane, isoflurane** (an isomer of enflurane), **desflurane** and **sevoflurane**. Desflurane and sevoflurane have low blood:gas solubilities which allow a more rapid postoperative recovery. Enflurane has some convulsant activity so is avoided in patients with epilepsy. Desflurane and isoflurane, but not sevoflurane, may irritate the airways.

Intravenous agents

The intravenous agents are most often short acting and used to induce anaesthesia, which will then be maintained by inhaled agents. Thiopental, etomidate and propofol are all very lipid soluble and cross the blood–brain barrier very quickly to produce unconsciousness in one arm-brain circulation time.

Thiopental

Thiopental, like other barbiturates, has no analgesic action and a low safety margin (cardiorespiratory depression). It is metabolized rather slowly (half-life 8–10 h) producing some CNS depression

Table 26.3 Perioperative Drugs

Use	Drugs
Reduction of anxiety	Benzodiazepine, e.g. diazepam, lorazepam, midazolam (+ useful amnesic action)
Reduction of parasympatho-mimetic effects: bradycardia, bronchial secretions	Atropine, scopolamine
Analgesia	Fentanyl, remifentanil (at induction)
Muscle relaxation	Vecuronium, succinylcholine (after induction)
Control of postoperative emesis	Metoclopramide, droperidol

postoperatively. However, the effect of a single anaesthesia-inducing dose lasts for only 5–10 min because the drug rapidly redistributes from the well-perfused tissues (including brain) to less well-perfused but higher capacity tissues (muscle initially, then fat).

Etomidate

Etomidate has some advantages over thiopental, causing less cardiorespiratory depression and less hangover. It has little analgesic action. It causes some involuntary movement and postoperative sickness, both of which may be controlled by other drugs. Adrenocortical suppression is possible.

Propofol

The widely used propofol is rapidly metabolized and so avoids the hangover effects of thiopental. Rapid recovery from its action also allows it to be used on its own as an intravenous (IV) infusion to maintain anaesthesia; this is particularly useful for day-case surgery.

Ketamine

Ketamine, given intramuscularly (IM) or IV, can produce surgical anaesthesia suitable for brief procedures on its own. The anaesthesia is, however, commonly referred to as dissociative, since it is possible for the patient to remain conscious, but with insensitivity to pain and with short-term amnesia. A high incidence of hallucinations and dysphoria restricts its use in adults, but a lower incidence in children makes it suitable for minor paediatric surgery.

Perioperative drugs

Anaesthetic agents alone do not usually provide optimal conditions for operations, so drugs may be given prior to inducing anaesthesia (premedication), after induction (e.g. neuromuscular blockers) or during recovery (Table 26.3).

Components of nutrition include water, carbohydrates, proteins (including essential amino acids that cannot be synthesized by the body in sufficient quantities), fats, vitamins, trace elements and indigestible fibres. Disorders of nutrition include excessive caloric intake leading to obesity, eating disorders such as anorexia nervosa and bulimia nervosa and various malnutrition disorders.

Malnutrition disorders are often directly related to diet deficiencies in vitamins (structurally unrelated organic compounds), trace elements and minerals. Whilst disorders of malnutrition can be serious or life threatening, they can usually by corrected by supplementing the diet with the otherwise diet-deficient mineral. Therefore the pharmacology of obesity and eating disorders is discussed below.

OBESITY

Obesity is caused by excessive caloric intake compared to energy expenditure over a prolonged period of time. The body mass index (BMI) is used to characterize individuals with a BMI >30.0 kg/m^2 (Table 27.1). Obesity is an increasing worldwide problem; for example one in three adults in the United States is classified as obese (BMI >30.0 kg/m^2) and another one in three adults is classified as overweight (BMI 25.0–29.9 kg/m^2).

Pathophysiology
Obesity may be caused by both lifestyle and genetic factors leading to increased total body fat in adipose tissues. Obesity increases the risk of cardiovascular diseases (atherosclerosis, sudden death due to cardiac arrhythmias), type 2 diabetes mellitus, cancers (endometrial, post-menopausal breast, prostate, colorectal), pulmonary function (sleep apnea), osteoporosis, gout, skin disorders (acanthosis nigricans, skin turgor) and endocrine disorders (irregular menstrual cycle, earlier menopause, thyroid metabolism).

Therapy and pharmacology
Combined approaches to treatment are recommended, and clinicians prefer patients to undergo behavioural modification, exercise and changes in diet for long term, controlled weight loss. Surgery by reducing gastric volume (stapling of stomach) is also effective, but a selected option for morbidly obese patients. Various pharmacological options are available and might be used in combination with lifestyle changes listed above. Typically these drugs induce modest (5%–10%) weight loss.

Peptic and gastric lipase inhibitors
Orlistat inhibits pancreatic lipases to decrease gastrointestinal absorption of fats. Orlistat can provide a modest 10% reduction in weight after 2 years prescription. Side effects are negligible due to minimal oral absorption and therefore systemic exposure. However gastrointestinal disturbances may occur. Orlistat is contraindicated with warfarin.

5-HT$_{2C}$ receptor agonists
5-Hydroxytryptamine (5-HT)$_{2C}$ receptors are found almost exclusively in the brain. **Lorcaserin** is therefore thought to promote weight loss through satiety by activating 5-HT$_{2C}$ receptors in the hypothalamus to activate proopiomelanocortin (POMC) that results in satiety through an opioid mediated negative feedback mechanism. Side effects include headaches, dizziness and nausea.

Sympathomimetic and GABA receptor modulation
Phentermine (a sympathomimetic amine) and **topiramate** (a γ-aminobutyric acid (GABA) receptor modulator) can be given in combination to suppress appetite and satiety. Side effects include constipation, dizziness, dry mouth and insomnia. They are contraindicated in patients with glaucoma and hyperthyroidism.

Opioid receptor antagonism and dopamine and noradrenaline re-uptake inhibition
Naltrexone (opioid receptor antagonist) and **bupropion** (re-uptake inhibitor of dopamine and noradrenaline) can also be given in combination. Bupropion might also activate POMC, and this effect can be augmented by naltrexone. Side effects include constipation, dizziness, dry mouth and nausea.

GLP-1 receptor agonists
Glucagon-like peptide 1 (GLP-1) receptor agonists (**liraglutide**) used in the treatment of type 2 diabetes reduce bodyweight by increasing satiety and slowing gastric emptying. Side effects include nausea, vomiting, diarrhoea and pancreatitis.

Table 27.1 Body Mass Index and Health

Undernutrition	Normal Weight	Overnutrition
Severe <15.9 kg/m^2		Overweight 25.0-29.9 kg/m^2
Moderate 16-16.9 kg/m^2	18.5-24.9 kg/m^2	Obesity 30.0-39.9 kg/m^2
Mild 17.0-18.4 kg/m^2		Morbid obesity >40.0 kg/m^2

From Page C, Curtis M, Walker M, Hoffman B. *Integrated Pharmacology*. 3rd ed. Philadelphia: Elsevier; 2006.

EATING DISORDERS

Anorexia nervosa (starvation due to an individual's distorted image of their body) and bulimia nervosa (binge eating to induce vomiting and use of laxatives) are classified as mental health conditions, and are best treated through psychotherapy, family therapy, counselling and dietary advice. Patients might be also be offered antidepressant drugs to help with other conditions such as anxiety, depression, social phobias and obsessive compulsion.

PHYSIOLOGY OF THE ORAL CAVITY

The teeth and supporting tissues provide the initial digestive process essential to all bodily activities. Chewing and swallowing are carried out by specialized oral tissues, such as the teeth, tongue, salivary glands and muscles of mastication. The maxillary and mandibular dentition articulate via the temporomandibular joint in a specific pattern to generate the forces needed for mastication. Chewing pressure and oral sensations are mediated by the trigeminal nerve in response to information provided by proprioceptive nerves in the oral tissues. The salivary glands produce more than a litre of saliva daily to lubricate the oral tissues, facilitate taste and initiate the digestive process.

THE TEETH AND OTHER ORAL TISSUES

Tooth structure, the oral mucosa and the salivary glands are important in health and in dental disease.

The tooth crown is composed of a crystalline and highly mineralized (96%) calcified tissue, the enamel. Dentin, a less-mineralized tissue, forms the bulk of the tooth structure and protects the vital tooth pulp throughout the root length. The dental pulp contains loose connective tissue, blood vessels and nerves. Odontoblasts, which produce the dentin, are found at the interface between the pulp tissue and dentin, with projections extending into the dentinal tubules. Finally, the root is covered with a calcified connective tissue structure, the cementum. Carious lesions expanding into the dentin, or surgical removal of enamel during treatment, expose the dentinal tubules to external stimuli and painful sensations. Teeth are attached to the maxillary and mandibular alveolar bone by the supporting structures of the teeth, which are termed the periodontium. Alveolar bone is unique because its primary function is to support the teeth and it will gradually disappear as teeth are lost. The periodontal ligament is located between the alveolar bone and cementum, and contains fibres specifically arranged to connect the teeth with alveolar bone. This arrangement allows for subtle tooth movement in response to the forces of mastication.

ORAL MUCOSA

The buccal mucosa is similar to other mucosal tissues, but the gingival mucosa in proximity to the teeth and covering the periodontium is a specialized mucosa. The mucosal attachment to the tooth, near the cemento-enamel junction, creates a ring of unattached gingival tissue, which forms a small space between the mucosa and tooth (i.e. the gingival sulcus or crevice). The depth of the gingival sulcus in relation to the height of the gingival attachment is important in the diagnosis and treatment of periodontal disease.

SALIVARY GLANDS

Adequate salivary flow and composition are essential for maintaining healthy oral tissues. Saliva consists of water and mucin combined with minerals, enzymes and immune components. It initiates digestion of some foodstuffs, functions as a lubricant to protect mucosal tissues and facilitates mastication. It is also involved in taste perception and caries prevention and as a factor influencing the microbial environment of the mouth.

DISEASES OF THE ORAL CAVITY

Dental plaque, caries and gingivitis
Most dental diseases are associated with microorganisms, infection and the resulting inflammatory response.

Dental plaque
Caries and gingivitis are common dental diseases and are related to the formation of dental plaque. Plaque is a soft nonmineralized deposit consisting of microorganisms in a glycoprotein matrix. It begins as a pellicle of salivary proteins adhering to the enamel surface. Oral microorganisms colonize the pellicle forming the plaque content. The varieties of plaque microorganisms play a key role in the development of dental disease. If plaque is removed or reduced through regular dental hygiene practice, the incidence of dental caries, gingivitis and periodontitis is significantly reduced. Plaque that has become mineralized is called dental calculus (tartar).

Dental caries
Dental caries or decay is probably the most universal and common of all reported dental diseases. Caries development is a time-dependent event involving a critical relationship between the host, plaque microorganisms, metabolic acid production and diet. *Streptococcus mutans* is generally regarded as the most cariogenic microorganism, but *Lactobacillus* species are also implicated in some types of carious lesion. Acid production associated with a combination of cariogenic microorganisms and a cariogenic diet including sucrose or other rapidly digestible carbohydrates furthers the progression of demineralization and the development of carious lesions. Factors that reduce saliva production can also contribute to the development of dental caries. Once caries reaches the dentinal tissues, it progresses in a more diffuse pattern.

Gingivitis (inflammation of the gingiva)
Gingivitis describes the inflammatory reaction of the gingival mucosa in close proximity to the teeth to a variety of etiologic agents including plaque microorganisms.
- Plaque-associated gingivitis is common, particularly in people with poor oral hygiene. It is usually asymptomatic except for localized bleeding during brushing. If plaque and calculus deposits expand into the gingival crevice, the nature of the microorganisms changes to an anaerobe-dominated bacterial population and leads to more serious infections of the periodontium.
- Acute necrotizing ulcerative gingivitis (ANUG) is an acute painful form of gingival infection associated with fusiform and spirochete organisms, with a clinical presentation very different from that of the inflammatory gingivitis of plaque. Ulcerated and highly inflamed gingival tissues are typically observed. Fever and lymphadenopathy may also be part of the acute presentation.

SYSTEMIC FACTORS MAY ALSO PLAY A ROLE IN GINGIVITIS

Management
Dental plaque, caries and gingivitis are three distinct presentations of dental disease but are uniquely linked as a focus for preventive dental medicine.

Removal of plaque and calculus (oral prophylaxis and scaling) from tooth surfaces is a major part of the overall preventive program.

Over-the-counter (OTC) mouth rinses have limited benefits in controlling plaque and calculus. Chlorhexidine gluconate oral rinse reduces plaque bacteria and gingivitis with twice daily use but must be used in conjunction with appropriate dental treatment. Its use in other oral mucosal diseases is discussed later. Dentifrices containing other antibacterial agents, including triclosan and fluoride, are also promoted for plaque control. Calculus-control toothpastes containing pyrophosphate or zinc salts are designed to prevent supragingival calculus formation and do not affect existing calculus.

Chlorhexidine gluconate is a biguanide, cationic agent with antibacterial action. The cationic portion of the molecule binds to negatively charged bacterial cell components altering cell osmotic dynamics with leakage of cellular ions. In higher concentrations, chlorhexidine is bactericidal as it causes precipitation of cellular contents. The spectrum of activity of chlorhexidine includes many Gram-positive and Gram-negative microorganisms which have been implicated in dental disease. Examples are *S. mutans, Porphyromonas gingivalis, Prevotella intermedia, Bacteroides forsythus* and *Campylobacter rectus*. Chlorhexidine is indicated for use as adjunctive treatment to prophylaxis and scalding to reduce plaque formation and for control of gingivitis. It is administered as an oral rinse (0.12%–0.2%). Twice daily rinses (15 mL for 30 seconds and expectorated) are initiated after prophylaxis and scaling for use between dental appointments. Up to 30% of chlorhexidine is retained in the oral cavity after rinsing and is slowly released over 12 hours. The sustained action is believed to be related to binding to oral tissues, namely the hydroxyapatite of tooth enamel, the pellicle, the oral mucosa and salivary proteins. Rinsing with water, eating or drinking must be avoided for at least 30 minutes after use. Because chlorhexidine is used topically, systemic side effects are rarely noted as limited amounts will be swallowed. Repeated use of chlorhexidine rinses is associated with discoloration of teeth and alteration of taste in some patients. The discoloration is superficial and easily removed by professional tooth polishing. Chlorhexidine is contraindicated in patients with a positive history of hypersensitivity to the drug.

Treatment and prevention of dental caries includes plaque control and the use of systemic and/or topical fluorides.

Fluoride in the water supply and in a multitude of dental products has significantly reduced the incidence of dental caries in children in developed countries, but dental caries in areas where fluoride is not available remains a major dental concern. Treatment and prevention of dental caries includes removal of all carious lesions, oral hygiene to reduce dental plaque, dental sealants to cover pits and fissures in the tooth structure, cariogenic diet control and the use of systemic or topical fluorides.

The beneficial effect of fluoride in caries prevention was initially recognized in the 1930s. In many countries, multiple fluoride preparations are available for systemic or topical application to prevent dental caries. Maximum benefits accrue when fluoride use is coupled with a program of regular preventive dental care. Other uses of fluoride include a reduction in tooth sensitivity due to exposed dentinal or cemental surfaces, remineralization of incipient carious lesions, and some reduction in gingivitis. Fluoride interacts with the hydroxyapatite of enamel to produce fluorohydroxyapatite. This latter compound is less soluble in acids originating from sugar metabolism by plaque bacteria. Fluoride has also been shown to decrease the population of *S. mutans* and to interfere with metabolism in plaque bacteria. Fluoride can be administered as fluoride rinses, dentifrices, gels and stannous fluoride solutions, all of which are intended for topical application. Sodium fluoride tablets are also available to supplement systemic

fluoride ingestion in the presence of inadequate fluoridated water supplies. Fluoride is absorbed rapidly (80%–90%) from the upper gastrointestinal (GI) tract with peak blood levels occurring in approximately 30 minutes. Fluoride is widely distributed to calcified tissues, bone and teeth, with up to 50% of the daily intake deposited in calcified tissues. Renal clearance accounts for most of the excreted dose. Systemic fluorides are generally administered with water or juice as dairy products substantially reduce fluoride absorption. Systemic fluoride should not be prescribed when the water content of fluoride exceeds 0.6 ppm. Daily sodium fluoride doses, which vary among countries, are regularly published by various dental organizations. Fluoride supplementation must take into account the total daily amount of naturally ingested fluoride from all sources, the climate (in hot climates more water is consumed) and the patient's age, weight and physical status. Adverse effects of supplemental systemic or topical fluorides are usually limited to GI complaints and occur infrequently. However, the use of prescribed fluorides and topical home fluoride products in very young children should be supervised to avoid excessive ingestion. Side effects include nausea with or without vomiting, excessive salivation and abdominal pain. Severe toxicity, requiring medical attention, may occur with accidental ingestion of larger amounts (10–20 mg in children). Chronic ingestion of excessive fluoride can lead to the development of dental fluorosis, an unsightly staining of the teeth.

Acute dental pain

Pain as a general topic and the principles of its treatment are covered in detail in Chapter 13. Acute pain associated with dental disease is probably the most common complaint of dental patients. Any injury to the oral tissues leads to the release of inflammatory mediators and sensitization of trigeminal afferent nerve endings by prostaglandins and bradykinin. Acute oral pain is also a symptom of many orofacial diseases including acute infection, mucosal lesions, obstructed salivary gland ducts and tissue trauma. Early carious lesions are often associated with acute transient pain that is readily alleviated by dental treatment. However, untreated carious lesions can lead to destruction of tooth structure, allowing oral microorganisms to invade pulpal tissues. Pulpal infection leads to the development of painful inflammation or to an acute periapical abscess and persistent pain. If left untreated this infection can rapidly extend from the alveolar bone into adjacent soft tissues resulting in a cellulitis. Determining the aetiology of dental pain is sometimes complicated because pain can be referred from other tissues such as the sinuses and the ears, and from the temporomandibular joint.

Management of dental pain

Management of acute orofacial pain begins with diagnosis and appropriate dental treatment. Systemically administered drugs, or local anaesthetic drugs, either alone or in combination, are most frequently used for controlling acute orofacial pain, especially before and immediately after definitive dental treatment. Opioids with a favourable oral-to-parenteral effectiveness ratio are preferred, as is the oral route of administration. Acute orofacial pain of moderate intensity or greater can be effectively managed with opioid drugs. Opioids act centrally to modify pain perception by interacting with multiple opiate receptors and mimicking endogenous opioid peptides. Sedation and euphoria often accompany opioid analgesia as an added benefit in controlling the emotional component of pain. Opioids are rarely used alone for acute dental pain and are frequently combined with aspirin, nonsteroidal anti-inflammatory drugs (NSAIDs) or acetaminophen. Detailed discussion of these and related drugs and their use in acute pain syndromes is found in Chapter 13. Local anaesthetic drugs with or without vasoconstrictors such as adrenaline are essential for the control of pain during dental surgery and treatment. Vasoconstrictive drugs are used in combination with local anaesthetics to prolong the duration of action by dealing absorption of the local anaesthetic drug and to reduce bleeding during soft tissue surgery. Examples of local anaesthetics/vasoconstrictors commonly used in dentistry include the following:

Amide local anaesthetics:
- Lidocaine with and without adrenaline
- Mepivacaine with and without levonordefrin
- Prilocaine with and without adrenaline
- Etidocaine with adrenaline
- Bupivacaine with adrenaline
- Articaine with adrenaline

Ester local anaesthetics:
- Chloroprocaine with adrenaline
- Tetracaine (topical only)
- Benzocaine (topical only)

An alternative strategy for controlling postoperative dental pain has been advocated using combinations of NSAIDs and long-acting local anaesthetics. Of the latter, both etidocaine and bupivacaine provide analgesia well into the post-treatment period when the anticipated pain response is greatest. A normal dose of an NSAID is taken soon after treatment and before the return of normal oral sensations. This combination of drugs has been shown to reduce the intensity of pain in the immediate post-treatment period and reduce the need for opioid medications.

Chronic orofacial pain

Chronic orofacial pain can arise from:
- inflammation or internal derangements of the temporomandibular joint,
- myalgia associated with the oral and facial musculature, or
- lesions in the central nervous system (CNS).

NSAIDs are used for the symptomatic management of pain associated with injury or inflammatory processes and opioids should be limited to longer acting drugs, used only to initiate pain control or completely avoided because of the possibility of dependence, unless the pain is due to oral cancer. Tricyclic antidepressants may be used to alleviate pain and symptoms such as depression and altered sleep patterns. The pain arising from trigeminal neuralgia responds to the anticonvulsant drugs carbamazepine and phenytoin. Centrally acting skeletal muscle relaxants methocarbamol or cyclobenzaprine are sometimes useful if myalgia or muscle spasm is present.

Adverse effects of analgesic drugs
- The most common adverse effects of opioids are nausea, sedation and dizziness.
- The most common adverse effect of NSAIDs is gastrointestinal irritation.
- The most common adverse effects of local anaesthetics are usually psychogenic, such as syncope and anxiety, but they can cause arrhythmias if they become systemic.

Anxiety

A visit to the dentist can be an intimidating experience for many patients to the point some actually avoid dental care until the pain demands emergency attention. Dentists have long been portrayed as the harbingers of pain, so reinforcing the patient's anxiety. In such patients the use of anxiolytic drugs can help.

Management of anxiety

Sedation can be useful to control anxiety and mild anxiety can be effectively controlled with oral doses of benzodiazepines such as diazepam, triazolam, lorazepam and midazolam. Promethazine or hydroxyzine alone, or in combination with meperidine, is often used in sedation procedures for children. However, the quality of oral sedation is not always predictable and may be inadequate for an extremely anxious patient.

Inhalation sedation with nitrous oxide-oxygen can also be used to manage fear and anxiety in dental patients. Concentrations ranging from 25% to 50% nitrous oxide in oxygen, administered by nasal mask, are commonly used to provide sedation sufficient for the mildly anxious dental patient. Patients are responsive to commands and remain conscious throughout the procedure with intact protective reflexes. Limited analgesia may be evident in some patients. The pharmacokinetics of nitrous oxide dictate the advantage of this technique including rapid onset, ease in regulation of sedation depth, and rapid recovery. Local anaesthetics are used in combination with nitrous oxide conscious sedation to ensure adequate pain control. Nitrous oxide sedation is sometimes combined with orally administered anxiolytic drugs for the more anxious patient. This requires careful attention to drug doses and patient monitoring as excessive CNS depression and toxicity can result especially in paediatric patients.

Intravenous (IV) sedation is ideal for the very anxious patient and for more extensive dental procedures. Again, midazolam or diazepam alone or in combination with meperidine has been extensively used. Other drugs suitable for IV administration include the rapid-acting barbiturates or opioids such as fentanyl. IV administration of sedative drugs allows for controlled induction and dose titration for adjustment to a desired sedation level.

Acute odontogenic infections

The general principles of treatment of viral and bacterial infections are described in Chapters 29 and 30, respectively. Dental caries, periodontal disease, acute periapical abscesses, salivary gland infections and many other oral infections are caused by microorganisms that are part of the normal oral flora. Other oral infections are caused by microorganisms introduced into the oral cavity by trauma (*Staphylococcus*) or other means (herpes). Separate microenvironments within the oral cavity account for the growth of aerobic and both facultative and obligate anaerobic microorganisms existing in a commensal relationship. As a result, most odontogenic bacterial infections are caused by a mix of pathogens with significant involvement of both facultative and obligate anaerobes. Aerobic streptococci and, to a lesser extent, staphylococci along with fungi (yeast) are also part of the normal oral flora and are potential pathogens.

Odontogenic oral infections cause fever, malaise, swelling, pain and pus formation

Odontogenic oral infections can present with acute symptoms of fever, malaise, swelling and pain. Redness and pus formation may be evident, depending on the site of the infection. Pulpal infection often expands to the periapical tissues, with involvement of alveolar bone if dental treatment is delayed. At this point, pain will usually prompt the patient to seek dental care, but the abscess may continue to spread from the alveolar bone until it opens onto a soft tissue surface as an intraoral fistula. With an avenue of drainage for the abscess, either through the tooth or soft tissue fistula, acute symptoms often abate and the infection assumes a chronic status. However, the infection may also spread diffusely in soft tissues with resulting cellulitis. Rarely, the infection will spread from a mandibular site, dissecting along the facial planes into the neck or from a maxillary site, spreading to the cavernous sinus of the brain. These latter infections can create life-threatening situations and require aggressive treatment.

Management of acute dental infections

Acute odontogenic infections are best managed with a combination of dental intervention and antibiotic therapy.

- Recognize the cardinal signs of infection.
- Consider the integrity of the patient's immune system.
- Know which are the potential oral pathogens.
- Match the antibiotic's spectrum to the causative pathogens.
- Incise and drain any abscess that is pointing.
- Self-limiting infections may respond to dental treatment without the use of antibiotics.

For most dental infections, antibiotic drug selection is based on the presenting symptoms, the location of the infection, a knowledge of the microorganisms usually associated with the type of infection and experience. Antibiotic drugs selected for acute odontogenic infections should have a spectrum that includes streptococcal species and anaerobic bacteria. Fortunately, most microorganisms that cause common oral infections have remained sensitive to traditional antibiotic drugs. However, laboratory culturing and sensitivity tests should be performed if the infection fails to respond as expected, when sampling without contamination can be accomplished and in osteomyelitis. The antibiotics often used in the treatment of oral infections include penicillins such as penicillin V potassium, amoxicillin, amoxicillin with clavulanate or ampicillin; tetracyclines such as tetracycline, doxycycline or minocycline; cephalosporins such as cephalexin or cefaclor; macrolides such as erythromycin, azithromycin or clarithromycin; and clindamycin or metronidazole.

Penicillin V potassium is bactericidal and remains the drug of first choice for the treatment of many odontogenic infections as it has a spectrum that includes the streptococcal and anaerobic organisms frequently encountered in acute infections. Amoxicillin is also favoured as a first choice because of its oral bioavailability and its effectiveness against some Gram-negative organisms. Penicillin G or ampicillin is preferred for parenteral administration. Erythromycin and related macrolides are used as alternative drugs for the penicillin-allergic patient and if the infection is less severe. However, clindamycin has a favourable Gram-positive and anaerobic spectrum of action and is considered by many as the alternative choice of penicillin. Cephalosporins are seldom drugs of first choice, but are used when staphylococcal organisms are involved, for example in case of osteomyelitis or oral trauma. Metronidazole, which has an anaerobic spectrum, is rapidly becoming a drug of choice for selected periodontal infections. It is most often used in combination with another antibiotic with a desirable aerobic spectrum. Tetracyclines are generally limited to infections associated with the periodontium but are also used as an alternative to penicillin V potassium in the treatment of actinomycosis. The role of the quinolone antibiotics for common dental infections remains to be established. There are recent data to suggest limited use in some oral infections where culture and sensitivity testing indicate a favourable clinical outcome.

Adverse effects of antibiotics

- All antibiotics can cause GI adverse effects and diarrhoea.
- Allergic reactions occur more frequently with the penicillins.
- Anti-infectives alter the normal flora causing a risk of opportunistic candidiasis, especially in immunosuppressed patients.
- Tetracycline use in children causes permanent grey-yellow mottling of teeth.

Periodontal infections

Periodontitis (infection of the periodontium) can present in several acute or chronic forms and with different etiologies. In adults it is typically chronic with symptoms limited to an erythematous-appearing gingiva that bleeds on probing or brushing. The distinguishing feature of periodontal disease is a continuing infection of the supporting tissues of the teeth, resulting in a progressive loss of gingival attachment and alveolar bone. It is the most common cause of tooth loss in adult patients. Periodontitis often goes undetected until the patient presents bleeding gums or blood on the toothbrush, in which case the patient should be referred for dental evaluation. In the younger age group it can present as a juvenile periodontitis.

Management of periodontal infections

Controlling periodontal disease involves a variety of treatment approaches such as the control of plaque and gingivitis as a way of reducing the number of supragingival microorganisms, and bacteria in plaque contribute to the inflammatory aspect of periodontal disease. However, if there is microbial invasion of the deeper tissues of the periodontium, systemic anti-infective drugs, irrigation with anti-infectives, and surgical debridement may be required to control the disease. Systemic anti-infective drugs should include drugs that are effective against multiple anaerobic organisms. Selection depends on the causative organisms and antibiotic sensitivity. Tetracyclines and amoxicillin alone or in combination with metronidazole or even ciprofloxacin have been used. Recently, a low dose (20 mg, twice daily) doxycycline product has been introduced. It appears that this dose has no antimicrobial activity; rather it acts by inhibition of crevicular bacterial collagenase responsible for injury to the periodontium. In addition, specialty doses forms, including a tetracycline-containing monofilament fibre, a doxycycline polymer gel, a metronidazole gel, minocycline powder and a chlorhexidine resorbable chip have been developed for adjunctive treatment in refractory periodontal disease. The gels, fibre, powder or chip are placed into the periodontal pocket around the tooth while the drug is slowly released over several days. Contraindications to the use of specialty doses forms include the presence of an acute periodontal abscess or hypersensitivity to the individual drug component.

Prophylactic use of anti-infective drugs in dentistry

The prophylactic use of antibiotics in dentistry is not generally required for routine dental treatment in patients without risk factors and with a normally functioning immune system. However, selected patients with pre-existing myocardial or valvular pathology may be at risk for endocarditis secondary to a bacteraemia. Certain dental procedures, including extractions, oral and maxillofacial surgery, periodontal therapy, deep scaling and other dental procedures are associated with a transient bacteraemia that usually lasts less than 15–20 minutes. Selected oral microorganisms have been implicated as a cause of infective endocarditis in patients at risk. Advisory groups throughout the world have established guidelines for antibiotic prophylaxis for patients at risk. Amoxicillin, penicillin V potassium or another suitable alternative drug (clindamycin, a macrolide or cephalosporin) is usually recommended for prophylactic use immediately prior to the dental procedure.

There is considerable debate about the risk and benefits and drug choice for patients with joint prostheses; however, prophylaxis may be considered for patients with a compromised immune system. Recommended guidelines cannot address every patient situation, and consultation between the physician and dentist is advised.

At-risk patients with poor oral hygiene, extensive caries, gingivitis or periodontitis should be placed on a dental treatment program that includes elimination and prevention of dental disease.

COMMON DISEASES OF THE ORAL MUCOSA

Candida infections

Candida albicans is the most common cause of an oral yeast infection. The incidence of oral candidiasis has increased in recent years and is particularly common among people with human immunodeficiency virus (HIV) infection or other causes of immunosuppression. Decreases in saliva flow associated with Sjogren's syndrome or the use of drugs that decrease salivary flow contribute to the risk of candidiasis. The lesions of candidiasis are seen on the buccal and palatal oral mucosa and the tongue and can produce an angular cheilitis. Erythematous mucosa lesions appearing on a tissue-bearing surface for a denture prothesis are typically the result of a *Candida* infection.

Management

Antifungal drugs used for the treatment of candidiasis include the following:

- The topical agents nystatin, clotrimazole, amphotericin B and chlorhexidine
- The systemic agents fluconazole, itraconazole and ketoconazole

Nystatin is the drug of choice for acute candidiasis

The drug of choice for acute candidiasis is nystatin, which can be used as a topical rinse, ointment or lozenge. Chlorhexidine rinse is also effective. Candidiasis in denture wearers can also be treated with topical nystatin, but resolution of the infection can be difficult because the organism attaches to the denture base and is a potential source of re-inoculation. Soaking the denture in nystatin or chlorhexidine solutions or remaking the denture is usually required. Patient compliance for a topical regimen can become a problem. Systemic ketoconazole or fluconazole maybe required for:

- the noncompliant patient,
- the treatment of chronic atrophic candidiasis, or
- candidiasis in the immunocompromised patient.

Herpes viruses cause most oral viral infections

An initial herpes infection can manifest in an adult or child as an acute herpetic gingivostomatitis or in the adult as pharyngotonsillitis. Both are associated with fever and lymphadenopathy with significant pain and ulcerative-like acute lesions. However the most common manifestation of herpes infection is recurrent herpes labialis (cold sore, fever blisters). It appears with a prodromal onset of tingling or burning, which is usually followed by vesicle formation and rupture, pain and finally crusting. Other members of the herpes virus group such as herpes zoster, Epstein-Barr virus, and rarely, coxsackie viruses can also produce oral lesions. Hairy leukoplakia, which is observed in patients with HIV, is associated with the Epstein-Barr virus.

Management of initial herpetic infections is usually symptomatic and includes topical local anaesthetics, systemic analgesic, and chlorhexidine rinses. Repeated episodes of recurrent herpes labialis can sometimes be controlled with systemic acyclovir. Topical acyclovir or penciclovir applied during the early prodromal stage may reduce the pain and duration of the lesion. Valacyclovir could also be used for systemic administration.

Acute aphthous ulceration

Recurrent aphthous stomatitis (canker sores) is probably one of the most prevalent oral mucosal diseases, with a general population incidence of 20%. Minor aphthous ulcers are the most common and appear as small (5 mm diameter or less) painful ulcerative lesions covered with a grey pseudomembrane. They are seen on the nonkeratinized oral mucosa and the lateral borders of the tongue. Major aphthous ulcers occur less frequently but are larger (over 1 cm in diameter) and extremely painful. Herpetiform ulcers occur as clusters of ulcers on the palate but are rarely observed. Their etiology remains unknown, but emotional stress, trauma and nutritional deficiencies have been implicated. Oral ulcers are also associated with malabsorption diseases.

Treatment is symptomatic, usually with topical local anaesthestics although systemic glucocorticoids are sometimes required for frequent and repeated episodes.

Lichen planus and benign mucous membrane pemphigoid cause inflammation of the oral mucosa as well as other tissues. Pemphigoid is an autoimmune disease. The acute symptoms of lichen planus are usually treated with topical anti-inflammatory glucocorticoids. Treatment objectives include eradicating the ulcerative lesions and controlling symptomatic exacerbations. High potency topical glucocorticoids in gel form seem to produce the most favourable response and least risk of systemic absorption. If the lesions are not responding, higher potency topical glucocorticoids are used and sometimes systemic prednisone is indicated. An intralesional injection of triamcinolone is sometimes given. Pemphigoid generally responds well to topical anti-inflammatory glucocorticoids. However, severe refractory pemphigoid requires more aggressive treatment with prednisone or the use of an immunosuppressive drug such as azathioprine. Dapsone has occasionally been used. The long-term use of systemic glucocorticoids or the use of immunosuppressive drugs should be managed by a physician as the adverse effects can be more severe and need to be carefully monitored. The use of topical glucocorticoids for any of these lesions may suppress the immune system and lead to the development of candidiasis, which should then be treated with nystatin or chlorhexidine oral rinses.

Drug-induced oral disease

Many dental patients will be taking one or more prescribed medications, which may produce adverse effects that can manifest as painful oral mucosal reactions (stomatitis). Such adverse effects include mucositis and oral ulcerations associated with cancer chemotherapy, lichenoid drug reactions, lupus erythematosus-like reactions, pemphigus-like drug reactions and erythema multiforme. Contact allergic reactions may also be observed but occur with less frequency. Angioedema has been observed with some drugs and cinnamon-based ingredients in dentifrices. Dental materials, including metals and acrylic polymers, have also been implicated in soft tissue allergic reactions. Phenytoin, cyclosporine and the calcium ion (Ca^{2+}) antagonists can cause gingival hyperplasia, which develops in approximately 40% of patients who take phenytoin. Among the Ca^{2+} antagonists, some data suggests that isradipine is less likely to cause gingival hyperplasia. The gingival mucosa begins to enlarge and cover the teeth. In severe cases the overgrowth will almost entirely cover the teeth and must be surgically reduced. Drugs with anticholinergic effects frequently reduce salivary flow, leading to a drug-induced xerostomia. A dry mouth can also be due to systemic disease and must be considered in these cases.

Management

Management of drug-induced oral adverse effects includes the following:

- Identifying the suspect drug
- Working with the physician and patient to seek an alternative drug whenever possible

Otherwise, palliative care and efforts to improve dental hygiene and control plaque are needed. Acute inflammatory symptoms often respond to topical or systemic anti-inflammatory glucocorticoids. An antifungal agent such as nystatin or a chlorhexidine rinse can be used for opportunistic candidiasis. Local anaesthetic rinses may be beneficial for stomatitis associated with cancer chemotherapy. A dry mouth presents a significant challenge as there are no suitable artificial saliva substitutes. And drug-stimulated salivary flow is less than satisfactory. Oral pilocarpine may produce some benefit in patients who have a reduced salivary flow following head and neck radiation. Cevimeline, a cholinergic agonist, was recently introduced for treatment of dry mouth symptoms associated with Sjogren's syndrome.

Viruses consist essentially of DNA or RNA in a protein coat. They have no ribosomes or protein-synthesizing apparatus, although some contain enzymes. They replicate by taking over the metabolic processes of the host. Because a virus virtually (and in some cases, actually) becomes part of its host cell, selective chemotherapy is difficult.

The human immunodeficiency virus (HIV) – an RNA retrovirus – will be taken as an example of viral infection of a host cell (Fig. 29.1). Antiviral drugs will be dealt with under two headings: anti-HIV drugs and other antiviral agents.

Viral infection of a cell

The binding sites on the host cell to which the virus attaches are normal membrane constituents: receptors for cytokines, neurotransmitters or hormones, ion channels, integral membrane glycoproteins, etc. Thus the virus that causes infantile diarrhoea attaches to the β-adrenoceptor; the rabies virus attaches to the acetylcholine receptor on skeletal muscle. With many viruses, the receptor-virus complex enters the cell by receptor-mediated endocytosis during which the virus coat may be removed. Some viruses bypass this route.

On entering and infecting a host cell, the virus genome itself acts as – or is transcribed into – virus-specific messenger RNA, which then directs the synthesis of new virus particles. DNA viruses enter the host cell nucleus to accomplish this. Most RNA viruses replicate without involving the host cell nuclear material. RNA retroviruses (e.g. HIV, responsible for the acquired immunodeficiency syndrome (AIDS)) have an enzyme, reverse transcriptase, that makes a DNA copy of the viral RNA; this DNA copy is integrated into the host genome and directs the generation of new viral particles (Fig. 29.1).

Anti-HIV drugs

The two main groups of anti-HIV drugs are reverse transcriptase inhibitors (RTIs) and protease inhibitors. Combinations of these is essential in treatment to prevent the development of tolerance.

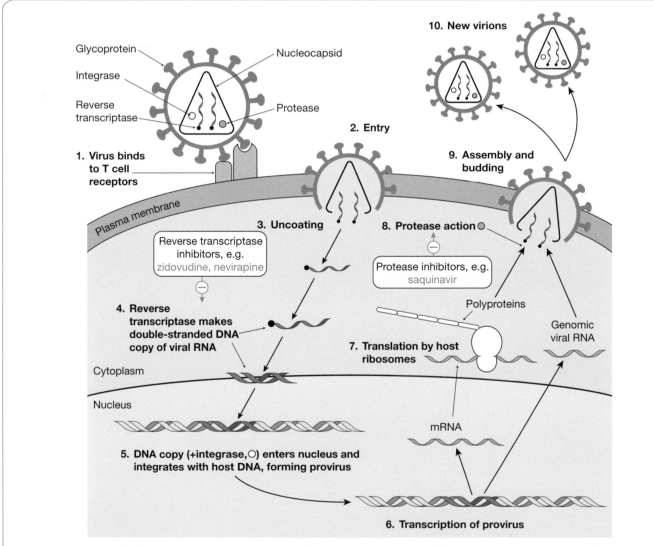

Fig. 29.1 Schematic diagram of the infection of a T cell with the human immunodeficiency virus (HIV) retrovirus, showing the principal viral structures, the main steps in viral replication (1–9) and the sites of action of anti-HIV drugs.

Reverse transcriptase inhibitors

Nucleoside RTIs

Nucleoside RTIs (NRTIs) inhibit the action of the viral reverse transcriptase. The drugs are analogues of endogenous nucleosides and are phosphorylated by host cell enzymes to give a false 5'-trisphosphate. This competitively inhibits the equivalent trisphosphates of the host cell needed by the reverse transcriptase for the formation of the viral DNA. Examples are **zidovudine**, abacavir, didanosine, lamivudine, zalcitabine and stavudine.

Zidovudine (AZT, azidothymidine) This analogue of thymidine is usually given orally but can be given by intravenous (IV) infusion. The cerebrospinal fluid (CSF) concentration is 65% of the blood level and the half-life of the false trisphosphate is 3 h. Most of the drug is metabolized in the liver, but 20% is excreted via the kidney. *Unwanted effects* with long-term use include blood dyscrasias, gastrointestinal (GI) tract disorders, central nervous system (CNS) disturbances, myopathy, rashes, fever and a flu-like syndrome. Short-term use in fit individuals usually causes only minor, reversible adverse effects. *Resistance* is likely to occur in late-stage HIV disease.

Abacavir This guanosine analogue is given orally; it is well absorbed and inactivated in the liver. The CSF concentration is one-third that of the plasma. *Unwanted effects* include skin rashes, GI tract disturbances and, rarely, a serious general hypersensitivity reaction.

Non-nucleoside RTIs

The non-nucleoside RTIs (NNRTIs) are chemically diverse compounds that denature the catalytic site of the reverse transcriptase. Examples are nevirapine and efavirenz.

Nevirapine This drug is given orally and its CSF concentration is 45% of that in the plasma. It is metabolized in the liver. *Unwanted effects* include rash and, rarely, Stevens–Johnson syndrome. Drug interactions can occur. This drug can reduce mother-to-child transmission of HIV by about 50%.

Protease inhibitors

In the final stage of assembly and budding, a viral protease cleaves precursor polyproteins to give the structural and functional proteins of the new virions. Protease inhibitors prevent this step. Examples are **saquinavir**, indinavir and nelfinavir. All are given orally, saquinavir being subject to first-pass metabolism. All inhibit the P450 liver enzymes so drug interactions are possible. In general, these drugs are well tolerated. *Unwanted effects* include GI tract disturbances, insulin resistance and hyperlipidaemia. With long-term use, redistribution of fat is seen (some fat accumulation, some fat loss).

Treatment of HIV/AIDS with anti-HIV drugs

A combination of several drugs is used (known as highly active antiretroviral therapy (HAART)) consisting of two nucleoside RTIs (NRTIs) with either a non-nucleoside RTI (NNRTI) or one or two protease inhibitors. Recently the human immunodeficiency virus (HIV) integrase inhibitor raltegravir has been introduced for the treatment of patients with HIV who are resistant to other drug classes. Maraviroc is another new drug that blocks the interaction between HIV-1 and the chemokine receptor CCR5 on host cells. None of these drugs cure HIV infection, but they can slow progress of the disease and prolong life. They have to be taken indefinitely and a balance must be struck between the therapeutic and adverse actions. Patients with acquired immunodeficiency syndrome (AIDS) will also be taking numerous other drugs for the inevitable intercurrent infections, so drug interactions are a hazard.

Other antiviral drugs

The antiviral agents for infections other than HIV can be classified according to their mechanism of action.

Inhibition of attachment or penetration of host cell

Amantadine

This drug blocks a primitive ion channel (M2) in the viral membrane, preventing the fusion of the virion to host cell membranes and thus inhibits the release of newly synthesized viruses from host cells. Amantadine is used in the prophylaxis and treatment of acute influenza A in high risk groups, although it is not effective against influenza B. Amantadine is less widely used with the introduction of influenza vaccines as there is quite a high level of resistance with this drug and because neurological side effects and renal failure can occur.

Zanamivir

This is a neuraminidase inhibitor and prevents the release of new virions. It is given as a powder by inhalation and is well tolerated.

Palivizumab

This is a humanized monoclonal antibody raised against a specific surface glycoprotein of the respiratory syncytial virus; it neutralizes the virus. It is given intramuscularly (IM).

Inhibition of transcription of the viral genome

Acyclovir

The drug is inactive until converted to the trisphosphate. The first phosphorylation is only effectively carried out by the viral kinase (so the step can only occur in infected cells); subsequent steps are catalysed by host cell kinases. Acyclovir selectively inhibits viral DNA polymerase. It can be given orally, intravenously (IV) or topically and is degraded fairly speedily within host cells. It has minimal unwanted effects. Resistance can occur.

Ganciclovir

This also undergoes phosphorylation and suppresses DNA replication in a similar manner to acyclovir. It is given IV or orally and persists in the host cell for approximately 20 h. *Unwanted effects* include myelosuppression, which occurs in 40% of patients and is potentially carcinogenic.

Foscarnet

This non-nucleoside analogue of pyrophosphate inhibits viral DNA polymerase by attaching to the pyrophosphate binding site. It is given by IV infusion and can cause serious renal toxicity.

Ribavirin

This is a synthetic nucleoside that is given by aerosol for respiratory viral infections.

Immunomodulators

Peginterferon-alfa-2a

The cytokine interferon-α (IF-α) induces host cell enzymes that have antiviral activity. Peginterferon-alfa-2a is IF-α conjugated with polyethylene glycol (PEG) which increases its persistence in the plasma. It is given IV or IM. Blood dyscrasias, GI tract disturbances and flu-like symptoms may occur.

Immunoglobulins

Normal pooled plasma contains immunoglobulins that can neutralize some viruses. *Hyperimmune* immunoglobulins specific for particular viruses can be effective against the viruses that had infected the donors.

Clinical uses of non-anti-HIV antiviral agents

- **Zanamivir**: influenza A and B.
- **Acyclovir**: herpes viruses.
- **Ganciclovir**: cytomegalovirus (CMV) infection, especially CMV retinitis in patients with acquired immunodeficiency syndrome (AIDS).
- **Ribavirin**: respiratory syncytial virus, influenza, possibly Lassa fever.
- **Foscarnet**: CMV (fairly effective).
- **Interferons**: hepatitis B; may also be useful in AIDS.
- **Hyperimmune immunoglobulin**: hepatitis B, varicella zoster, CMV, rabies, tetanus.
- **Palivizumab:** respiratory syncytial virus.
- **Raltegravir and maraviroc:** AIDS resistant to other treatment approaches.

Antibacterial drugs are used to treat bacterial infections. Many species of bacteria cause disease in humans; these are termed *pathogens*. It was once thought that these pathogenic bacteria had a special ability to cause infections whereas bacteria that lived happily and innocuously within the mammalian organism, termed *commensals*, lacked this ability. It is now known that commensals – and also bacteria in the environment that are normally harmless – are virtually all capable of being pathogenic. In the healthy host, the immune/inflammatory response prevents these inoffensive organisms from giving rise to infections; however, if the immune system is compromised, as in patients infected with human immunodeficiency virus (HIV) or after the use of immunosuppressant drugs, these bacteria can be opportunistic and cause disease.

Antibacterial drugs can be *bactericidal*, i.e. they kill the bacterium, or they can be *bacteriostatic*, i.e. they stop the bacterium growing. With these latter drugs, the enfeebled organism is easier for the host's defence mechanisms to eliminate the bacteria. If these mechanisms are impaired, only bactericidal drugs are effective.

The term *antibiotic*, originally developed to describe a chemical agent produced by one microorganism that killed or prevented the growth of another microorganism, is now subsumed in the term *antibacterial drug*. Antibacterial drugs, to be effective, need to manifest selective toxicity, i.e. they should be toxic to the bacterium but innocuous in the human host. However many of the biochemical processes are common to both bacterial and mammalian cells. Nevertheless, there are components and metabolic processes in the bacterial cell that are sufficiently different from those in humans to be targets for antibacterial drugs.

Targets for Antibacterial Drugs
Fig. 30.1 describes the potential targets for selective antibacterial drugs.

The terms Gram-positive and Gram-negative
Many organisms are classified as Gram-positive or Gram-negative. These terms refer to whether the bacteria stain with Gram's stain, but it has more significance than that of an empirical reaction to a stain. Gram-positive and Gram-negative bacteria differ from each other in several important respects that have implications for the effects of antibiotics.

One important difference is in the structure of the cell wall, which provides support for the plasma membrane and is subject to an internal pressure of approximately 5 atmospheres in Gram-negative organisms and 20 atmospheres in Gram-positive organisms. The bacterial cell wall must, therefore, be able to resist these pressures. Its main constituent is peptidoglycan (Fig. 30.1). Gram-negative bacteria have a single layer of peptidoglycan that in Gram-positive bacteria can be up to 40 layers thick. Each peptidoglycan layer consists of numerous backbones of amino sugars, some having short peptide side-chains that are cross-linked to form a lattice (Fig. 30.2).

There are other differences between the cell wall in Gram-positive and Gram-negative bacteria that are pharmacologically relevant.

The cell wall of *Gram-positive organisms* is a relatively simple structure, 15–50 nm thick of which 50% is peptidoglycan and about 40% consists of acidic polymer. The latter, being highly polar, favours the penetration of positively charged antibacterial drugs, such as streptomycin, into the cell.

In *Gram-negative organisms*, the cell wall is thinner but more complex, and it also has an outer membrane (similar in some respects to the plasma membrane) that connects to the single layer of peptidoglycan. The outer membrane contains transmembrane water-filled channels, termed *porins*, through which hydrophilic antibacterial drugs can move freely. In addition, complex polysaccharides on the outer surface comprise the *endotoxins* that determine the antigenicity of the organism. *In vivo*, these can trigger various aspects of the inflammatory reaction.

The lipopolysaccharide of the cell wall is also a major barrier to penetration by benzylpenicillin, methicillin, the macrolides, rifampicin, fusidic acid and vancomycin.

Difficulty in penetrating this complex outer layer is probably the reason why some antibiotics are less active against Gram-negative than Gram-positive bacteria and is the basis of the extraordinary insusceptibility to most antibiotic drugs of *Pseudomonas aeruginosa*, a pathogen that can cause life-threatening infections in neutropenic patients and in patients with burns and wounds.

Resistance to antibacterial drugs
The genetic determinants of resistance
Chromosomal determinants Mutations of the chromosomal genes in the bacterium are important in methicillin-resistant staphylococci, and in infections with mycoplasma and organisms causing tuberculosis.

Extrachromosomal determinants Many bacteria have, lying free in the cytoplasm, genetic elements that can replicate on their own. These are closed loops of DNA (termed *plasmids*) that can carry resistance genes – often with resistance to several antibiotics. Some stretches of plasmid DNA can be transposed from one plasmid to another and from a plasmid to the chromosome. These stretches are called *transposons* and they can spread resistance between plasmids (Fig. 30.3).

Transfer of resistance genes between bacteria This occurs mainly by conjugation, in which protein tubules called *sex pili* connect two bacteria, allowing transfer of plasmids between them. Genes can also be transferred by phages (bacterial viruses).

The biochemical mechanisms of resistance
There are a number of mechanisms whereby bacteria can become resistant to antibiotics.

Production of enzymes that inactivate the drug Examples are β-lactamases, which inactivate many penicillins, acetyltransferases, which inactivate chloramphenicol and kinases and other enzymes that inactivate aminoglycosides.

Modification of the drug-binding sites This occurs with aminoglycosides, erythromycin and penicillin.

Decreased accumulation of the drug in the bacterium Plasmid-mediated efflux of the drug causes tetracycline resistance in both Gram-positive and Gram-negative organisms and fluoroquinolone resistance in *Staphylococcus aureus*. Reduced penetration can cause resistance to aminoglycosides, chloramphenicol and glycopeptides.

Alteration of the target enzymes An example is the plasmid-mediated synthesis of a dihydrofolate reductase that is insensitive to trimethoprim, or of a dihydropteroate synthetase with low affinity for sulphonamides, but unchanged affinity for *p*-aminobenzoic acid (PABA).

Resistant pathogens
Many pathogenic bacteria have developed resistance to the commonly used antibiotics; important examples include the following:
- Some strains of staphylococci (methicillin-resistant *Staphylococcus aureus* (MRSA)) and enterococci are resistant to virtually all current antibiotics; these organisms can cause virtually untreatable nosocomial (acquired in hospital) infections.

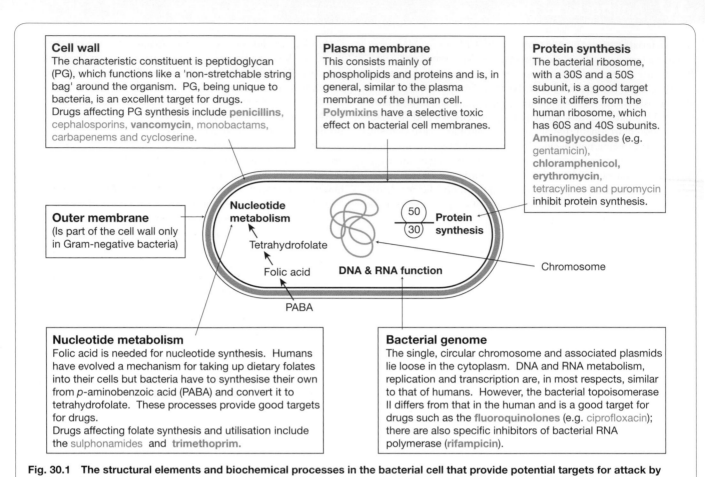

Cell wall
The characteristic constituent is peptidoglycan (PG), which functions like a 'non-stretchable string bag' around the organism. PG, being unique to bacteria, is an excellent target for drugs. Drugs affecting PG synthesis include **penicillins**, cephalosporins, **vancomycin**, monobactams, carbapenems and cycloserine.

Plasma membrane
This consists mainly of phospholipids and proteins and is, in general, similar to the plasma membrane of the human cell. **Polymixins** have a selective toxic effect on bacterial cell membranes.

Protein synthesis
The bacterial ribosome, with a 30S and a 50S subunit, is a good target since it differs from the human ribosome, which has 60S and 40S subunits. **Aminoglycosides** (e.g. gentamicin), **chloramphenicol**, **erythromycin**, tetracylines and puromycin inhibit protein synthesis.

Outer membrane
(Is part of the cell wall only in Gram-negative bacteria)

Nucleotide metabolism

Tetrahydrofolate

Folic acid

50 / 30 Protein synthesis

DNA & RNA function

PABA

Chromosome

Nucleotide metabolism
Folic acid is needed for nucleotide synthesis. Humans have evolved a mechanism for taking up dietary folates into their cells but bacteria have to synthesise their own from *p*-aminobenzoic acid (PABA) and convert it to tetrahydrofolate. These processes provide good targets for drugs.
Drugs affecting folate synthesis and utilisation include the sulphonamides and **trimethoprim**.

Bacterial genome
The single, circular chromosome and associated plasmids lie loose in the cytoplasm. DNA and RNA metabolism, replication and transcription are, in most respects, similar to that of humans. However, the bacterial topoisomerase II differs from that in the human and is a good target for drugs such as the **fluoroquinolones** (e.g. ciprofloxacin); there are also specific inhibitors of bacterial RNA polymerase (**rifampicin**).

Fig. 30.1 **The structural elements and biochemical processes in the bacterial cell that provide potential targets for attack by antibacterial agents.**

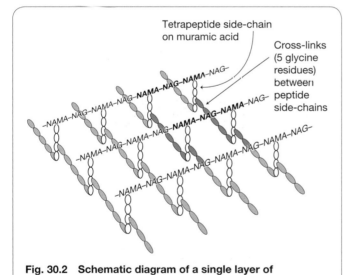

Tetrapeptide side-chain on muramic acid

Cross-links (5 glycine residues) between peptide side-chains

—NAMA—NAG—NAMA—NAG—

Fig. 30.2 **Schematic diagram of a single layer of peptidoglycan such as might be found in *Staphylococcus aureus*.** The darkened area at top right is used to explain the action of β-lactam antibiotics in Figs. 30.5 and 30.6. *NAG*, *N*-acetylglucosamine; *NAMA*, *N*-acetylmuramic acid.

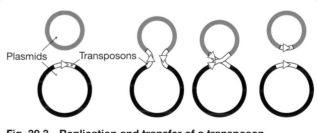

Plasmids   Transposons

Fig. 30.3 **Replication and transfer of a transposon between plasmids.**

- Drugs that affect bacterial protein synthesis
- Drugs that affect bacterial DNA and RNA synthesis and function
- Drugs that affect bacterial folate synthesis and utilization
- Antituberculosis drugs
- Antileprosy drugs

Drugs that affect peptidoglycan synthesis
These drugs include the penicillins, cephalosporins, monobactams, carbapenems and glycopeptides. The first four are termed β-lactam antibiotics because they all have a β-lactam ring in their structure (Fig. 30.4).

Mechanism of action
The β-**lactams** inhibit the synthesis of the peptidoglycan corset by inhibiting the enzyme that inserts the cross-links to the peptide

- Some strains of *Mycobacterium tuberculosis* have developed resistance to most antituberculosis drugs.

Antibacterial Drugs
There are many different classes of antibacterial drugs:
- Drugs that affect bacterial peptidoglycan synthesis

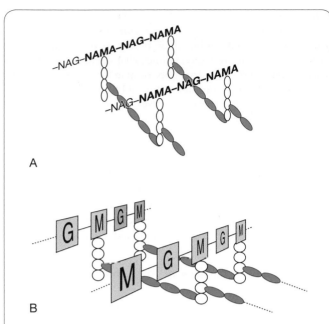

A

B

Fig. 30.4 Structures of penicillin and clavulanic acid. Substituents at R^1 determine the pharmacological characteristics of different types of penicillin. *A,* Thiazolidine ring; *B,* β-lactam ring.

chains that are attached to the peptidoglycan backbone (Figs. 30.5 and 30.6). **Glycopeptides** (e.g. vancomycin) inhibit an earlier reaction. The effect is to weaken the corset enclosing the bacterium. Since the internal osmotic pressure within the organism is high, this leads to rupture of the bacterial cell. These drugs are thus *bactericidal.*

Penicillins

The main types of penicillin are given in Table 30.1 and their basic structure in Fig. 30.4. All act by binding to penicillin-binding proteins before interfering with cell wall synthesis. They then inactivate an inhibitor of autolytic enzymes in the cell wall, leading to rupture as the corset gives way. Many organisms are now resistant to penicillins.

Resistance to penicillins The main mechanism of resistance is the production of β-lactamases, which disrupt the β-lactam ring. The concomitant use of a β-lactamase inhibitor that binds to the bacterial enzyme may overcome this (e.g. clavulanic acid; Fig. 30.4). Other mechanisms of resistance are modification of the binding sites and reduced permeability of the outer membranes.

Pharmacokinetic aspects The drugs pass into all body fluids: joints, pleural and pericardial cavities, bile, saliva and milk. They cross the placenta, but not the blood–brain barrier (unless the meninges are inflamed). Excretion is via the urine and can be blocked by **probenecid.**

Unwanted effects The penicillins are not directly toxic (though they can cause convulsions if injected intrathecally) but can cause

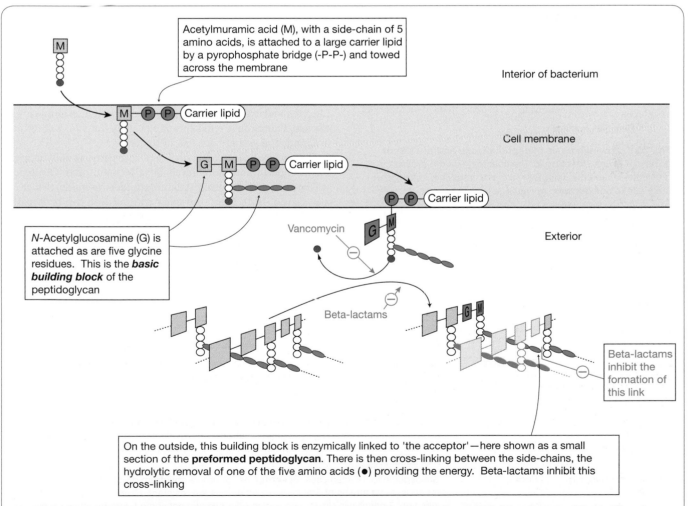

Fig. 30.5 A section of the peptidoglycan corset. This was shown darkened in Figs. 30.2 and 30.6. It has been modified in (A) and modified again in (B) to show the segment depicted in Fig. 30.6. *G,* N-acetylglucosamine (NAGA); *M,* N-acetylmuramic acid (NAMA).

allergic reactions in some people: skin rashes (common) and anaphylaxis (rare but life threatening).

Clinical uses of the penicillins

- First choice drugs for many infections, particularly for bacterial meningitis and infections of bone, joints, skin, soft tissues, throat and urinary tract.
- Gonorrhoea and syphilis.
- Note that many organisms (particularly staphylococci) may be resistant.

Cephalosporins and cephamycins

These are chemically related to penicillin. Examples are **cefaclor, cefadroxil** and cefotaxime.

The *mechanism of action* is the same as for the penicillins: interference with cell wall synthesis. Many Gram-negative bacteria now produce a β-lactamase that inactivates these drugs.

Unwanted effects Mainly hypersensitivities.

Pharmacokinetic aspects Cefaclor is given orally; others are given intramuscularly (IM) or intravenously (IV). They pass into all body fluids: joints, pleural and pericardial cavities, bile, saliva and milk, and also cross the placenta. They cross the blood–brain barrier poorly unless the meninges are inflamed. They are excreted mainly in the urine, but partly in the bile.

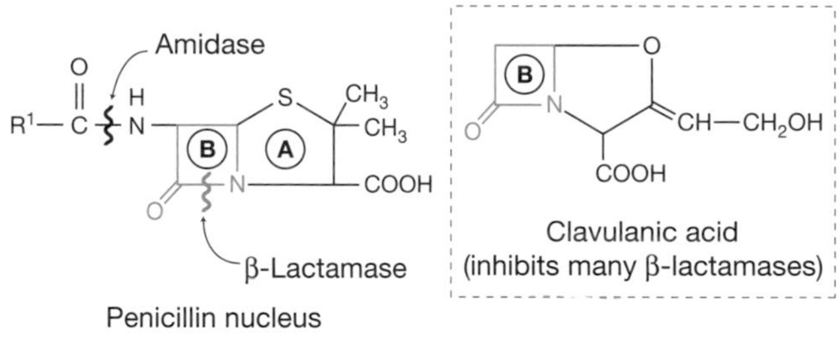

Fig. 30.6 The synthesis of peptidoglycan and the site of action of drugs affecting it. The figure shows the process of biosynthesis and the establishment of a cross-link in a segment such as the one depicted in Fig. 30.2 for a bacterium such as *Staphylococcus aureus*.

Other β-lactams

Carbapenems These broad-spectrum antibiotics (e.g. **imipenem**; used with **cilastatin**, which blocks its breakdown by the kidney) are resistant to many, but not all, β-lactamase-producing drug resistant bacteria, and are important in the treatment of infections resistant to other antibiotics. Given IV and excreted in urine.

Monobactams Aztreonam is active only against Gram-negative aerobic bacteria and is resistant to most β-lactamases.

Glycopeptides

Examples are **vancomycin** and teicoplanin. The glycopeptides act by interfering with cell wall synthesis (Fig. 30.6). Vancomycin is not absorbed from the gastrointestinal (GI) tract. It is given IV, is widely distributed and is excreted by the kidney. It is used only for multiple-resistant staphylococcal infections and is given by mouth for local effect within the GI tract in pseudomembranous colitis.

Clinical use of cephalosporins and cephamycins

Second choice for many infections such as septicaemia, meningitis, pneumonia, biliary tract and urinary tract infections if these are caused by susceptible organisms.

Drugs that inhibit bacterial protein synthesis

The main drugs that inhibit protein synthesis are the aminoglycosides, chloramphenicol, tetracyclines, macrolides, fusidic acid and clindamycin. Figs. 30.7 and 30.8 show bacterial protein synthesis and sites of action of drugs.

Aminoglycosides

These are bactericidal, broad-spectrum agents whose action is enhanced by inhibitors of cell wall synthesis. They are given by injection and excreted in the urine. An important example is **gentamicin**. Excretion is renal and poor kidney function will result in accumulation and greater risk of toxicity.

Dose-related ototoxicity and nephrotoxicity, usually irreversible, can occur and blood levels must be monitored. Ototoxicity will be exacerbated if given with furosemide (frusemide) (which can also be ototoxic). Neuromuscular transmission can be impaired and the drugs are contraindicated in myasthenia gravis.

Table 30.1 The Main Types of Penicillin

Type of penicillin	Absorption in gastrointestinal tract	Main properties and similar agents
β-Lactamase sensitive, e.g. benzylpenicillin (penicillin G)	Poor	The first choice for many infections but destroyed by β-lactamases; many staphylococci now resistant. Given intramuscularly (IM) or intravenously (IV) but not intrathecally. Active against most Gram-positive cocci and Gram-negative bacteria. Phenoxymethylpenicillin is well absorbed in the gastrointestinal tract but is less potent.
β-Lactamase resistant, e.g. flucloxacillin, methicillin	Reasonable	Active against the same organisms as benzylpenicillin but less potent. Used mainly for infections with organisms that produce β-lactamase. Many staphylococci now resistant.
Broad-spectrum: amoxicillin	Very good	Active against more organisms than benzylpenicillin but less potent; destroyed by β-lactamases but can be given in combination with clavulanic acid. Given orally, IM or IV. Many bacteria now resistant. Skin reactions can occur. (Ampicillin is similar but less well absorbed.)
Antipseudomonas, e.g. piperacillin	Poor	Susceptible to β-lactamases. Spectrum as for broad-spectrum drugs, plus pseudomonads. Most strains of *Staphylococcus aureus* are resistant. Given IV or by deep IM injection. Ticarcillin is similar and is also effective against some Gram-negative organisms (e.g. *Proteus*); it can be combined with clavulanic acid.

Tobramycin is another aminoglycoside that can be administered by inhalation to treat pseudomonas infections in the lungs of patients with cystic fibrosis.

Resistance – due to plasmid-controlled inactivating enzymes – is increasing. The enzymes have less effect on **amikacin**. Streptomycin is reserved for treatment of tuberculosis.

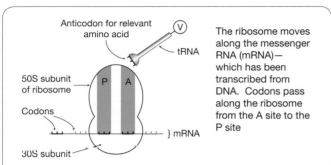

Fig. 30.7   Outline of the basic structure and function of the bacterial ribosome.

The 'P site' contains the growing peptide chain attached to a molecule of transfer RNA (tRNA). The next amino acid residue to be added—linked to its specific tRNA, with its distinctive anticodon—moves into the A site, being bound to the site by codon:anticodon recognition

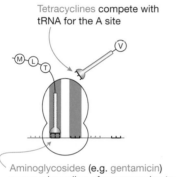

Transpeptidation occurs, linking the peptide chain on the tRNA at the P site to the amino acid on the incoming tRNA at the A site

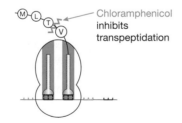

The tRNA denuded of its peptide chain is ejected and the tRNA (with peptide attached) in the A site is translocated to the P site. The ribosome then moves on one codon on the mRNA (a new tRNA with attached amino acid can now move into the A site)

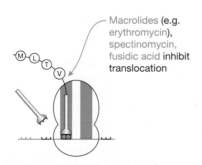

Fig. 30.8   The main steps in protein synthesis and the mechanism of action of drugs. Recent information about the E site has not been included.

Macrolides

The main macrolide is **erythromycin**, which has an antibacterial spectrum fairly similar to penicillin and has been used as an alternative drug. It is also active against mycoplasma and chlamydial infections. It is used for respiratory tract infections, *Campylobacter enteritis* and legionnaires' disease. Its use for penicillin-resistant staphylococcal infections has been compromised by the development of plasmid-controlled resistance due to alteration of its binding site for the ribosome. Clarithromycin and azithromycin are active against *Haemophilus influenzae* and azithromycin kills *Toxoplasma gondii* cysts. Given orally or by IV infusion. Azithromycin is often used to treat exacerbations of patients with chronic obstructive pulmonary disease (COPD) and like other macrolides also possesses some anti-inflammatory actions in addition to antibacterial effects.

Tetracyclines

Examples are **tetracycline** and **doxycycline**. These are orally active, bacteriostatic, broad-spectrum antibiotics and are the drugs of choice for rickettsial, mycoplasma and chlamydial infections, brucellosis, cholera, plague and Lyme disease. However, many organisms are now resistant to these drugs. Absorption is decreased in the presence of food. Doxycycline is excreted in the bile. GI tract disorders are commonly seen. These drugs are deposited in growing bone and are contraindicated in children and pregnant women.

Chloramphenicol

Chloramphenicol is a potent broad-spectrum antibiotic given orally or IV. It can cause serious idiosyncratic depression of the bone marrow, a rare but severe pancytopenia or fatal aplastic anaemia. Poor inactivation and excretion in the newborn can cause grey baby syndrome, which has a 40% mortality rate.

Its use is reserved for *H. influenzae* infections resistant to other agents and meningitis in patients in whom penicillin cannot be used. It is also useful in the treatment of bacterial conjunctivitis. It is also effective in typhoid fever.

Clindamycin

Clindamycin acts against many penicillin-resistant staphylococci and some anaerobes such as *Bacteroides*. Its use can result in pseudomembranous colitis: a severe inflammation of the colon caused by toxins produced by clindamycin-resistant faecal organisms.

Drugs affecting DNA synthesis

The main drugs in this class are the fluoroquinolones.

Fluoroquinolones

Examples are **ciprofloxacin**, norfloxacin and cinoxacin. These are broad-spectrum antibacterial drugs that are particularly effective against Gram-negative organisms. They are also active against chlamydia and mycobacteria.

Mechanism of action   The drugs inhibit topoisomerase II (DNA gyrase), the enzyme that produces the supercoil in the chromosome (Fig. 30.9), which is essential for transcription and replication.

Pharmacokinetic aspects   Ciprofloxacin is given orally or by IV infusion. It is well absorbed from the GI tract, except in the presence of magnesium and aluminium. It accumulates in the kidney, prostate and lung and concentrates in phagocytes. Elimination is partly by metabolism in the liver and partly by excretion in the urine.

Unwanted effects   GI tract disorders and skin rashes can occur, as can joint pains, allergic reactions and photosensitivity.

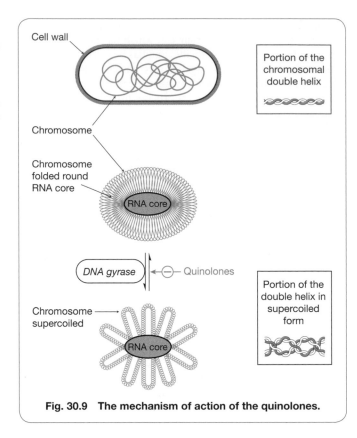

Fig. 30.9 The mechanism of action of the quinolones.

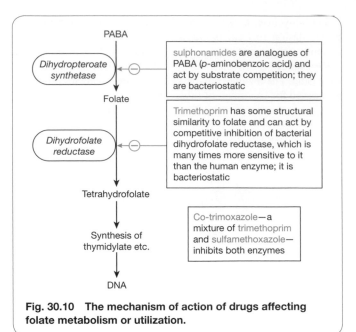

Fig. 30.10 The mechanism of action of drugs affecting folate metabolism or utilization.

As the drugs can inhibit γ-aminobutyric acid (GABA) binding to GABA receptors in the central nervous system (CNS), convulsions may occur.

Clinical use of the fluoroquinolones

- Complicated urinary tract infections
- Gonorrhoea
- Cervicitis
- Prostatitis
- Typhoid fever
- Septicaemia caused by sensitive organisms
- Respiratory tract infections (but not if caused by pneumococci)

Drugs affecting bacterial folate synthesis and utilization

The main drugs in this class are sulphonamides, trimethoprim and co-trimoxazole. The mechanism of action is shown in Fig. 30.10.

Sulphonamides

Examples are **sulfamethoxazole** (short acting), **sulfalene** (sulfametopyrazine; long acting) and sulfadiazine.

Sulphonamides are given orally, pass into inflammatory exudates and cross the placenta. They are inactivated in the presence of pus.

Unwanted effects Allergic reactions (rashes, fever), bone marrow depression and crystalluria can occur. (Alkalinizing the urine and giving plenty of fluids prevents the last of these).

Resistance Common and plasmid mediated.

Trimethoprim

Trimethoprim is active against most common pathogens. It is given orally, is well absorbed and widely distributed; it is excreted in the urine.

Unwanted effects GI tract disturbances, blood disorders and skin rashes.

Clinical uses of trimethoprim, co-trimoxazole and the sulphonamides

- Trimethoprim on its own is used for urinary tract and respiratory infections.
- Co-trimoxazole is used only for *Pneumocystis carinii* pneumonia, nocardiasis and toxoplasmosis.
- Sulphonamides are now only used:
  - with trimethoprim for a few special conditions,
  - for respiratory nocardial infections, and
  - for sexually transmitted chlamydial infections and chancroid.

Antituberculosis drugs

Tuberculosis is now the world's main cause of death from a single agent and treatment has become a problem because of the development of multidrug-resistant strains of *Mycobacterium tuberculosis*:
- *First-line drugs* used in treatment are isoniazid, rifampicin, ethambutol and pyrazinamide.
- *Second-line drugs* are capreomycin, cycloserine, ciprofloxacin and streptomycin.

To reduce the emergence of resistant organisms, combination therapy is used: first a 2-month phase of isoniazid, rifampicin and pyrazinamide; then a 4-month phase of isoniazid and rifampicin.

Isoniazid

Isoniazid acts only on mycobacteria, being bacteriostatic on resting organisms and bactericidal on proliferating ones. Its mechanism of action is not understood.

Pharmacokinetic aspects It is given orally and is well absorbed. It is widely distributed, passing into the cerebrospinal fluid (CSF) and into necrotic tuberculous lesions. It enters into mammalian cells and is taken up by tubercle bacilli. It is acetylated in the liver – slowly in some individuals (slow acetylators), fast in others – the former responding more efficiently to therapy. Elimination is partly by acetylation and partly by excretion unchanged in the urine.

Unwanted effects These are dose related, the most frequent being allergic reactions. Adverse effects in liver, blood, joints and blood vessels can occur. Isoniazid decreases the metabolism of several antiepileptic drugs.

Resistance   This does occur, but importantly does not cause cross-resistance with other antimycobacterial drugs.

Rifampicin

Mechanism of action   Inhibition of the bacterial, but not the human RNA polymerase. Rifampicin enters phagocytic cells and kills the intracellular tubercle bacilli. Rifampicin has very potent antimycobacterial action and is also effective against most Gram-positive and many Gram-negative species.

Pharmacokinetic aspects   It is given orally, widely distributed and excreted in urine and bile. It imparts an orange tint to saliva, sweat and tears. Induction of hepatic metabolizing enzymes results in decreased action of warfarin, narcotic analgesics, glucocorticoids and oral contraceptives.

Unwanted effects   They are not common, but include skin rashes, fever, GI tract disturbances and, rarely, serious liver damage. CNS symptoms, allergic reactions and a flu-like syndrome can occur.

Resistance   Modification of the bacterial RNA polymerase to give rise to resistance has been reported.

Ethambutol

Ethambutol acts only against mycobacteria, being taken up by them and inhibiting their growth. It is given orally and can cross into the CSF. It is partly metabolized and partly excreted unchanged in the urine.

Unwanted effects   These are uncommon, but optic neuritis can occur, as can GI tract disturbances and joint and CNS symptoms.

Resistance   This is likely to occur if the drug is used on its own.

Pyrazinamide

Pyrazinamide is active against intracellular organisms in phagolysosomes in macrophages. It is well absorbed and can cross into CSF; it is excreted by the kidneys.

Unwanted effects   Include gout, GI tract upsets and fever.

Resistance   Develops quite readily, but cross-resistance with isoniazid does not occur.

Capreomycin

Capreomycin is a peptide antibiotic given IM.

Unwanted effects   Kidney damage, deafness and ataxia can occur.

Cycloserine

Cycloserine is a broad-spectrum antibacterial agent affecting not only tubercle bacilli but many other organisms. It acts at an early stage of cell wall synthesis. Given orally, it is widely distributed in tissues and body fluids (including the CSF) and is excreted in the urine.

Other drugs

Streptomycin is an aminoglycoside (see above for mechanism of action) now rarely used for treatment of tuberculosis. Ciprofloxacin is dealt with above.

Antileprosy drugs

There are two forms of leprosy: paucibacillary leprosy, in which few bacilli are present and in which the lesions are tuberculoid; and multibacillary leprosy, in which numerous bacilli are present and the lesions are termed *lepromatous*.

The drugs available are dapsone, clofazimine and rifampicin.

Dapsone

Dapsone is related chemically to the sulphonamides and probably acts by a similar mechanism. It is given orally and is widely distributed through body water and tissues. It undergoes enterohepatic cycling, but some is acetylated and excreted in the urine.

Unwanted effects   These are fairly common and include methaemoglobinaemia, GI tract disturbances, allergic skin rashes, neuropathy and, occasionally, exacerbation of lepromatous lesions.

Resistance   This is increasing and necessitates combined treatment with other drugs.

Clofazimine

Clofazimine is a dye that is given orally and is taken up by macrophages. Its effect only starts after 6–7 weeks of treatment and it has an 8-week half-life.

Unwanted effects   Include reddening of the skin and urine, and GI tract disturbances.

ANTIFUNGAL DRUGS

The incidence of fungal infections has been increasing with the spread of acquired immunodeficiency syndrome (AIDS) and the increased use of broad-spectrum antibiotics that reduce the non-pathogenic bacteria which normally compete with fungi. Fungal infections can occur on the surfaces of the body or, more seriously, within the body; the latter are seen more frequently in immunocompromised patients such as those receiving chemotherapy for the treatment of cancer.

Amphotericin

Amphotericin has a very wide spectrum of antifungal activity. It interacts with ergosterol and forms a transmembrane ion channel in the fungal membrane. It affects only fungi because cholesterol, not ergosterol, is the main sterol in human cells. Given orally, it is not well absorbed but acts in the gastrointestinal (GI) tract. It can be given by intravenous infusion and intrathecally. It is eliminated very slowly (over weeks) in the urine. Unwanted effects with parenteral amphotericin are common and can be serious and include renal toxicity, hypokalaemia, anaemia and anaphylactic reactions.

Flucytosine

Flucytosine is converted to 5-fluorouracil, an anti-metabolite, within fungal cells. It has a narrow spectrum of action affecting mainly yeast and cryptococcal infections. It is given orally or by intravenous infusion and is widely distributed in the body. Unwanted effects are infrequent.

Azoles

This group includes imidazoles and triazoles; these are effective in the treatment of a wide range of fungal infections.

Mechanism of action

Azoles inhibit the fungal P450 enzymes that are necessary for the synthesis of ergosterol – an essential component of the fungal membrane. Examples are fluconazole, itraconazole and clotrimazole.

Fluconazole is given orally or intravenously and is widely distributed, passing into the cerebrospinal fluid (CSF) and other bodily fluids. Itraconazole is given orally and undergoes extensive first-pass metabolism.

Unwanted effects of fluconazole are mild; itraconazole can cause GI tract disturbances.

Terbinafine

Terbinafine inhibits the synthesis of ergosterol, a crucial component of fungal cell membranes. Given orally, it is selectively taken up by the nails, skin and fat. Unwanted effects are mild.

Caspofungin

This compound disrupts fungal cell walls. It is given by infusion. Unwanted effects are GI tract disturbances, rashes, fever and tachycardia.

Clinical uses of antifungal drugs

- Amphotericin (+ flucytosine in severe cases), or fluconazole on its own: used for invasive candidiasis, cryptococcosis and mucormycosis; amphotericin infusion: used for invasive aspergillosis and histoplasmosis.
- Azoles: clotrimazole or itraconazole: used for ringworm and athlete's foot. Itraconazole is also used for histoplasmosis.
- Terbinafine: used for fungal nail infections.
- Caspofungin: used for invasive candidiasis and invasive aspergillosis unresponsive to amphotericin or itraconazole.

The main protozoans that produce disease in humans are those causing malaria, amoebiasis, pneumocystis infection, trypanosomiasis and leishmaniasis.

MALARIA

Malaria, a mosquito-borne disease caused by various *Plasmodium* species, is a major killer in the developing world and sporadic cases occur elsewhere as a result of air travel. The female anopheline mosquito injects sporozoites during a blood meal. Fig. 32.1 shows the subsequent sequence of changes in the parasite and their relation to the bouts of fever.

The main malarial parasites are *Plasmodium vivax* and *Plasmodium falciparum*, both of which cause fever every third day (tertian malaria), *P. vivax* causing benign and *P. falciparum* causing malignant tertian malaria (malignant because it is a very severe form of the disease and can be fatal). *P. vivax* gives rise to hypnozoites in the liver; these lie dormant and can produce relapses months or years later. *P. falciparum* does not form hypnozoites and thus has no exo-erythrocytic stage. *P. malariae*, which is rare, has a 72-h cycle (quartan malaria) and also has no exo-erythrocytic stage.

Clinical use of antimalarial drugs

	For the clinical attack	For chemoprophylaxis
All infections except chloroquine-resistant *Plasmodium falciparum*	Oral chloroquine; then primaquine to attack the hypnozoites and prevent relapse	Oral chloroquine or proguanil
Chloroquine-resistant *P. falciparum*	Quinine then doxycycline or proguanil + atovaquone	Doxycycline or proguanil + atovaquone

Antimalarial agents

Chloroquine reduces the necessary digestion of haemoglobin by the plasmodium and also inhibits the parasite's haem polymerase (the enzyme that inactivates the toxic free haem generated by the organism, which is fatal for it). It is usually given orally (half-life 0.5 h) but can be given by injection. It is widely distributed in the body, but much is concentrated in the parasite-infected red cells. Unwanted effects include nausea, vomiting and dizziness. Large doses cause retinopathy and bolus injections can cause dysrhythmias. *P. falciparum* is resistant in most parts of the world and *P. vivax* is resistant in some places.

Halofantrine is given orally; the parent drug has a half-life of 1–2 days and the active metabolite 3–5 days. Unwanted effects include gastrointestinal (GI) tract disturbances and, occasionally, cardiac dysrhythmias.

Quinine is given orally (half-life 10 h) but can be given by intravenous (IV) infusion. It is usually followed by doxycycline (see below) and either dapsone (given orally, half-life 24–48 h) or sulfadoxine, a long-acting sulphonamide (half-life ~ 8 days). Quinine causes GI upsets, tinnitus, headache, blurred vision and allergic reactions. Large doses affect the heart (dysrhythmias) and/or the central nervous system (CNS) (delirium). Blackwater fever may be associated with the use of this drug.

Mefloquine is given orally (half-life 30 days) and has a slow onset of action. Like chloroquine, it inhibits the plasmodial haem polymerase. It can cause GI tract disturbances and is known to produce neuropsychiatric symptoms.

Pyrimethamine is a folate antagonist inhibiting folate utilization having greater affinity for the plasmodial than for the mammalian system. It is only used with sulfadoxine. It is given orally and is slow acting (half-life 4 days). It has few unwanted effects.

Proguanil has a similar action to pyrimethamine. It is a slow-acting schizonticide (half-life 16 h) with some action on the pre-erythrocytic stage of *P. vivax*. It is given orally.

Primaquine is given orally (half-life 3–6 h) and usually with chloroquine. It can cause haemolysis in individuals with genetic deficiency of red cell glucose 6-phosphate dehydrogenase.

Doxycycline is a broad-spectrum tetracycline antibiotic that acts by inhibiting plasmodial protein synthesis.

Artemether is a semi-synthetic derivative of artemisinin – a compound extracted from a shrub used in traditional Chinese medicine. Given orally, rectally or intramuscularly (IM). Mechanism of action: It is concentrated in parasitized cells where it generates reactive oxygen species and may inhibit a calcium transporter. It inhibits haemoglobin degradation in the parasite. Only used in combination therapy. Unwanted effects are few, but neurotoxicity can occur with high doses.

OTHER PROTOZOAL INFECTIONS

Amoebiasis

Amoebiasis is caused by the ingestion of the cysts of *Entamoeba histolytica*. The cysts develop in the GI tract into motile trophozoites which can invade the intestinal wall and, rarely, migrate to the liver. The presence of the organism in the GI tract usually causes dysentery; its presence in the liver causes amoebic abscesses. Some individuals remain symptom-free carriers, i.e. they excrete the cysts, which can infect others.

Clinical use of amoebicidal drugs

- Acute severe dysentery: metronidazole (or tinidazole) followed by diloxanide.
- Chronic amoebiasis: diloxanide.
- Hepatic amoebiasis: metronidazole followed by diloxanide.
- Treatment of carriers: diloxanide.

Drug treatment

Metronidazole kills the motile form of *E. histolytica*. It is given orally (half-life 7 h) but can also be given IV and rectally. It has few unwanted effects but has a bitter taste and interferes with alcohol metabolism. **Diloxanide** is given orally and has a direct action in the GI tract against the non-motile form of the amoebae.

Leishmaniasis

The leishmania parasite has two forms, a flagellated form in the sandfly (the insect vector) and a non-flagellated form that occurs in the bitten human. Infected humans develop cutaneous and/or visceral leishmaniasis. The protozoan is ingested by mononuclear phagocytes and it remains alive intracellularly.

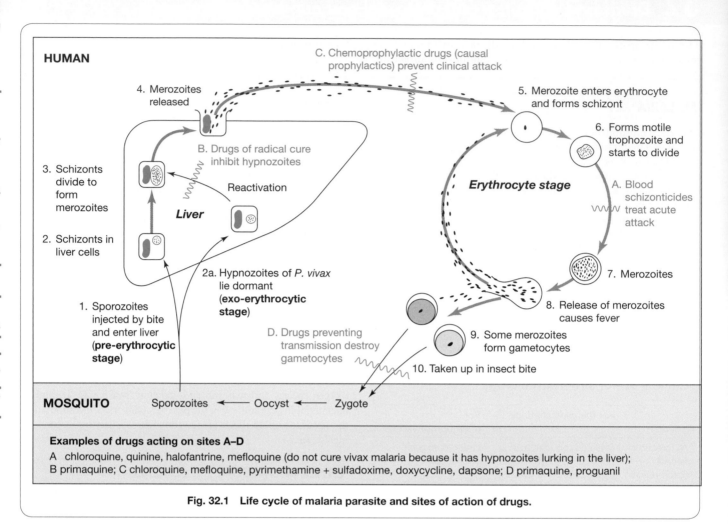

Fig. 32.1 Life cycle of malaria parasite and sites of action of drugs.

Drug treatment
The main drug used is **sodium stibogluconate**, which is given IM or by slow IV injection daily in a course lasting 10–20 days. Coughing may occur during injection. Unwanted effects are GI tract disturbances, muscle pain and cardiovascular disturbances.

Other drugs used are amphotericin and pentamidine isethionate.

Pneumocystis infection
Pneumocystis carinii is widely distributed in the mammalian kingdom but only causes disease (pneumocystis pneumonia (PCP)) in individuals who are immunosuppressed. It is a common presenting symptom and a leading cause of death in patients with acquired immunodeficiency syndrome (AIDS).

Drug treatment
The drug of choice is **co-trimoxazole**, which is a mixture of trimethoprim (a folate antagonist related to pyrimethamine) and sulfamethoxazole (Fig. 30.10 in Chapter 30). Together these interfere with thymidylate synthesis and, therefore, with DNA synthesis. It is given orally in high doses. Other drugs are atovaquone, trimethoprim-dapsone and pentamidine.

Trypanosomiasis
The trypanosomes *Trypanosoma gambiense* and *Trypanosoma rhodesiense* cause sleeping sickness.

Drug treatment: **suramin** or **pentamidine**. Suramin is endocytosed by the parasite and damages it; the parasite is then cleared by host responses. The drug is given IV very slowly. It is relatively toxic, especially to the kidney. Optic atrophy, blood dyscrasias and skin rashes can occur. Pentamidine is taken up by the parasites and rapidly kills them. It is given IM daily for 10–15 days.

Trichomoniasis
Trichomonas vaginalis causes vaginal infection in females and, sometimes, urethral infection in males. It is treated with **metronidazole**.

Toxoplasmosis
Toxoplasma gondii is a protozoal infection of cats. Oocysts from cat faeces can cause disease in humans. Treatment (which should be left to experts) is with **pyrimethamine-sulfadiazine**.

Anti-helminthic drugs
These are drugs used to act on parasitic worms and the main groups of helminths that infest humans are:

Cestoda (tapeworms)
Nematoda (roundworms)
Trematoda (flukes)

To be effective anti-parasite drugs need to be able to penetrate the cuticle of the worm or be able to enter the GI tract.

Anti-helminthic drugs achieve their effects on parasites through a number of mechanisms:

Damaging or killing the worm directly
Paralyzing the worm
Damaging the cuticle of the worm, rendering the worm more susceptible to host defence mechanisms
Interfering with worm metabolism

The main anti-helminthic drugs are the following:

Niclosamide: A salicylamide derivative used to treat tapeworm infestations. It blocks glucose uptake that leads to damage to the scolex (the attachment end of the worm) causing the worm to detach from the wall of the GI tract to be expelled in the faeces. Niclosamide is a safe drug as it is poorly absorbed. Patients need to fast before treatment and purgatives are used to expel the dead worm segments (proglottids).

Praziquantel: This increases the permeability of the helminth plasma membrane to calcium. Low concentrations lead to contraction and spastic paralysis, with higher concentrations leading to vesiculation and vacuolization, with subsequent damage to the tegument of the worm. Praziquantel is orally active and is the drug of choice for all schistosome infections and for cysticercosis. This drug can cause mild GI disturbance and headache.

Piperazine: A reversible neuromuscular blocker that leads to flaccid paralysis in worms so that they can be expelled with normal peristalsis into the faeces. Piperazine is an orally active drug used to treat roundworm and threadworm infestations of the gut which has a good safety profile.

Benzimidazoles: This class of drug includes mebendazole, thiabendazole and albendazole that bind with high affinity to tubulin dimers and thus prevent polymerization of microtubules. This effect of benzimidazoles is selective for parasites as they are 250–400 times more effective against the target in the parasite compared with the target in mammalian cells. These drugs are orally active and are used to treat hydatid diseases, nematode infestations and single doses can be used to treat pinworm infestations. Benzimidazoles should not be given to pregnant women as they are teratogenic and embryotoxic. They can also rarely lead to hepatotoxicity.

Diethylcarbamazine: This is the drug of choice to treat lymphatic filariasis caused by *Wuchereria bancrofti*, *Loa loa* and *Brugia malayi*. It kills microfilariae in the peripheral circulation and adult worms in the lymphatic system through a poorly understood mechanism of action. Diethylcarbamazine can cause GI disturbance, headache and lassitude, as well as more serious side effects from dead worm materials such as lymph gland enlargement and tachycardia. To minimize these effects of a sudden release of dead worm material, the initial dose of diethylcarbamazine is started low and then increased over 21 days.

Ivermectin: This immobilizes the tapeworm *Onchocerca volvulus* by causing tonic paralysis by potentiating the effect of γ-aminobutyric acid at the neuromuscular junction. Ivermectin is administered orally and is the treatment of choice for river blindness and for the treatment of chronic *Strongyloides* infection.

It can cause ocular irritation and immediate immune reaction to dead microfilariae (the so-called Mazzotti reaction), which can be severe.

Levamisole: A **nicotinic** receptor agonist at the neuromuscular junction which leads to spastic paralysis resulting in the worm being easily expelled in the faeces. It is orally active and used to treat roundworm infestations and causes mild nausea and vomiting.

A summary of the main uses of anti-helminthic drugs is shown in Table 32.1 (see Table 12.6 in *Crash Course: Pharmacology*).

Table 32.1 Classification of Medically Important Helminth Infections and the Main Drugs in Their Treatment

	Helminth species	Drug used in treatment
Cestodes		
Beef tapeworm	*Taenia saginata*	Niclosamide, praziquantel
Pork tapeworm	*Taenia solium*	Niclosamide, praziquantel
Fish tapeworm	*Diphyllobothrium latum*	Niclosamide, praziquantel
Hydatid tapeworm	*Echinococcus granulosus*	Albendazole
Nematodes		
Intestinal species		
Common round worms	*Ascaris lumbricoides*	Mebendazole, piperazine
Threadworms/ pin worms	*Enterobius vermicularis*	Mebendazole, piperazine
Threadworms (US)	*Strongyloides stercoralis*	Thiabendazole, albendazole
Whipworms	*Trichuris trichiura*	Mebendazole
Hookworms	*Necator americanus*	Mebendazole
	Ancylostoma duodenale	Mebendazole
Tissue species		
Trichinella	*Trichinella spiralis*	Thiabendazole
Guinea worm	*Dracunculus medinensis*	Mebendazole
Filarioidea	*Wuchereria bancrofti*	Diethylcarbamazine
	Loa loa	Diethylcarbamazine
	Brugia malayi	Diethylcarbamazine
	Onchocerca volvulus	Ivermectin
Trematodes		
Blood flukes/ schistosomes	*Schistosoma japonicum*	Praziquantel
	Schistosoma mansoni	Praziquantel
	Schistosoma haematobium	Praziquantel

From Page C. *Crash Course: Pharmacology*. 5th ed. Philadelphia: Elsevier; 2019.

The term cancer refers to a malignant tumour. Cancer cells can manifest, in greater or lesser degree, uncontrolled proliferation, invasiveness, the ability to metastasize and/or infiltrate normal tissues and loss of function due to lack of the capacity to differentiate. Benign tumours manifest only uncontrolled proliferation.

PATHOLOGY

The two main alterations in DNA underlying cancerous change in a cell are (1) mutation/inactivation of tumour suppressor genes and (2) mutation/activation of *proto-oncogenes*. Proto-oncogenes are genes that normally code for the growth factor-induced and apoptotic pathways, and thus control the cell cycle and cell proliferation. Oncogenes code for cancerous changes. The development of cancer, however, is a multistage process, involving not only more than one genetic change, but also other non-genetic factors (hormonal effects, presence of carcinogens) that increase the likelihood that the mutation(s) will result in cancer. The formation of new blood vessels (angiogenesis) is required for the growth of the tumour, the infiltration of cancer cells into nearby tissue and their metastasis to other organs.

Most anticancer drugs are cytotoxic, i.e. they damage or kill cells; they do not affect the underlying pathogenetic mechanisms, namely the changes in growth factors and/or their receptors, in the cell cycle and apoptotic pathways, in telomerase expression or in tumour-related angiogenesis. Most are mainly antiproliferative, acting primarily on dividing cells (Fig. 33.1) and have no specific inhibitory effect on invasiveness, the loss of differentiation or the tendency to metastasize. As these cytotoxic drugs inhibit cell proliferation, they will also affect rapidly dividing normal cells. Therefore they can depress the bone marrow, impair healing, depress growth, cause sterility and hair loss and be teratogenic; most cause nausea and vomiting and detrimental effects on the mucous lining of the gastrointestinal (GI) tract.

There are also now many new immunotherapeutic approaches to the treatment of cancers that use the body's own immune system to attack cancer cells. Other new approaches include targeting receptor mechanisms upregulated in cancer cells and targeting these with biologics (Table 33.1).

ANTICANCER DRUGS

Most currently used anticancer drugs have the adverse effects specified above; only the adverse effects particular to each drug are given below. Cells damaged by cytotoxic anticancer drugs undergo apoptosis.

Alkylating agents and related drugs
These agents directly interfere with DNA synthesis.

Cyclophosphamide
This alkylating nitrogen mustard agent can form covalent bonds with bases (usually guanine) in the DNA. It has two alkylating groups and can cross-link the two strands, interfering with cell division and triggering apoptosis. It is given orally or intramuscularly (IM) and is metabolized in the liver tissues to give *phosphoramide mustard* (the active moiety) and *acrolein*, which is responsible for

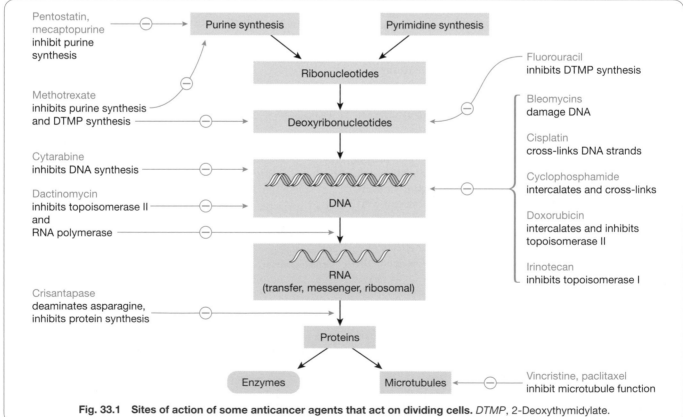

Fig. 33.1 **Sites of action of some anticancer agents that act on dividing cells.** *DTMP*, 2-Deoxythymidylate.

Table 33.1 Summary of Cancer Therapies

Class of drug	Drug	Mechanism of action	Use	Important side effects
Alkylating agent	Cyclophosphamide	Pronounced effect on lymphocytes Immunosuppressant Intrastrand cross-linking of DNA	Haematological malignancy	N&V Bone marrow depression Haemorrhagic cystitis
Alkylating agent	Procarbazine	Inhibits DNA and RNA synthesis Interferes with mitosis	Hodgkin's disease	Hypertension Flushing reaction
Platinum compound	Cisplatin	Intrastrand cross-linking of DNA	Solid tumours (especially testes and ovary)	Nephrotoxic Severe N&V
Antimetabolite	Fluorouracil	Inhibition of DNA synthesis	Basal cell carcinoma	Gastrointestinal upset Myelotoxicity
Antimetabolite	Cytarabine	Pyrimidine analogue—inhibits DNA polymerase	Acute myeloid leukaemia	Gastrointestinal upset Myelotoxicity
Cytotoxic antibiotic	Doxorubicin	Inhibits DNA and RNA synthesis, through interference with topoisomerase II	Bladder cancer	N&V Myelosuppression Hair loss Cardiotoxic in high doses
Vinca alkaloids (mitotic inhibitor)	Vincristine	Bind to tubulin and inhibit its polymerization, causing arrest at metaphase inhibiting mitosis	Haematological malignancy	Mild myelosuppression Neurotoxic → paraesthesia and weakness Abdominal pain
Mitotic inhibitor	Etoposide	Inhibits DNA synthesis by action on topoisomerase II Inhibits mitochondrial function	Haematological malignancy	Vomiting Alopecia Myelosuppression
Monoclonal antibody	Rituximab	Binds to CD20 protein → lyses B lymphocytes	Lymphoma	Hypotension Chills and fever Hypersensitivity reaction
Monoclonal antibody	Trastuzumab (Herceptin)	Binds to oncogenic protein human epidermal growth factor receptor 2 (HER2)	Breast cancer that overexpress HER2	
Protein kinase inhibitor	Imatinib	Inhibits oncogenic cytoplasmic kinase (BCR/ABL) & platelet-derived growth factor	Chronic myeloid leukaemia	Gastrointestinal upset Headaches Rashes (can get resistance)

DNA, Deoxyribonucleic acid; N&V, nausea and vomiting; RNA, ribonucleic acid.
From Page C. *Crash Course: Pharmacology.* 5th ed. Philadelphia: Elsevier; 2019.

bladder toxicity. Unwanted effects include nausea and vomiting and acrolein-mediated haemorrhagic cystitis. The last effect can be ameliorated by giving the sulfhydryl donor mesna. Another alkylating nitrogen mustard is chlorambucil.

Cisplatin

This platinum coordination compound can cross-link DNA and trigger apoptosis. It is given by infusion. It causes very severe nausea and vomiting (which can be ameliorated by the anti-emetic 5-hydroxytryptamine (5-HT)$_3$ antagonist ondansetron) and can result in kidney damage unless copious fluids and diuretics are given. It has low myelotoxicity.

Antimetabolites

Antimetabolite agents interfere with DNA synthesis. For most, the unwanted effects are bone marrow depression and damage to the intestinal epithelium with resultant GI tract disturbances.

Methotrexate is a folate antagonist; it inhibits the enzyme dihydrofolate reductase, competing with dihydrofolate in the generation of tetrahydrofolate, thus inhibiting the formation of thymidylate. It is given orally and taken up into cells, where it persists for weeks in the form of polyglutamate derivatives. High-dose regimens must be followed by rescue with folinic acid (a form of tetrahydrofolate). *Fluorouracil*, a pyrimidine analogue, is converted to a fraudulent

nucleotide which interferes with thymidylate synthesis. It is given by injection. *Cytarabine*, pyrimidine analogue, is converted in the cell to the trisphosphate which inhibits DNA polymerase. *Fludarabine*, purine analogue, has a similar mechanism of action to cytarabine. It is given intravenously (IV). *Pentostatin*, a purine analogue, inhibits adenosine deaminase, an enzyme important in the generation of inosine – an early stage of ribonucleotide synthesis.

Cytotoxic antibiotics

Certain antibiotics can exhibit anticancer activity and act directly on the nucleic acids. *Doxorubicin* intercalates in the DNA and inhibits the action of topoisomerase II. It is given by infusion and the unwanted effects include dose-related cardiac damage. *Bleomycins* cause DNA fragmentation and the unwanted effects include pulmonary fibrosis and allergic reactions. They have low myelotoxicity. *Dactinomycin* intercalates in the DNA and inhibits RNA polymerase and topoisomerase II.

Plant derivatives and miscellaneous agents

These act by a variety of means. *Vincristine* is a vinca alkaloid; it binds to tubulin and interferes with spindle formation in dividing cells. It is given IV often in conjunction with a glucocorticoid. It is relatively non-toxic, having low myelotoxicity, but can cause sensory changes and muscle weakness. *Paclitaxel*, a taxane, stabilizes microtubules in the polymerized state and interferes with spindle formation. It is given by IV infusion. Unwanted effects may include serious myelosuppression and cumulative neurotoxicity. Hypersensitivity is common and necessitates pretreatment with glucocorticoids. *Etoposide* inhibits mitochondrial function and topoisomerase II action. *Irinotecan* inhibits topoisomerase I and interferes with DNA function. It has fewer unwanted effects than most cytotoxic anticancer drugs.

In hormone-sensitive tumours, inhibition of tumour growth can be brought about by antagonists or synthesis inhibitors of those hormones, or by hormones with opposing action. Some examples are **glucocorticoids** (see Chapter 16), which inhibit lymphocyte proliferation and are used for leukaemias, **tamoxifen**, an anti-oestrogen effective in hormone-dependent mammary cancer and flutamide, an androgen antagonist used in prostate cancer.

Multikinase inhibitors

Many growth factors activate cells via activation of tyrosine kinase receptors (e.g., vascular endothelial growth factor and platelet derived growth factor). Pazopanib, sunitinib, sorafenib and imatinib are examples of kinase inhibitors that inhibit cell signalling in cells and are used in the treatment of chronic myeloid leukaemia and acute lymphoblastic leukaemia, as well as advanced renal cell carcinoma.

Immunotherapy and monoclonal antibodies

A number of new immunological approaches have been developed involving treatments to boost the body's own immune system which has been called immunotherapy. Such approaches include the use of vaccines (e.g. bacillus Calmette-Guérin (BCG)) to provide immunostimulation to treat bladder cancer, vaccination against the human papilloma virus (HPV) as certain strains have been associated with cervical cancer and the use of cytokines such as interferon gamma, interleukin 2 (IL-2) and tumour necrosis factor. Aldesleukin is an IL-2 drug used to treat metastatic renal cell carcinoma and is administered by subcutaneous (SC) injection. There have also been a number of so-called checkpoint inhibitors introduced for the treatment of cancer that interfere with key signalling pathways, such as nivolumab, an anti-programmed death ligand 1 (PDL1) antibody for the treatment of advanced melanoma. A number of other monoclonal antibodies have also been introduced for the treatment of various cancers that target specific proteins expressed on cancer cells that can either trigger the body's immune system to kill the cancer cell or that may be attached to a radioactive substance or a cancer drug. Examples include: trastuzumab (Herceptin) that targets tumours overexpressing epidermal growth factor 2 (HER) 2 receptor and is used for the treatment of metastatic breast cancer; cetuximab (that also targets HER2) which is used in combination with irinotecan for the treatment of colorectal cancers overexpressing HER2; basiliximab and daclizumab directed against T lymphocytes; rituximab that targets B lymphocytes and is used in the treatment of diffuse large B lymphocyte non-Hodgkin's lymphoma; and bevacizumab that neutralizes vascular endothelial growth factor and prevents angiogenesis used in the treatment of colorectal cancer.

Treatment regimens with anticancer drugs

The detailed clinical uses of anticancer drugs are the province of the oncologist. Anticancer drugs are usually given in combinations that increase anticancer action without increasing toxicity. For example, methotrexate, which depresses the bone marrow, can be given with a drug that has low myelotoxicity (e.g. cisplatin or bleomycin). Drugs are usually given in large doses intermittently, in several courses, with 2–3 weeks between courses, because this permits the bone marrow to regenerate during the intervals. Resistance can occur to most anticancer drugs and will complicate treatment.

Variation in drug responses between individuals can be affected by ethnicity, age, gender, pregnancy, disease and drug interactions. Thus the practitioner must take these factors into account for effective and safe drug treatment. Advances in mapping individual genetic information have led to the concept of introducing individualizing drug therapy to best suit likely receptive patients (personalized medicine). (Rang & Dale's *Pharmacology*, 8th edition, Chapter 11 provides an expansion on this topic which is condensed below).

Responses to some drugs (e.g. vaccines, oral contraceptives) are robust and predictable to allow standard dose calculations to be used. Other drugs (e.g. antihypertensives, anticoagulants) require individual monitoring to ensure efficacy is reached and safety concerns are managed or minimized.

AGE, GENDER AND ORIGIN

An individual's metabolism of drugs will change several times with age. The expression pattern of drug-metabolizing enzymes is different in the foetus and in infants compared to adults. In particular, premature infants can be deficient in some enzymes compared to full-term infants; coupled with a still developing renal system, this means attention must be given to these babies in terms of their ability to metabolize and eliminate drugs.

However, as the child develops, his or her ability to metabolize (oxidize) many drugs is more rapid than in adults. The dosing regimen may reflect this increased activity, until children reach puberty and the rate of drug metabolism converges to that of an adult.

Aging then causes further changes in the absorption, distribution, metabolism and excretion (ADME) of drugs:
- Chronic, complicated diseases sometimes require the use of multiple drug treatments, and the likelihood of drug interactions becomes more probable, and competition for cytochrome P450 isoforms is more pronounced.
- Serum albumin concentration decreases, increasing the likelihood of saturable drug binding and increased availability of circulating free fraction of a drug.
- Lean body mass decreases, leading to changes in the volume of distribution.
- Liver weight decreases, and cytochrome P450 has a reduced capacity to oxidize drugs, therefore affecting metabolism and elimination to certain drugs.

The influence of gender has been explored to a lesser extent, with a few instances of variations in drug disposition reported.

Ethnicity is understood to affect drug metabolism. For example, population differences in the expression of P450 isoforms have been reported in Caucasian versus Asian populations, as well as the rate of drug acetylation.

DRUG INTERACTIONS

The administration of multiple drugs increases the probability of their interaction. These interactions might increase or decrease the actions of a drug, and the nature of the interactions can affect efficacy (as an additive or negative interaction) and bioavailability:
- The use of granulocyte colony-stimulating factor (G-CSF) and plerixafor produces synergistic mobilization of stem cells from the bone marrow in patients undergoing leukaemia transplant therapy (additive interaction with beneficial outcome).
- Selective serotonin reuptake inhibitors (SSRIs) can increase the risk of bleeding associated with anti-platelet drugs by further impairing platelet function (additive interaction with safety concern).
- The reversible binding of ibuprofen to cyclooxygenase (COX)-1 can prevent aspirin from acetylating the enzyme. Thus, long lasting inhibition of thromboxane A_2 (TXA_2) can be reduced, and the prophylactic benefit of aspirin in people at risk of thrombosis is diminished (negative interaction with safety concern).
- Nonsteroidal anti-inflammatory drugs (NSAIDs) can displace warfarin from blood albumin, making safety management of oral anticoagulant therapy harder because warfarin is normally highly bound.
- Nutrients sometimes interfere in drug efficacy. For example, calcium in milk reduces tetracycline antibiotic absorption from the stomach, thereby decreasing antimicrobial activity. Grapefruit juice can delay the metabolism of various medicines.
- Drugs can either be inducers or inhibitors of liver P450 enzymes and therefore affect the metabolism of other drugs acting on the same enzyme.

EFFECT OF DISEASE ON DRUG ACTION

Disease will have an impact on an individual's response to a drug. Kidney or liver disease in particular might require the dose to be reduced in order to prevent toxicity due to impaired elimination. Drug absorption can be affected in diseases that affect gastric stasis, malabsorption or oedema of the ileal mucosa. Furthermore, when a disease is associated with the target organ of a drug, the effect will clearly be compounded:
- Chronic renal failure, as well as causing renal-dependent effect of drug availability, significantly reduces non-renal clearance of drugs metabolized by the liver and intestine through suppression of cytochrome P450 activity. Morphine and nimodipine have a particularly decreased metabolism.
- Liver cirrhosis affects phase 1 elimination more than phase 2. Thus, drug choice might be a consideration if a choice between elimination steps exists.

GENETIC VARIATION

Mutations and polymorphisms to genes can lead to changes in response to drugs. Some examples would be the single gene pharmacokinetic disorders such as plasma cholinesterase deficiency, drug acetylation deficiency and aminoglycoside ototoxicity.

PERSONALIZED MEDICINES

Clinical pharmacogenomic tests can be used to predict drug responsiveness in individual patients. However there is often a scientific, economic and educational barrier to their effectiveness. Single nucleotide polymorphisms (SNPs) and their combinations (haplotypes) can be identified from tissue biopsies and blood. This is a branch of medicine that is still being established, yet practical examples include:
- *Human Leukocyte Antigen (HLA) gene tests* for anti-HIV drug **abacavir**, anti-epileptic drug **carbamazepine** (susceptibility to severe or life-threatening skin rashes) and the anti-psychotic drug **clozapine** (agranulocytosis).

- *Drug metabolism related gene tests* for **tamoxifen** and hepatic cytochrome CYP2D6; **5-fluorouracil** and dihydropyrimidine dehydrogenase (DPDYD).
- *Drug target-related gene tests* for **dasatinib** and **imatinib** where mutations to targeted chromosomes (e.g. the Philadelphia chromosome in chronic myeloid leukaemia or gene rearrangements for the platelet derived growth factor receptor) confer resistance to these drugs.
- Combined (metabolism and target) gene tests can be utilized, for example warfarin which is metabolized by CYP2C9 and its target, vitamin K epoxide reductase.

It is important to note that the scientific discovery of new medicines has often been derived from venoms, toxins, poisons and chemicals derived from plants. It is therefore important to understand how such molecules affect physiology. (Page et al., *Integrated Pharmacology*, 2nd ed, Chapters 29 and 30 provide an expansion on this topic which is condensed below.)

TOXICITY AND TARGET ORGAN DAMAGE

Exposure to venoms occurs through direct contact with a venomous animal, whereas ingestion is a common route of exposure for toxins and poisons from both animals and plants. Acute toxicity often arises from brief exposure to venoms or toxins, whereas chronic low-level exposure to chemicals in the environment (or food) can induce long term toxicity.

Organs that are particularly susceptible to damage from toxins and venoms include the kidneys, lungs and liver (Fig. 35.1). The reversibility of damage depends on the repair and regenerative potential of the target tissue. Liver damage is often reversible, whereas damage to the central nervous system (CNS) is more likely to be irreversible.

MEDICAL PROCEDURES FOR TREATMENT OF POISONING AND TOXICITY

Effective procedures involve removal of the source of exposure; limitation of absorption and increasing speed of elimination; and the use of antidotes, antivenoms and antitoxins to pharmacologically inhibit the mechanism of action by which the toxin or venom is thought to cause organ damage (Table 35.1).

NATURAL SOURCES

Venoms occur in all animal groups, and these are usually proteins or polypeptides. Furthermore, serious anaphylaxis can occur after repeated exposure. Examples are shown in Table 35.2. Plant toxins and poisons are usually small organic molecules and can be very diverse, as expected of a diverse and wide phylum. Examples are shown in Table 35.3, and the list reveals common names that students will recognize as forerunners to drugs described elsewhere in this book, because the active substances from plants has led to the serendipitous discovery of many important medicines that are either extracted directly from plants or synthetic derivatives of extracts.

INDUSTRIAL OR MAN-MADE TOXINS

Industrial and environmental poisons can include metals, air pollutants and gases, aromatic and aliphatic hydrocarbons,

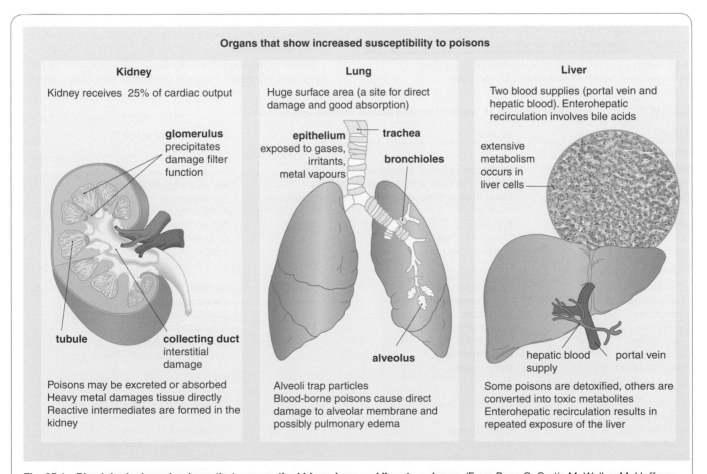

Organs that show increased susceptibility to poisons

Kidney

Kidney receives 25% of cardiac output

glomerulus
precipitates
damage filter
function

tubule **collecting duct**
interstitial
damage

Poisons may be excreted or absorbed
Heavy metal damages tissue directly
Reactive intermediates are formed in the kidney

Lung

Huge surface area (a site for direct damage and good absorption)

epithelium **trachea**
exposed to gases,
irritants, **bronchioles**
metal vapours

alveolus

Alveoli trap particles
Blood-borne poisons cause direct damage to alveolar membrane and possibly pulmonary edema

Liver

Two blood supplies (portal vein and hepatic blood). Enterohepatic recirculation involves bile acids

extensive
metabolism
occurs in
liver cells

hepatic blood **portal vein**
supply

Some poisons are detoxified, others are converted into toxic metabolites
Enterohepatic recirculation results in repeated exposure of the liver

Fig. 35.1 Physiological mechanisms that expose the kidney, lung and liver to poisons. (From Page C, Curtis M, Walker M, Hoffman B. *Integrated Pharmacology*. 3rd ed. Philadelphia: Elsevier; 2006.)

insecticides, pesticides and herbicides. Their full and varied toxicological profiles are beyond the scope of this book, but examples are provided below.

Heavy metals such as mercury, cadmium, lead and arsenic are often toxic due to their combination with essential macromolecules. Therapy after acute poisoning can involve the use of chelators that hold the metal ions in inactive forms suitable for mobilization and excretion.

Table 35.1 Principles for the Treatment of Poisoning

Remove the source of poison or the victim from the source (e.g. rescue)

Remove and limit the absorption of the poison (e.g. fresh air, wash, emesis, limit contact)

Supportive therapy (e.g. ventilation, external cardiac massage, saline/oxygen, drugs)

Specific therapies:
    Antivenins for animal venoms
    Antitoxins for bacterial toxins
    Chelators for heavy metals
    Gases (e.g. oxygen for carbon monoxide)

Other drug therapies:
    Ethanol for methanol
    Digoxin antibodies for digoxin
    Pyridoxine for isoniazid
    Nitrite and thiosulfate for cyanide
    N-acetylcysteine for acetaminophen

Specific antagonists:
    Atropine and oximes for organophosphate anticholinesterase inhibitor poisoning
    Flumazenil for benzodiazepine overdose
    Opioid antagonists (naloxone) for opiate overdose
    Anticholinesterases for neuromuscular blocking drugs

From Page C, Curtis M, Walker M, Hoffman B. *Integrated Pharmacology*. 3rd ed. Philadelphia: Elsevier; 2006.

Air pollutants can be particulate matter (1–5 μm) that are deposited in the lower airways and alveoli and are now known to enter the circulation. Examples include asbestos and products arising from the combustion of hydrocarbons: carbon monoxide, sulphur dioxide, nitrogen dioxide, aldehydes and acrolein (from burning tobacco). Direct effects on the lungs can include airway irritability, sneezing, coughing, excessive mucus production and in the longer term, lung cancer.

Industrial chemicals known to induce health problems include petroleum distillates, halogenated hydrocarbons, alcohols and aromatic hydrocarbons. Acute adverse effects include nausea, vomiting, dizziness and headaches. Long-term exposure to such chemicals can cause kidney and liver damage; some chemicals (aromatic hydrocarbons) are thought to induce cancer such as leukaemia.

Pesticides (insecticides, fumigants, rodenticides, herbicides and fungicides) can contaminate food and generally result in chronic low-level exposure, and normally acute poisoning only results from eating heavily contaminated foods or during crop spraying.

CARCINOGENSIS AND MUTAGENESIS

Some chemicals can increase the risk of certain cancers or induce mutagenesis and most drugs to be used chronically in the treatment of humans need to be tested to ensure they do not induce such a risk. The mechanisms of action of chemical mutagens and carcinogens include the following:

- Genotoxins induce genetic damage by covalently binding to DNA to produce mutations.
- Epigenetic compounds amplify cancer by affecting the bioavailability or metabolism of genotoxins, inhibiting DNA repair or acting as mitogens.
- Promoters increase the incidence of cancer induced by carcinogens and mutagens but do not interfere with DNA directly.

Table 35.2 Sources and Mechanisms of Action of Various Animal Venoms and Toxins

Toxin	Source	Mechanisms of action
Small molecules		
Tetrodotoxin	Puffer fish, octopus, salamander	Na$^+$ channel blocker
Saxitoxin	Shellfish contaminated with dinoflagellates	Na$^+$ channel blocker
Ciguatoxin	Large tropical fish contaminated with dinoflagellates	Actions on Na$^+$ channel
Cardiac glycosides	Toad skin	ATPase inhibitor
Batrachotoxin	Frog skin	Na$^+$ channel activator
Domoic acid	Shellfish (mussels)	CNS toxin
Palytoxin	Sea anemone	Ionophore
Proteins and polypeptides		
α bungarotoxin	Elapid snakes (kraits)	Nicotinic receptor blocker
β bungarotoxin	Elapid snakes (kraits)	Presynaptic cholinergic nerves
α conotoxin	Coneshells	Skeletal muscle Na$^+$ channel blocker
μ conotoxin	Coneshells	N-type Ca^{2+} antagonist
ω conotoxin	Coneshells	Direct acting cardiotoxin
Cardiotoxin	Elapid snakes	Cell membrane destruction
Phospholipases	Many snakes	
Bacterial toxins		
Botulinum toxin	*Clostridium botulinum*	Synaptin in cholinergic nerve endings
Cholera toxin		
Pertussis toxin	*Cholera vibrio*	Activation of G$_2$ protein
Endotoxin	*Bordetella pertussis*	Inactivates G$_0$/G$_5$ protein
Tetanus toxin	Gram-negative bacteria	Cell membranes
Staphylococcal toxin	*Clostridium tetani*	Cell membrane ionophore
	Staphylococcus spp.	Enterotoxin

From Page C, Curtis M, Walker M, Hoffman B. *Integrated Pharmacology*. 3rd ed. Philadelphia: Elsevier; 2006. CNS, central nervous system, ATPase, Adenosine triphosphatase enzyme.

HERBAL MEDICINES

As mentioned above, many important drug classes have been derived from chemicals found in plants (Table 35.4). However, isolating the active substance from a mixture of potential active chemicals with similar structural characteristics is a very difficult task. This has meant that throughout history many societies have used herbal medicines which often contain potentially several active ingredients (although perhaps not all with desirable properties). There is also a lack of stringent quantitative analysis of many herbal medicines such that standardization of constituents over time, and between batches from different manufacturers, is difficult and seldom accomplished. Thus predicting the pharmacology and toxicology of herbal medicines is often not possible with any degree of accuracy.

Table 35.3 Sources and Mechanisms of Action of Various Plant and Fungal Poisons

Poison	Source	Mechanism of action
Plant Poisons		
Atropine, scopolamine	Solanaceae (jimson weed, deadly nightshade)	Muscarinic receptor antagonists
Cardiac glycosides	Digitalis, strophanthus, oleander, convallaria	ATPase inhibitors
Aconitine	Hellebores	Cardiac Na^+ channel activator
Capsaicin	*Capsicum sp. (peppers)*	Substance P depleter
Ricin	Castor bean	Protoplasmic poison
Myristicin	Nutmeg and mace	Hallucinogenic
Emetine	*Ipecacuana spp.*	Vomiting centre stimulant
Pennyroyal oil	*Mentha spp.*	Hepatotoxic and oxytocic
Safrole	Sassafras tree	Animal carcinogen
Pyrrolizidine	Heliotropium, comfrey (herbal tea)	Hepatotoxic
Fungal toxins		
Muscarine	*Clitocybe, Amanita spp., Inocybe spp.*	Muscarinic agonist
Phallotoxins, amatoxins	*Amanita spp. (death cap, destroying angel)*	Hepatotoxic
Coprine	*Coprinus spp.*	Blocks aldehyde dehydrogenase
Ibotenic acid	*Amanita sp.*	Hallucinogenic
Psilocybin	*Psilocybe spp.*	Hallucinogenic
Aflatoxins	*Aspergillus spp.*	Hepatocarcinogenic
Ergot alkaloids	*Claviceps spp.*	Multiple actions
Orelline	*Cortinarius spp.*	Nephrotoxic

From Page C, Curtis M, Walker M, Hoffman B. *Integrated Pharmacology*. 3rd ed. Philadelphia: Elsevier; 2006.

Table 35.4 Examples of Drugs Obtained from Plants Traditionally Used as Herbal Remedies or Poisons

Botanical name of plant (common name)	Herbal products	Chemicals isolated: used as medicines
Atropa belladonna (deadly nightshade)	Belladonna leaf, belladonna tincture	Atropine, hyoscyamine
Datura stramonium (jimson weed, thorn apple)	Stramonium, stramonium tincture	Atropine, hyoscyamine
Hyoscyamus niger (henbane)	Henbane tincture	Scopolamine (hyoscine)
Cinchona ledgeriana (cinchona tree)	Cinchona bark, Jesuit's bark, cardinal's bark, cortex peruanus	Quinine, quinidine
Colchicum autumnale (autumn crocus, meadow saffron)	Colchicum seed fluid extract, colchicum seed tincture	Colchicine
Digitalis purpurea (purple foxglove)	Digitalis folia (powdered leaf), tincture of digitalis	Digitoxin
Digitalis lanata (woolly foxglove)	Digitalis folia (powdered leaf), tincture of digitalis	Digoxin
Strophanthus gratus	Strophanthus seeds	Ouabain
Ephedra sinica	Ma huang	Ephedrine, pseudoephedrine, phenylpropanolamine
Papaver somniferum (opium poppy)	Powdered opium, laudanum (tincture of opium alkaloids)	Morphine, heroin, codeine, papaverine
Physostigma venenosum (calabar or ordeal bean)	Whole beans	Physostigmine (eserine)
Pilocarpus jaborandi	Chewed leaves (induced sweating)	Pilocarpine
Rauwolfia serpentine	Rauwiloid, alseroxylon (Raudixin)	Reserpine
Salix alba (white willow)	Extract of willow bark	Salicylic acid
Strychnos toxifera, Chondrodendron tomentosum	Curare (arrow poison)	*d*-tubocurarine
Vinca rosa (periwinkle)	Alleged oral hypoglycemic	Vincristine, vinblastine

From Page C, Curtis M, Walker M, Hoffman B. *Integrated Pharmacology*. 3rd ed. Philadelphia: Elsevier; 2006.

Many drugs are taken for non-medical purposes, most commonly to generate a sense of well-being or to give pleasure. Drug dependence arises with centrally acting drugs producing a psychological reward and follows repeated administration. It is reinforced by a need to avoid unpleasant withdrawal effects and by the ritual of drug taking itself. Dependence (addiction) is characterized by:

- *psychological dependence*: craving, compulsive drug-seeking behaviour,
- *physical dependence*: habituation/tolerance associated with a withdrawal (abstinence) syndrome, and
- *tolerance*: the need to increase dose to maintain the desired effect.

Drug abuse is important because of the damage done to the individual's health and the cost to society – in healthcare costs, criminal behaviour, time out of productive work, etc. Drugs abused for their effects in the central nervous system (CNS) include opioids (see Chapter 13), stimulants/psychotomimetics (amphetamines, cocaine, lysergic acid diethylamide (LSD)), anxiolytics (benzodiazepines, see Chapter 12) and depressants (barbiturates (see Chapter 12), solvents). Here we specifically consider **nicotine, ethanol, cannabinoids, amphetamines** and **cocaine**. Apart from alcohol and tobacco, the important drugs of abuse are controlled under the Misuse of Drugs Act categories A to C (in the United Kingdom), reflecting their addictive power. Their unauthorized possession is a criminal offence. Drugs misused to improve performance (e.g. anabolic steroids in sports) are not considered here.

PATHOPHYSIOLOGY

Dependence-producing drugs enhance dopaminergic transmission in the important reward pathway from the midbrain to the limbic system and especially to the nucleus accumbens. Tolerance seems to involve adaptive changes to the effects of the drugs. Thus the inhibitory effect of opioids on adenylate cyclase activity in the brain is countered by a rise in the amount of enzyme synthesized. This increased enzyme activity can at least partially explain a rebound withdrawal effect when the drug is discontinued. Downregulation of receptors and receptor desensitization may also be involved. A genetic predisposition towards addictive behaviour has been identified.

Nicotine

Nicotine is taken mainly by tobacco smoking, or less often by chewing, and is strongly addictive. There has been a significant increase in nicotine addiction over recent years with the wide availability of e-cigarettes whereby the user 'vapes' uncontrolled amounts of nicotine.

Mechanism of action

Nicotine produces its effects through activation of nicotinic receptors normally activated by acetylcholine (ACh). Activation of nicotinic receptors by nicotine in the CNS leads to the desirable effects and regular use leads to desensitization of these receptors. The behavioural effects depend on dose and may be excitatory or depressant. Indeed smokers may seek either a calming effect or a stimulant effect. Nicotine is reported to enhance learning in rats. Long-term use is associated with a large increase in the number of nicotinic receptors in the CNS. (Tolerance might have been expected to correlate with a decrease in receptor density; the paradoxical increase is most likely due to a high proportion of receptors being in the desensitized state.) Slow release from nicotine patches is used with counselling to assist in quitting the habit of smoking cigarettes to obtain a 'fix' of nicotine and increasingly ex-smokers are using e-cigarettes to obtain their nicotine.

Pharmacokinetics and unwanted effects

Nicotine is rapidly absorbed from the lungs and also is well absorbed from patches applied to the skin. It is mostly metabolized by oxidation in the liver and has a half-life of 2 h. Peripheral side effects of nicotine are those expected of stimulation of nicotinic receptors in the autonomic ganglia and the adrenal medulla, e.g. tachycardia and a rise in blood pressure. Stimulation of the posterior pituitary causes antidiuretic hormone (ADH) release and, consequently, decreases urine flow. *Adverse effects of tobacco smoking* are mainly due to nicotine, tars and carbon monoxide (CO). (In heavy smokers, up to 15% of haemoglobin may be converted to carboxyhaemoglobin.) Lung, throat and bladder cancer are increased in tobacco smokers probably due to the carcinogens in the tars produced by smoking. Smokers also have an increased risk of bronchitis and chronic obstructive pulmonary disease (COPD) thought to mainly be caused by the tars. The increases in coronary heart disease and stroke in smokers are most likely caused by nicotine and CO. Nicotine and CO from smoking in pregnancy may be responsible for low birth weight.

Ethanol

Alcohol dependence is widespread and heavy drinking is a factor in many hospital admissions.

Pharmacological actions

Ethanol has CNS depressant actions similar to those of gaseous anaesthetics and the molecular mechanism is likely to involve enhancement of γ-aminobutyric acid (GABA)$_A$ receptor action, inhibition of N-methyl-D-aspartate (NMDA) receptors and inhibition of the opening of voltage-gated calcium ion (Ca^{2+}) channels. Ethanol has a relatively low potency and large quantities are needed to elicit pharmacological actions. Little effect is seen below a plasma concentration of 10 mmol/L and 100 mmol/L (500 mg/100 mL). Higher doses can lead to death (by respiratory depression). Activation of the reward pathways described above probably occurs by depression of an inhibitory input. Inebriation produces the well-known euphoria and increased self-confidence. Less-desirable effects are motor incoordination and aggressive behaviour. Cutaneous vasodilatation can cause heat loss and hypothermia. Ethanol inhibits ADH secretion from the pituitary gland, causing diuresis. Other hormonal effects are feminization of men due to reduced testosterone levels and a Cushing's syndrome-like action due to enhanced glucocorticoid action. It is suggested that a modest consumption of ethanol has a beneficial effect on coronary heart disease partly due to increasing plasma high-density lipoproteins. The abstinence syndrome includes tremors, nausea and sweating that in alcoholics may progress to delirium tremens (the DTs) characterized by confusion, hallucinations and aggression. DTs may be alleviated by benzodiazepines. In heavy drinkers, tolerance raises the plasma concentration at which performance deteriorates.

Pharmacokinetics and unwanted actions

Ethanol is well absorbed from the gut and is eliminated mainly (90%) by oxidation to acetaldehyde and acetic acid (Fig. 36.1). Metabolism is saturated at relatively low plasma concentrations due to the limited availability of oxidized nicotinamide adenine dinucleotide (NAD$^+$), leading to zero-order elimination with a fixed rate of approximately 10 mL/h. A small proportion (higher after enzyme induction in heavy drinkers) is oxidized by the P450 system. Limited amounts of ethanol are eliminated unchanged in the breath and urine and provide the basis for police tests of alcohol consumption. **Disulfiram** inhibits aldehyde dehydrogenase and thus elevates the plasma concentration of acetaldehyde. This produces a range of unpleasant symptoms and its use in chronic alcoholics is intended to discourage alcohol consumption. Long-term alcohol abuse can lead to brain damage, dementia and severe liver damage. The poor diet of alcoholics also contributes to their poor health. The *foetal alcohol syndrome*, characterized by facial deformities and slow mental development in the baby, follows heavy ethanol consumption in pregnancy.

Cannabinoids

Cannabinoids are taken for relaxation and enhancement of sensory perception. They are only weakly addictive and produce mild withdrawal symptoms. The most active compound in cannabis (hashish, marijuana) is Δ9-tetrahydrocannabinol (THC).

Pharmacological actions

These compounds act on G-protein-coupled cannabinoid receptors (CB). CB$_1$ receptors are responsible for the CNS effects, coupling

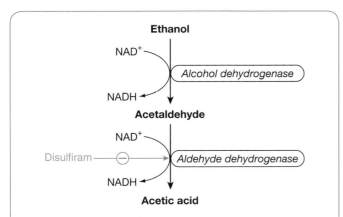

Fig. 36.1 The main pathway for metabolism of alcohol.
Disulfiram causes a build-up of acetaldehyde. *NAD+*, Oxidized nicotinamide adenine dinucleotide; *NADH*, reduced nicotinamide adenine dinucleotide.

to G$_i$, to inhibit adenylate cyclase, activate potassium ion (K$^+$) channels and inhibit Ca^{2+} channels. (CB$_2$ receptors are found in the periphery and affect immune responses.) Anandamide, derived from arachidonic acid, is an endogenous agonist at cannabinoid receptors.

Clinical use

Cannabinoids (e.g. nabilone) improve appetite and have a useful anti-emetic action, which is made use of in cancer chemotherapy. Trials are currently investigating the use of cannabinoids in treating severe pain (particularly neuropathic) and have been approved for the treatment of symptoms of multiple sclerosis.

Pharmacokinetics and unwanted actions

Cannabinoids are usually taken by smoking, though oral absorption from cannabis cakes occurs readily. Cannabinoids are very lipid soluble and strongly protein bound. Distribution to adipose tissue causes them to be retained in the body for several days. THC is mostly metabolized to inactive products by microsomal oxidation, though a small proportion of a more active metabolite is produced. Biliary excretion is greater than urinary excretion. A single dose of THC acts for 2–3 h. Learning, memory and motor control may be adversely affected. Cannabinoids may also aggravate schizophrenia and depression. Sympathomimetic actions such as tachycardia occur. Unlike alcohol, heroin and amphetamine, they are relatively safe in overdose.

PSYCHOMOTOR STIMULANTS

These include amphetamine (dexamphetamine is its D-isomer), methylamphetamine, methylphenidate, fenfluramine, methylene-dioxymethamphetamine (MDMA, ecstasy), cocaine and methylxanthines. (Nicotine has some similar effects.) The amphetamines, cocaine and the methylxanthines are used clinically. Table 36.1 has details of psychotomimetics (hallucinogens/psychedelics).

Amphetamines and cocaine
Mechanisms of action

These raise the synaptic concentrations of noradrenaline (NA), dopamine (DA) and 5-hydroxytryptamine (5-HT). Four processes contribute to this action:

- Stimulation of release into the synaptic cleft
- Inhibition of neuronal reuptake

Table 36.1 Central Nervous System (CNS) Stimulants and Psychotomimetic Drugs

Type	Examples	Mechanisms	Actions	Clinical uses	Unwanted actions
Methylxanthines	Caffeine, theophylline	Phosphodiesterase inhibition Antagonism of adenosine receptors	Bronchodilatation, diuresis, cardiac stimulation Improved motor tasks, wakefulness	Asthma (theophylline ethylenediamine (aminophylline)) (see Ch. 25)	Cardiac dysrhythmia, tremors Agitation, anxiety, rapid breathing, insomnia
Analeptics	Doxapram	Stimulation of neurons in respiratory centre		Apnoea in premature babies, respiratory depression (not often used nowadays)	Convulsions
Hallucinogens (psychotomimetics)	Phencyclidine, **ketamine**	NMDA receptor block, activation of σ-receptors	Stereotyped behaviour	Dissociative anaesthesia (ketamine)	
	LSD, mescaline, psilocybin, DMT, MDMA	Elevation of synaptic 5-HT, activation of 5-HT receptors	Altered perception, delusions	None	Nausea and vomiting (mescaline). Long-lasting psychopathological effects (LSD)

DMT, Dimethyltryptamine; *LSD*, lysergic acid diethylamide; *MDMA*, methylenedioxymethamphetamine; *5-HT*, 5-hydroxytryptamine.

- Inhibition of monoamine oxidase (MAO)
- Inhibition of vesicular uptake

Stimulants affect NA, DA and 5-HT transmission to different extents, resulting in different patterns of action. Amphetamines are substrates for the reuptake transporter for catecholamines and, by an exchange process, cause transmitter release. Cocaine potently inhibits the transporters but is not itself transported and does not stimulate release. The rise in synaptic NA concentration at sympathetic nerve endings with cocaine and amphetamines confers sympathomimetic activity (e.g. pupil dilation). Cocaine also blocks neuronal Na^+ channels to produce local anaesthesia.

Actions

These include euphoria,* elation, improved concentration, appetite suppression, stereotyped behaviour, inhibition of REM sleep and sympathomimetic actions.

Pharmacokinetic aspects

Amphetamines are generally well absorbed from the gut and cross the blood–brain barrier easily. (Crack cocaine, the free base form of the drug, is volatile and is usually smoked). Amphetamine is mostly excreted unchanged in urine; as a base, its excretion is enhanced in acidic urine (see Chapter 5). Cocaine, an ester, is readily hydrolysed and has a short half-life (around 1 h).

Addiction

Amphetamines and cocaine are very addictive though physical withdrawal symptoms are not pronounced. Actions on DA pathways seem to be particularly involved (see Chapter 11).

Unwanted actions

Psychosis, hallucinations, addiction, insomnia, anorexia, anxiety, aggressiveness, hypertension, dysrhythmias, hyperpyrexia, neurotoxicity, muscle damage (MDMA), teratogenicity (cocaine).

Clinical uses of amphetamines

(Note that amphetamines and other uptake inhibitors are appetite suppressants but are not recommended for treatment of obesity.)
- Attention deficit and hyperactivity disorder (ADHD). The use of stimulants in treating ADHD, a condition characterized by excessive motor activity, may seem paradoxical. However, the increase in mental alertness and concentration subdues the hyperactivity. **Methylphenidate** is recommended for ADHD. Some amphetamine analogues are used for narcolepsy.

Methylxanthines

More detail on xanthines is given in Table 36.1 and in Chapter 19.

Mechanisms of action

By inhibiting phosphodiesterase, caffeine and theophylline increase cellular concentrations of cyclic adenosine monophosphate (cAMP) and potentiate responses mediated by β-adrenoceptors and D_1 receptors. This effect occurs only at high doses. The behavioural effects probably involve antagonism of adenosine receptors. Postsynaptic adenosine receptors reduce the firing rate of neurons and presynaptic receptors inhibit transmitter release. Caffeine, by blocking presynaptic receptors, can enhance transmitter release. Caffeine will reverse the sleep-inducing and behavioural depressant actions of adenosine, improving wakefulness and mental alertness.

Pharmacokinetics

Caffeine is well absorbed from the gut and is metabolized (mainly by demethylation) in the liver (plasma half-life approximately 6 h).

---

*The euphoria is likely to involve enhanced activity in the DA pathway projecting from the midbrain ventral tegmental area to parts of the frontal cortex and limbic system, in particular to the nucleus accumbens. Increased activity of the NA projections from the locus ceruleus to parts of the cerebral cortex and limbic system is involved in the increased arousal and vigilance induced by these drugs.

Note: Page numbers followed by "f" indicate figures and "t" indicate tables, and "b" indicate boxes.